ALPHA MALE CHALLENGE

The **10**-Week Plan to
BURN FAT, GAIN MUSCLE & BUILD TRUE ALPHA ATTITUDE

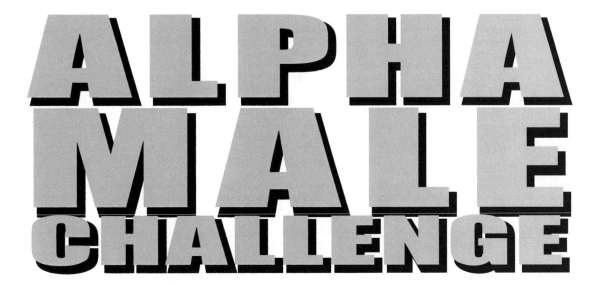

ALPHA MALE CHALLENGE

JAMES VILLEPIGUE, cscs
author of *The Body Sculpting Bible for Men*
AND
RICK COLLINS, jd, cscs

RODALE

© 2009 by James Villepigue and Rick Collins
Photographs © 2009 by Rodale Inc.

MaleScale is a registered trademark.

Rodale books may be purchased for business or promotional use or for special sales. For information, please write to:
Special Markets Department, Rodale Inc., 733 Third Avenue, New York, NY 10017

Printed in the United States of America
Rodale Inc. makes every effort to use acid-free ♾, recycled paper ♻.

Photographs by Thomas MacDonald/Rodale Images

Book design by Christopher Rhoads

Library of Congress Cataloging-in-Publication Data

Villepigue, James C.
    Alpha male challenge : the 10-week plan to burn fat, gain muscle, and build true alpha attitude / by James Villepigue and Rick Collins.
        p.   cm.
    Includes index.
    ISBN-13: 978–1–59486–931–0   hardcover
    ISBN-10: 1–59486–931–6   hardcover
    1. Bodybuilding.   2. Exercise.   3. Physical fitness for men.   I. Collins, Rick.   II. Title.
GV546.5.V528 2004
613.7'13—dc22   2009026798

Distributed to the trade by Macmillan

2   4   6   8   10   9   7   5   3   1   hardcover

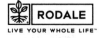

LIVE YOUR WHOLE LIFE™

We inspire and enable people to improve their lives and the world around them
For more of our products visit **rodalestore.com** or call 800-848-4735

Rick Collins
To Kathy, Lauren, and Caitlin, my A-Team,
and to all my wonderful family and friends

James Villepigue
For my wife, Heather; my daughters, Sienna James and Kaiya; my mom, Nancy; my sister, Deborah;
and my beloved father, James R Villepigue, a genuine True Alpha.
To my heavenly Father above, I thank you for blessing my life with love, happiness, and health.

CONTENTS

ACKNOWLEDGMENTS

Just as no individual man is an island, neither is a writing duo. In many ways, *Alpha Male Challenge* was a team effort. We are most grateful for the invaluable contributions of Jud Dean, Jack Darkes, Jay Cohen, David Sandler, Jill Jitomir, and Colette Nelson. We also wish to thank Mike DiMaggio, Hector Lopez, Doug Kalman, Jose Antonio, Marie Spano, Mark Myhal, Will Brink, Steve Fleck, and Stew Smith, to name but a few, for their helpful input on the book's content. We also extend our gratitude to all those who have assisted us with the mechanics of bringing our broader "True Alpha" vision to realization, including Alan Feldstein, Will Brink, Mike Nelson, Justin Miller, Tony Serge, John Romano, Dai Tran, Kim Albert, Eric Hillman, Christopher Oliver, Steve Blechman, and Fairfax Hackley. Our research assistants, including John Ray, Matt Stock, Ara Basmajian, and Diana Vargas, among others, provided welcome support. Additionally, we wish to thank all of those whose quotes and contributions within the pages that follow have helped to make this book even better. We'd also like to acknowledge the best-selling Body Sculpting Bible franchise, as its historic success helped pave the way for this collaborative endeavor. Perhaps most of all, our wives, Heather and Kathy, and our families deserve special thanks, as do Marc Gann, Bob McDonald and the hardworking staff of the law firm of Collins, McDonald, and Gann. Without their collective patience and understanding, this book would not have been possible.

CHAPTER ONE
THE DECLINE AND FALL OF MANLINESS

Okay, guys, it's time to take an honest look at yourself. Make sure the shades are down and you have privacy in the house. Stand in front of the mirror in your underwear. Do you like what you see? How does it compare to what you looked like a few years ago, or when you were in your mid 20s? Somewhere in the tornado of stress and obligations, between finishing school and today's hard look in the mirror, your body probably changed. If you're like most guys, tight became loose; hard became soft.

Your body may not only look different but may also *perform* less impressively as the years go by. Endurance, strength, and power all diminish. The knees, shoulders, and lower back all begin voicing complaints. The kinetic energy you radiated back when you could burn the candle at both ends is increasingly difficult to find. Your engine has stalled. The only thing moving fast and furious may be your hairline.

You've likely changed on the inside, too. Not surprisingly, there's a direct relationship between your appearance and your attitude—how you *feel* about yourself and your place in the world around you. Are you past your peak or just hitting your stride? Do you have the confident edge of a winner? Are you a strong leader and capable protector of your loved ones? Are you in charge of your life and in control of your destiny?

If you're not at the very top of your game, physically and mentally, you're not alone. Although modern American life is more "comfortable" than it was in generations past, many men are fatter, sicker, more stressed, and less rested than ever before. They're less rugged, less robust, and more likely to have a "muffin-top" spilling over their belts. It doesn't help that we live in a changing social environment in which it's harder than ever to figure out what a man is supposed to be and act like in order to be his best. Men are supposed to be "manly," aren't they? But somewhere along the way, "manliness" went from a virtue to a memory.

You are holding in your hands the key to a revolutionary transformation of your body and mind. Only 70 days from today, you can reclaim the muscular, masculine glory of being the best man you can be. Everything you need you'll find within these pages. The 10-week Challenge that begins on page 126 is the assembly manual for constructing the true Alpha Male—the ideal of masculine excellence.

So much of modern life is a challenge; we face daily struggles of so many kinds. Our use of the term *Challenge* is both a positive and empowering call to action and a recognition that nothing worthwhile typically occurs without hard work and sacrifice. And so, *we challenge you* to take control of your life by taking control of your health, your body, and even your thoughts and behaviors.

If you think conventional weight lifting is boring, we agree. That's why few guys stick with it. But we created a program to excite you! If you think "diets" involve bland, tasteless foods, we hear you. But our food plan—the perfect fuel for true Alpha Males—is both nutritious and absolutely mouthwatering! And if you're walking around with the same old attitude as the rest of the empty suits around you, prepare for a shock of inspiration that will change everything! If you accept this Challenge and follow it faithfully with us for the next 10 weeks, we promise you will reach a paradise of rich rewards.

But before we get you there, let's look at how you got where you are now.

NO TIME TO SPARE

Today's society is always on the go, 24 hours per day, 7 days a week. Many of us work long hours, and our schedules are often irregular and unpredictable. We seem to be working harder than ever even though many guys have less and less confidence in their financial forecasts. A good night's sleep is a rare luxury for many guys.

Long work hours don't leave much time for anything else. Add on social expectations within the dating scene, and not much spare time is left for single guys. For married men, shared household responsibilities dip even further into the pool of disposable minutes. Between 1965 and 1995, men's average weekly housework time doubled— from 4.9 to 10 hours—based on a survey of four national studies published in 2000 by University of Maryland researchers. And for guys with families, like us, the joys of parenting are offset by an ever-lengthening list of responsibilities

and seemingly impossible time pressures. Each stage of child rearing carries its own unique demands, from the bottle and diaper days to the endless chauffeur duties of the parents of socially active teens.

Our collective pool of available time sometimes seems to have dried to a puddle. Despite ubiquitous television and newspaper reports urging us to get more exercise, less than half of guys age 35 meet the American College of Sports Medicine's recommendation of at least 30 minutes of moderate physical activity on most days and preferably on all days. More than 70 percent of guys ages 25 to 34 don't do regular resistance training. If there's any spare time at the end of the day there's no energy left to do anything but vegetate in front of the TV or computer screen. The result? A metabolic and psychological vicious cycle that becomes ever more difficult to break out of with each passing year.

FAST TIMES AT STRESSFUL HIGH

The 24-hour television news cycle provides a never-ending stream of stressful visual and auditory information. Danger and risk, real or imagined, seem to be all around us. It's taking a toll on us. A few years ago, researchers led by an associate professor of psychology at Merrimack College studied the effects of 9/11-linked television viewing on dream content, concluding that each additional hour of viewing raised a viewer's stress level by 6 percent.

Meanwhile, it's not uncommon in many professions to be expected to be available at any and all times. Cell phones and PDAs are nagging, insistent companions demanding our constant attention. Business travel has its own menu of pressures and uncertainties, with canceled flights, lost luggage, and missed appointments. Perhaps even more sadly, we seem to have come to think that this is how life should be, and to expect this kind of lifestyle.

Research shows that stress affects our hormones. Testosterone is the primary male sex hormone and the biological marker for maleness—and manliness—itself. The right amount of it in the womb makes a fetus a boy. A surge of it during adolescence makes a boy a man. For the rest of your life, testosterone has profound effects on both your body and your brain, impacting your performance virtually everywhere—in the gym, on the job, and in the bedroom. We all know that testosterone is essential for building muscles. Higher testosterone levels are associated with more lean muscle. But testosterone also influences psychological factors, including mood, memory, libido, assertiveness, and confidence, and physiological factors, such as cholesterol levels, sperm production, and blood sugar. Healthy testosterone levels are essential to male health, and low testosterone is associated with a number of maladies and decreased quality of life.

In a 2002 article examining stress and hormones, Swedish researchers concluded that repeated exposure to stress can harm a man's testosterone production both in the short term and the long term. The result: depressed spirits and increased fatigue.

GETTING FATTER . . .

Many guys feel crushed by the stress and time demands of 21st-century life and start doing away with activities that seem nonessential. Studies show that physical exercise is one of the first things to go. For 2 years, researcher Ethan Hull and his colleagues at the University of Pittsburgh tracked the habits of 525 physically active subjects. At the start of the study, the childless male subjects averaged almost 8 hours of weekly exercise. Men who remained childless lost only a half hour of physical activity per week over the course of the study. Those who became parents cut back *a whopping 4½ hours per week*. Yes, the demands of those adorable little bundles of joy have a powerful reducing effect on our exercise habits. If guys who are hard-core enough to spend almost 8 hours per week exercising cut back by more than half when they become parents, you can only guess what happens to less-active guys.

Make no mistake: Lack of regular exercise is devastating to our health. According to a November 2007 report from the U.S. Centers for Disease Control and Prevention, one out of every three American men over age 20 is obese, and approximately 40 percent of men ages 40 to 59 are obese. Since 1999, the percentage of obese men has increased faster than the percentage of obese women. No doubt, lack of exercise and poor diet are major contributing factors, although, as we'll see, there's a hormonal factor as well.

Yes, the American male "couch potato" population is getting fatter, and having way too much body fat is no friend to manliness. With enough flab, the pectorals can take on an alarmingly feminine look. And getting fatter

---

TESTOSTERONE: THE GOOD, THE BAD, AND THE MANLY

"Testosterone, for all the good and bad publicity about it, is the hormone that makes males what they are. It not only changes us physically, but affects us psychologically as well and, contrary to much publicity, those changes are pretty much all for the better when it comes to men; they relate to better cognitive function as we age as well as our dominant (not aggressive) attitude. It is the 'take charge and get things done' hormone, and who doesn't need that kind of approach sometimes?"

—Jack Darkes, PhD, Assistant Professor of Psychology, University of South Florida

means getting sicker. Obesity is a major risk factor for cardiovascular disease, certain types of cancer, and type 2 diabetes. Lack of exercise contributes to the prevalence of strokes, high cholesterol, high blood pressure, blood clots, cognitive decline and dementia, diminished strength and muscle mass, osteoporosis, and depression. Men ages 45 to 64 today are three times more likely to suffer fatal heart attacks than they were 30 years ago. The price for being a couch potato can be very steep indeed, for the potatoes themselves and for those who depend on them. The burning question for women: What kind of shape is *your* husband in?

GETTING OLDER . . .

Even for guys who aren't carrying excess adipose baggage, the simple process of getting older can undermine your virility. Eugene Shippen, MD, a renowned expert on male health and hormones and the coauthor of *The Testosterone Syndrome*, introduces the problem this way:

Think back to when you were young. If you were like most people, you reached your physical peak in your late teens or early twenties. It was a time of rambunctious energy that resisted every effort to squander it away. Late nights, too much work and too much play, and, for many of us, far too much eating and drinking—all this produced very little in the way of untoward effects. For many twenty-year-olds, burning the candle at both ends is not a danger; it's an art form. Pushing past every reasonable limit, we recharged our cellular batteries as fast as we drained them. How were our organ systems and, indeed, every cell in our bodies able to keep up with the brutal pace? Hormones! We were in hormone heaven.

Ah, hormone heaven. Those were the days. But as the years start to slip away, so do those hormones. According to Mark Gordon, MD, a medical hormone expert, and owner of Millennium Health Centers in Encino, California, male testosterone levels decline at an average rate of 1 to 2 percent a year, starting at around 35 years of age. By the time you hit 40, your testosterone levels can be down by 5 to 10 percent. From the purely hormonal standpoint, you may become less and less "manly" every year.

Research published in 2006 in the *International Journal of Clinical Practice* suggests that more than *one-third of men over 45* may have clinically low testosterone levels, and that the odds of having low testosterone are 2.4 times higher for obese men. So, as our testosterone levels wane with age, our energy, muscle mass, and strength go down, our sex drive peters out, our body fat level rises, our good cholesterol goes down, our bad cholesterol goes up, and we have an increased susceptibility to depression and disease.

Testosterone improves muscle metabolism, which helps your body reduce blood sugar levels. With less sugar in the blood, the body doesn't need to release as much insulin, a storage hormone that moves glucose from the blood and stores it as body fat. Less testosterone means more body fat; conversely, more natural, healthy testosterone means less body fat. In fact, research led by Dr. Jean-Marc Kaufman at Ghent University Hospital in Belgium and published in a 2008 edition of *Clinical Endocrinology* shows that a man's percentage of body fat and circulating levels of testosterone are partly controlled by the very same set of genes.

Interestingly, not only does testosterone decrease as we age, but estrogen, the primary female hormone, increases as we age. Too much estrogen feminizes a man. Now, it's natural for certain enzymes in your body to convert some of your testosterone into estrogen at any age. However, as you get older, changes in enzyme and trace nutrients lead your body to convert a higher and higher proportion of your testosterone into estrogen. So, you can have a higher proportion of female hormone to male hormone than you did when you were younger. That's the age-related double whammy to your manliness, says Will Brink, health, fitness, and medical writer (www. BrinkZone.com).

So being fat and getting older both adversely affect the hormone responsible for your manliness. And get what else: According to studies published in *Social Forces* and in *Evolution and Human Behavior*, testosterone levels decline when you get married, and decline even further when you become a father. Why? "Testosterone is about competition, for dominance, and for mates," suggests Jack Darkes, PhD, an assistant professor of psychology at the University of South Florida. "Married men are no longer 'competing' for mates, and are even less so when they have children." Of course, testosterone isn't the be-all and end-all of manliness. It's just the biochemical marker for it—one physical standard for measuring it. At least as important are the *social* markers and standards. And that's where things get even more interesting.

A BRAVE NEW WORLD

Times have changed, and, overall, for the better. Women, who have struggled for equality in what had been a male-dominated environment, have made well-deserved leaps forward. According to the U.S. Department of Labor, by 2004 half of all management, professional, and related occupations were held by women. Increased gender equality has improved many areas of American life. Now grown-up guys are expected to learn how to cook a meal and diaper a baby, even if some are still reluctant to do so.

But workplace equality is no excuse for the new breed of androgynous men that emerged over the past 2 decades. Many guys just lost their solid footing, and they have nobody but themselves to blame. For whatever reasons, just as society opened the door to interchangeable work and play responsibilities, we found ourselves face-to-face with a stranger—a new kind of gender-neutral man. These metaphorically "low testosterone" men would rather watch *The Young and the Restless* than a Three Stooges movie.

Mark Simpson at Salon.com popularized our new, "softer" gender representative in 2002's "Meet the Metrosexual." "The typical metrosexual is a young man with money to spend, living in or within easy reach of a metropolis—because that's where all the best shops, clubs, gyms and hairdressers are." Shops? *Hairdressers?* Aren't guys supposed to see *barbers,* with manly names like "Vito," or "Max"? Clearly, the traditional attributes that make men just plain "male" were blurring. The problem applies to *any* guy who thinks the route to modern male self-improvement lies in a hair gel bottle, fancier pants, and a pedicure.

In *The Metrosexual Guide to Style,* Michael Flocker proclaimed that "there is a certain power and mystery in ambiguity" and crowed that "the peacock has reemerged" (although he mercifully suggested that "most men will want to stop well short of sarongs and nail polish"). Although the term *metrosexual* started getting thrown around so loosely that any guy who cared about his appearance got the label, that's not what we're talking about. The problem was that men were becoming "masculinity-challenged." A quote from the HBO series *Six Feet Under* announced, "Men are the New Women." A couple of years later, the line "Men. We're the new women" heralded the series *Big Shots* as a male version of *Sex and the City.* If tough-guy icons like John Wayne, Lee Marvin, or Robert Mitchum were still alive today, they'd never stop scowling. Is male self-improvement really all about the size and variety of your collection of facial moisturizers? Have we become, as *Muscle & Fitness* editor-in-chief Chris Lockwood wryly suggests, an "estrogen nation"?

BETA AIN'T BETTER

The situation is spreading beyond the United States. In October 2007, the *Sunday Times* of London headline proclaimed: "What modern women want: a beta male; Men are surrendering in the sex war, taking on the supporting role." As traditional gender roles erode and capable women march off to the gender-neutral corporate or professional battlefields describing themselves as "alpha females," more and more men are finding themselves filling the supportive role in relationships. Supportive is good. But do women really *want* men to surrender in the "sex war"? Do they really want soft, submissive mates? UrbanDictionary.com defines a beta male as "An unremarkable, careful man who avoids risk and confrontation. Beta males lack the physical presence, charisma, and confidence of the Alpha male." Ask the ladies: does the idea of a "beta boyfriend" really sound so good?

Is this man's destiny—to shrink down to naught but a passive supporter? All was not well. And it wasn't the men who first sensed something just wasn't right. It was the women. Take, for example, the comment posted online by Kate from San Diego in response to the *Sunday Times* article:

"... I am a strong alpha female (raised by alphas—and my sister is marrying a beta male who is happy to be beta). I have a hard time respecting men who are less alpha than I am. I'm forced to do all the work, and wonder if it's worth it in the end. I have tried the supportive, less dominant approach—and I ended up with a condescending boy-

friend who, when he realized I was smarter than he thought, more competent than he was and not going to take his crap got dumped. When I am completely myself men who show an interest hear what I do and the schedule I keep and get scared off. Where is the balance? I keep hoping to find the alpha that wants a partner—and to be honest—recognizing that a woman is a stronger organizing presence in the home shouldn't make the man feel like a beta. That actually seems to be what partnership is about . . . I will keep searching for my own alpha male hopefully one day I'll find him."

In "Why I Left My Beta Husband," an essay published recently in *Marie Claire* magazine, journalist Amy Brayfield explained why her marriage tanked. Here was the story of a driven businesswoman who left her stay-at-home-dad–husband despite his dutiful accommodations to her career. For all his housework and commendable parenting efforts, she realized one day that it had been almost a year since they'd made love and that just the thought of his touch made her "recoil." Had she changed, or had he? We know from the research that guys' testosterone levels drop after marriage and children, and that they also decrease when we stop accepting competitive challenges. Had his taken a nosedive? Clearly, he lost his edge, maybe even became depressed (associated with low testosterone). And in his wife's mind, he'd been cut down from the "sexiest man in the world" to no man at all . . . and with no *sex* at all. He'd been neutered. As she explained, "The truth is, I wasn't attracted to him anymore. . . . I'd neutralized him as a sexual being. I wanted to be overwhelmed by the sheer power of his masculinity in the bedroom, but I wasn't. Because I felt like the man in our relationship." And, it would seem, he didn't. There you have it. Gender role reversal followed through to completion—check, please! If you're like most guys, you're fine with today's ideas of gender equality and equal partnership; and if you're fortunate enough to have a dual career household—and double income—in today's tough market, you're grinning from ear to ear. But you're not interested in gender neutrality—you still want to feel like the man in a relationship. You still want to feel like a man, period. And she wants you to be a man, too.

Passive, submissive, and uncharismatic men who lack confidence or self-esteem aren't sexy. Beta isn't better. No disrespect, but somebody had to say it.

LESS THAN OUR FATHERS WERE

Most of us have been listening for years to the tales of our elders about how past generations were more manly than guys today. Our fathers and grandfathers would supposedly work 25 hours a day, wake up 2 hours before they went to bed, exist on a diet of sawdust and turpentine, and walk 500 miles shoeless through the blinding snow to get to school or work. Many guys took such claims of rugged manliness with a grain of salt. Were our predecessors *really* manlier?

From a biological standpoint, the answer appears to be a resounding "Yes!" As we've said, we've long known that testosterone levels drop with age, but nothing could have prepared us for the earth-shattering, mind-blowing revelation published in the *Journal of Clinical Endocrinology and Metabolism* in January 2007. This study provided evidence of a new physiological component to the de-masculinization of the modern man. The researchers looked at testosterone levels of groups of Boston men ranging in age from 45 to 79 taken in three waves: 1987 to 1989, 1995 to 1997, and 2002 to 2004. They found something quite troubling.

They examined the age-matched testosterone levels of each wave. For example, the researchers compared the men who were 65 years old in 1987 with the men who were 65 in 1995 and in 2002. They found that when they compared age-matched subjects, the men of the '80s had higher average testosterone levels than the men of the '90s, and the men of the new century have on average the least testosterone of all. Testosterone levels are going down.

That's right: Typical American men are becoming less manly and less "male" than their fathers and grandfathers were, *biologically*. And it's happening pretty fast, and for reasons that scientists can't identify. How bad is the crisis? It's open to debate, but Daniel Gwartney, MD, a medical researcher and columnist for *Muscular Development* magazine, points out that the data suggest that the average man's testosterone levels will drop by 14.4 percent between the ages of 45 and 54. Obviously, some of that can be chalked up to natural aging. However, for men of the 1990s, that substantial hormonal drop would have taken a full 3 to even 4 decades. "Consider the magnitude of this difference," says Dr. Gwartney, extrapolating from the data. "The hormonal change experienced in men today from age 45 to 54 is the same as the difference between men age 45 to 81 just ten years ago." Ouch! Yes, that puts the situation in perspective. And yes, you can pick your jaw up off the floor now.

THE *TRUE* ALPHA MALE

Stepping back and looking at the whole picture from a combined sociocultural and biological perspective, it's time to sadly admit that Arnold Schwarzenegger may soon be right if he calls us a nation of "girly men." What's happening to American men? Is it just coincidence that we are now importing leading men from Australia to play many of our heroic American film roles?

We like being men, and we think you do, too.

Let's be candid, we wouldn't have it any other way. Not preening girly men, but not "macho" men, acting (or overacting) on some kind of warped overblown image of what it is to be a man. It hasn't got anything to do with being better than anyone else, be they male or female; we are born with what we have, and what we choose to make of it is up to each and every one of us.

We think being healthy, strong, and confident is a great way for a man to live his life, and we think women appreciate us for being men and not being more feminine than they are. We're talking about *gentlemen,* not aggressive oafs. The kind of man that is not often talked about these days. Our desire to help build—or rebuild—that kind of man is why we wrote this book. Hopefully you're reading it because you see the value of that kind of man, too, both for yourself and for those in your life. What are the qualities that comprise the ideal contemporary man at the pinnacle of his development? How can we be the men that we want to be, that we enjoy being, that we were meant to be, taking responsibility for our own welfare and the welfare of those who depend on us?

Move over Mr. Beta, and make way for the arrival of the *true* Alpha Male. We're not talking about taking a step backward to the negative stereotypes of yesteryear; we're talking about moving forward toward the promise of the very best of what our gender can be.

It's never too late for second chances. It is time to reclaim masculine excellence. You won't have to visit a sweat lodge or form a man-hug circle to express your primal grief. This is a 10-week

instruction manual to build a whole new kind of man: one who is brimming with confidence and who integrates traditional rugged manliness with modern enlightenment. Not just a guy who looks like a heroic work of Alpha Architecture, but one who strives to *be* heroic. This is the road map to achieving the look, life, and winning attitude needed to not only compete and survive in today's jungle, but also to maximize your success and improve your health. It's not about twisting you into someone you're not. It's about developing the physical and mental aspects of what makes *you* a man.

When some people think of an "alpha male" they think of clashing antlers in the woods and guys who act like knuckle-dragging nimrods. We agree that stupid displays of territorial machismo should be relegated to the dark ages of our past. But we do not believe that the fiery passion and fortitude to stand up for ourselves and our principles or to fight for victory in the ultra-competitive world we inhabit should be extinguished. If you really think "kinder and gentler" means withdrawal from the struggle for excellence, justice, achievement, and success, then just let the other guy have the next promotion at work. Then explain it to your family.

The benefits of alpha male status in the animal kingdom are obvious: first dibs on food, territory, sexual partners, and virtually everything else of value. It's like winning the Darwinian raffle. In return, the alpha male provides leadership and protection of the collective. Overall, he has it good. In human society, true Alpha Males also have a similar increased potential for success. They make

MALE INFERTILITY

Not only testosterone but sperm counts are taking a dive. Studies around the globe have shown sperm quality and quantity are in serious decline. A critical reanalysis of earlier research was published in *Environmental Health Perspectives* in 1997, confirming that sperm density is significantly down in both the United States and Europe. In 2000, the same authors examined 47 more studies done between 1934 and 1996 and again found that semen quality was in significant decline throughout the Western world. Is man the next endangered species?

great leaders; they are better protectors and better providers. You can achieve true Alpha Male status by *choice*: by hard work and force of will, and by following a practical system for both physical and personality development to transcend the ordinary and achieve the extraordinary. And it's precisely in line with what contemporary women *really* want— a strong and sexy partner who's caring, chivalrous . . . and not a wet dishrag.

THE ULTIMATE "MAN-UAL" FOR GUYS

Are you ready to face the 10-week Challenge to get on top of your game? You'll get into the best shape of your life, improving your strength, power, speed, endurance, and overall health. You'll acquire an arsenal of techniques to strengthen commitment and boost confidence, preparing you to be an enlightened warrior facing life's battles and crises with heightened courage and bouncing back from adversity with greater resiliency. You'll learn principles that will improve your relationships with those around you. And you'll even be able to measure and track your progress from start to finish using a tool we'll introduce shortly: the revolutionary MaleScale. We bring you a unique presentation of fitness and lifestyle elements that reaches back into our ancestral past and forward into the latest groundbreaking research. It's based on what we've learned over the course of our decades in the trenches, and from successful people who've lived by the principles contained in this book. We have each successfully applied every individual component in this book over a span of years, and for the first time ever the strategies are assembled into one program.

We've brought together a completely unprecedented a combination of elements. Our unique access to the best and brightest exercise and fitness authorities, scientists, psychologists, nutritional experts, and diverse researchers has packed this book chock-full of the most cutting-edge information dissected and translated for quick comprehension and immediate use.

The truth is that every man has the power to make dramatic changes to his life. Our goal is to help you construct a muscular, masculine work of architecture that shouts volumes about how you see yourself. You can *look* more powerful, *feel* more powerful, and *be* more powerful—even as you restore *balance* to your life. This is a revolutionary approach to building muscle and reducing body fat, supported by both scientific and empirical evidence from the top gurus in strength training, resistance training, and exercise physiology. It harnesses the awesome power of your own hormones, including testosterone and growth hormone, and the fire of

MORE THAN MONKEY MUSCLE

Among all primates, it helps if the alpha male is bigger, stronger, and smarter to hold his own—or better—amid the groups and hierarchies he's part of. But at the same time, he must lead and work with others to protect the collective interests of his group. Social-brain theory explains it from an evolutionary perspective: As tree-dwelling primates moved outward from the deep forests in search of food and faced threats from savannah predators, they adapted by developing more powerful bodies and by living in larger groups to better keep watch and provide strength in numbers. But the bigger groups imposed a new job requirement: The members, especially alpha male leaders, had to be smart enough to balance their individual needs with those of the pack. Today, every true Alpha Male should recognize and honor his evolutionary role as a guardian and defender. Concern for others is integral to the true Alpha Male.

your own metabolism to ignite rapid change. It utilizes the incredible capacity of your mind to catapult you to greater success. We offer you an incredible opportunity. No matter what shape you're in now, you will look, feel, and perform better at the end of only 10 weeks on this program. That's right, just give us 70 days to prove it to you. *Alpha Male Challenge* is the *only* book men need to maximize their health, performance, and appearance. It's the road map to masculine excellence. It's based on research, not on fad ideas or on what some Hollywood trainer claims worked on a rich celebrity.

Well, there you are, with this book in your hands. Maybe you're still wondering whether this is the right book for you. Sure, you've tried some of the other books out there, and somehow most of them always end up lacking when it comes to real results. Maybe when that happened you started to wonder whether it was really possible for you to be different, to make improvements, to do better. If this sounds familiar, then you are in the right place. We're going to tell you how to do the right things to build a stronger, leaner body than you may ever have thought possible. And, more than that, we're going to tell you how to take those thoughts, the ones you have had after each of the "other" books didn't quite deliver, and put them away. It's time for you to find out what you're made of during our 10-week journey together—10 weeks that will begin a whole new chapter of your life. In case you haven't figured it out by now, this is a very different kind of diet and fitness book. So fasten your seat belt, rev your engine, and push the pedal to the floor!

FINDING MY TRUE ALPHA MALE

I WOKE UP ON THE MORNING OF MY 38TH BIRTHDAY and, as I did on most days for many years, promised myself that I would make some positive changes in my life. Two decades earlier, I'd been an athlete. I had weighed 225 pounds, and I was as strong as a bull. I felt great when I looked in the mirror. I felt confident everywhere I went. But the years had changed me. Now I was pushing 40 and tipping the scales at 307 pounds at 5'8". I was pretty much a couch potato when I wasn't working. My diet was awful, and I lacked the willpower to change it. My waist circumference measured just a few inches short of *five full feet*. I looked terrible. I felt miserable. And I was on a fast track to disability or the morgue. My father had a heart attack at 48. My mom died of cancer at the same age. Here I was, exactly 10 years away from that age, with four sons under the age of 9 and a beautiful wife, Kathleen. What would happen to them if I got sick, or worse? I knew I had to change my course. I knew my life depended on it.

But there were so many convenient excuses to stick with the same old routine, so many obstacles in the path. Over the years, I'd tried virtually every diet plan on the market, but they didn't work for me. I would join a gym every few years, stay with it for a month, but then give up. Nothing worked. I'm a busy attorney with a demanding solo practice and a family at home. I'm also the president of the local soccer league which runs three seasons a year, and I coach three different teams. There were never enough hours in a day to do it all. Whatever free time I had left, if any, I'd spent mostly in stupefied recuperation. I was 38 and exhausted. I had no energy. I felt over-the-hill. I was a mess. I wanted to eat healthier. But with all the pressure and demands and rushing around, it was just easier to eat whatever was fastest and most filling. I was eating all the worst foods, and as much of them as I could get my hands on.

It had to stop. That's what I said to myself. I went back to the gym on the day I turned 38, and a few times over the next week. I went through the motions of the same old exercise routines that I had done when I was 15, and again tried all my previously failed attempts to get back into a sustained exercise routine. But, deep down, I doubted I could dig out of the rut I'd created for myself. Within 2 weeks, I was worried that I would fail. Maybe it was just too late for me? Maybe I was past the point of no return?

I was sharing my frustration with my friend Mike, a young lawyer who was into bodybuilding and nutrition. I told Mike that I'd failed again and again at sticking to a diet or at staying with an exercise routine. Maybe I just didn't have it in me anymore, I admitted. Maybe it was time to give up.

Then Mike made a suggestion that would change my life. He urged me to come to his office for a few minutes to see something I'd find interesting. That "something" was a presentation of before-and-after pictures of men my age and older who had completed a 10-week program called the Alpha Male Challenge. Mike's boss is Rick Collins, a lawyer. Rick is older than me, but in awesome shape. The 10-week program was the brain-child of Rick and his co-author, internationally known fitness guru James Villepigue, a popular author whose previous books had sold nearly a million copies. I stared at the photos. I was speechless. The physical results achieved in only 10 weeks were incredible. And as awesome as the photos were, that was only part of the transformation that these men had undergone. Each man had been assessed, both before and after the program, on the Male-Scale™—a revolutionary tool that measures the physical and mental traits that define the True Alpha Male. Their improvements in strength, power, and conditioning were startling. But even more shocking were their improvements in *attitude*. They had measurably improved traits like their willpower, their courage, and their confidence! They weren't just thinner or stronger. They were *better*, overall!

I loved the whole idea. Who wouldn't want to be their best? Who wouldn't want to exude confidence and feel ready to meet any challenge? Who wouldn't want to be a True Alpha Male? If these men transformed themselves, maybe I could, too. For the first time in many years, I felt a sense of hope. The program itself, and its comprehensive goals, were different than anything else I'd ever heard of. I wanted *in*.

After obtaining my medical clearance, I underwent the various physical and mental assessments of the MaleScale™. My baseline scores were, well, less than pretty. My score on the MaleScale™, called my Alpha Factor, was 40. Not great, but I was determined to improve it, ready to start, and committed to take the Pledge and face the Challenge. And I did.

The first week of the Challenge was a complete shock for me. I'd spent many hours in the gym in the past, mostly unproductive. But nothing I'd ever experienced was like this. Alpha Wave Basic Training called for my body to move in new ways. There was jumping, and pulling, and pushing, and reaching—the likes of which I'd never done before. The Challenge incorporated various tests of strength and endurance, which forced me to dig deep to find the very best in me. And, crucially for me, it valued my time as if it were made for a lawyer or for any profession where time is money. It requires sticking to strict time limits—no wasting time talking at the water fountain between sets. Every moment was carefully planned and important. Every exercise was thoughtfully sequenced, and every single workout was different from the others. It made working out actually exciting—something totally new for me!

The rest of the Challenge is just as unique. I could go on and on about each aspect of the program but—I think half the fun is finding it out for yourself. The Work Heart/Play Heart cardio system, the Alpha Attitude drills and the Alpha Fuel Solution bring new twists and surprises over the 10 weeks. You won't be bored, but you also won't be overwhelmed. It's all doable, even for a guy with very limited time.

Of course, as brilliantly as James and Rick have crafted the Challenge, you have to expect that not everything always goes as planned. For me, it happened 3 weeks into the program when I was hospital-

ized for a kidney stone. I was discharged at about one in the morning. I had an Alpha Wave Basic Training workout the next morning at seven. In the past, I would have canceled the workout and taken some time to recuperate and let the stone pass. Maybe you would have, too. But the Challenge was changing me—not just on the outside, but on the inside. There was no doubt in my mind now that I'd be at the gym the next morning. And I was. That was my responsibility to myself. The Challenge had become my *personal* challenge, and one I wouldn't back down from.

I had made excuses for and to myself for a long time. What are your excuses? No time? Too busy? Bad knees? Bad back? Too old? Whatever they are, I urge you to throw them aside and face the Challenge. I did. And guess what? In my first 2 weeks on the Challenge I lost 12 pounds. In the full 10 weeks, I lost *52 pounds*. Me, a guy for whom nothing worked before! But I didn't just lose weight. I lost *fat*. I lost over 10 inches of fat off my waist! And I gained muscle and re-gained an athleticism I haven't had in 20 years. I am stronger and faster and more agile than I ever remember being. I added over 4 inches to my vertical jump, and I shaved 33 seconds off my 300-yard shuttle run! And I've changed on the inside, too. I have a whole new attitude about myself, about my work, about my life. Everything looks different, feels different. I have a sense of control over the world around me, and my place in it. I have a confidence that seems to radiate from me. I feel that I am capable of succeeding where I would have failed before. My new Alpha Factor: 73!

What's the time commitment needed to turn your life around? Much less than you think. I spent about 4 hours in the gym each week. Is that really so hard to do? As far as cardio, I integrated it into my daily life, just like the book suggests, and I engaged in fun aerobic activities like racquetball and basketball.

Now I'm a True Alpha Graduate of the Alpha Male Challenge. But I'm not stopping. I'm starting the Challenge all over again, pushing myself even harder this time. I'm 2 weeks into it and I am already down to 246 pounds—a mind-blowing *61 pounds* down from where I started. And I feel awesome! So last week I did something I never thought I'd ever do—I signed up for a triathlon. Why not? I know what I'm capable of and I won't set goals that don't challenge me. I did that for too long. Somewhere in these past 20 years, I started playing it safe, stopped pushing myself, and came up short of my goals. But not anymore. Whether it's promising myself that I'll run to a certain point and then doing it, promising myself I'll lift a certain weight and then doing it—I've been reminded of the lessons we're taught as children that we somehow forget as the years roll by; that we can do what we imagine, if we only keep the promises we make to ourselves.

Remember when you felt invincible? Remember your late teens, or college, or your mid-twenties, when you hit your stride? Maybe you did, or maybe you haven't hit it yet. That's what the philosophy of the Alpha Male Challenge is all about. It's not just about the simple Fuel Rules or the revolutionary training program. It's about setting you up for success in the gym, at the table, and for the rest of your life.

Both James and Rick have substantial followings in the bodybuilding and fitness communities. Both guys are blessed with tremendous success. James has written some of the most popular and best-selling books in the fitness genre. In addition to his law practice, Rick has had a career as an actor and has friends in high places in Hollywood. They could have endorsements from a choice of celebrities. But that's not what this book is about, or who it's for. This is a book for you and me. It's for every guy out there who knows, deep down, he could be more than he is, better than he is now—both inside and out. James and Rick have crafted the best road map ever created to take you there. They're amazing guys, and they've written a book like no other.

I'm humbled and moved that they have asked me to write this testimonial for them. And it's with heartfelt gratitude that I thank them for saving my life. I trusted them to shepherd me to become the man I always knew I could be, and they have done it beyond my wildest expectations. Just as they trusted me to articulately share my story, I urge you to put your trust in them. Take the Pledge. Face the Challenge. Just like me, you have the potential to be so much more than you ever imagined.

—ALEXANDER E. SKLAVOS, ESQ.

Go to www.AlphaMaleChallege.com to view the amazing videos of the True Alpha Males whose testimonials appear in this book.

CHAPTER TWO
ENTER THE MALESCALE

ALPHA MALE BONDING

Since we're going to be spending some time together, we ought to get to know each other. You already know why we wrote this book. Why did you buy it? What's most important to you over the next 10 weeks? Feeling healthier? Looking younger and more buff? Would you like more speed, endurance, functional strength, and power? Do you want to tackle life with renewed vigor, mental toughness, and confidence? To prime yourself for success? To feel *heroic*? We'd guess that building up your muscles and burning your excess fat ranks pretty high up there, huh? Some of you may still be in your twenties, perhaps; others will be quite a good deal older than that. Some of you will have lots of weight-training experience and some of you will have none. Some of you will be close to target body composition and others will be far from the mark. There's a place for every one of you within the *Alpha Male Challenge*.

Try something for us. Imagine yourself a year from now. Imagine yourself 5 years from now, and 10 years from now. What do you see? If you see an older, fatter version of yourself, it will probably come to pass. Mentally, you haven't committed yourself to the Challenge. If you see yourself as the successful product of the next 10 weeks, and the weeks and months beyond, then you see

someone quite different. You see a much better body. And you see a better man.

Ten weeks is only 70 days! A brief enough span for any guy to handle this program, but sufficient for you to effect radical changes on the way you look and feel. How do you want to be different 10 weeks from now? Let's pretend that you could wake up tomorrow morning with your wish granted. How would things be different? Put this book down and think about where you want to go. After all, most guys spend pretty much their whole lives running on the same old track. You're about to shake things up and change direction for the 10 weeks that will change your life. If you're going to do that, you ought to have a destination in mind.

So, let's put the Destination in your mind's eye. Let's say you want to gain 5 pounds of lean muscle and lose 10 pounds of unsightly fat over the next 10 weeks, as well as go from an ordinary mind-set to one of extraordinary confidence, willpower, and courage. Focus vividly on how you're going to look and feel with 10 fewer pounds of fat and with 5 new pounds of solid muscle. You might visualize how that favorite shirt or pair of jeans looks on you, generating some awe and envy from your coworkers or neighbors. Envision the incredible new confidence, ruggedness, and discipline that you exude and how your attitude positively affects you in every aspect of your life. It's all ahead for you if you face the Challenge.

DESTINATIONS, ROADBLOCKS, AND MOTIVATIONS

Are you serious about being the best you can be? We'll give you all the tools you'll need and walk you through the Challenge every step of the way, but you will need to do the work. If you're truly serious, grab a pen and paper and prepare to answer three questions. Trust us: Writing things down will strengthen your commitment to them over the next 10 weeks.

- **Question 1:** How do you want to improve yourself, inside and out? More strength and muscle? A leaner waist and better abs? More courage and confidence? Make a list and write it down, under "Destination." Be realistic. When you're done, you'll have your Destination right there in black and white.

- **Question 2:** Why haven't you reached your Destination goals long before now? What gets between you and regular exercise? What stops you from eating smarter? Think about all the roadblocks you've faced before and all the new ones you can envision—and write them down under "Roadblocks." Be honest with yourself. Take a look around; you are certainly not alone in your struggles.

- **Question 3:** Now that you know the "where" of your Destination and why you haven't gotten there yet, what motivated you to choose it? For example, what is it about losing weight, building strength and muscle, or improving your health that's important to you? What about it is important to the members of your family or others who depend on you? How would reaching your Destination improve your life?

Which is more persuasive to you, the list of fears and obstacles or the motivations to change? If the list of roadblocks is more persuasive, then you're not ready to embark on the *Alpha Male Challenge*. Put the book down, and try again tomorrow. Modern men are getting fatter and less healthy and manly and it's only going to get worse. But according to experts on successful personal change, none of that matters if it doesn't matter to you. Unless *you*, reading this right now, feel moved to take action, the revolutionary system presented in these pages will pass you by.

All animals, humans included, respond strongly to immediate rewards. So eating junk food is reinforcing; it may be easy, fast, sugary, full of fat, gooey, crunchy, or whatever floats your boat. Whatever it is, it is an immediate payoff, even if it will cost you later. Vegetating on the couch with a pizza, a cigarette, or a few cold beers each night after a long day's work certainly has its allure and is much more immediately rewarding than getting into the car and heading to the gym or going out for a rugged hike, even though the gym or the hike will pay off for you in the end.

If you're ready to forgo instant gratification for long-term and long-lasting gratification, then you're primed and ready, just like we want you to be. Our goal is to turn things around for you, to help you chart a course for masculine excellence as only you can define it for yourself. It's never too late for second chances. If you make a commitment to us, we'll make a commitment to you. Together, we will deliver you to your Destination. You will greatly benefit from the support of your loved ones and the help of some of the world's brightest medical, fitness, psychology, nutrition, and exercise physiology experts (who all happen to be our good friends). This is a manual to build the best "you." Do you want to get your winning edge back? Discover an edge and indomitable warrior's spirit you never even knew you had? Do you want a stronger, leaner body? More health and energy? Married or single, white collar or blue collar, from the bedroom to the boardroom and whatever your walk of life, you will find this book is dedicated to bringing out the very best man in you.

MEASURING MANLINESS

How do you measure the qualities of the true Alpha Male? Can someone's manliness be quantified? We spent a lot of time thinking about that question and researching the subject.

Guys love numbers. Our brains often think in terms of mathematical values. We compare scores and stats and rankings and understand things best with graphs and scales. Whether it's NASDAQ or MLB, it's all about numbers for many guys. But don't worry if actually doing the math isn't your thing; we've done all the tough math for you. Enter the MaleScale. We designed a revolutionary assessment tool that guys can use to quantify the matrix of skills and characteristics of the true Alpha Male. We didn't create it alone. We recruited an accomplished multidisciplinary team to help construct a convenient test that works. It combines physical and functional measuring tests with questions about thoughts and behaviors; the MaleScale measures both inner and outer qualities. While the MaleScale doesn't *directly* assess your current diet because what you're eating now doesn't directly bear on your ranking, your current food choices are *indirectly* measured by the assessments, as they should be. What you've been eating is reflected, often to a large degree, by the current state of your body and mind.

The MaleScale doesn't determine whether you're a true Alpha Male or not, because there is no yes or no answer. The MaleScale shows you where you rank on the true Alpha Male continuum. We call this ranking your Alpha Factor. The scale ranges from a score of 10 to 100. Some guys will have higher or lower Alpha Factors than others. What is important is that you can determine where you stand on the scale right now, and then take action to improve your ranking. You will find your baseline place on the MaleScale before you start the Challenge. Then you will embark on the revolutionary Challenge that begins on page 126 of this book. Ten weeks from now, you will measure again and compare. If you commit to the Challenge, you will be amazed by your progress.

You need to be absolutely 100 percent *honest* in *all* of your answers or you will only shortchange yourself later. The answers about your thoughts and behaviors must come from you, but we recommend that after writing your answers, you discuss them with a trusted friend or loved one. This will add an objective perspective.

The MaleScale consists of two parts. There are 10 measures of Alpha Attitude—your beliefs about yourself and your outlook on the world around you. There are 5 assessments of Alpha Architecture—the strength, health, and appearance of your body. In only 20 minutes or so, you will know, perhaps for the first time in your life, precise details about your current state of physical and psychological conditioning. The only tools you will need are a bathroom scale, a pencil, a calculator, cloth or vinyl tape measure, a watch with a second hand, a piece of chalk, a standard weight bench, and a barbell. You'll need an area where you can run a bit. You'll also need a willing accomplice to assist you to ensure that the 5 assessments of Alpha Architecture are performed safely and accurately. For photos for the 5 assessments of Alpha architecture, see www.alphamalechallenge.com.

Are you ready to see where you stand?

The MaleScale

We can't impress on you strongly enough the importance of being completely honest. For the 10 measures of Alpha Attitude, circle the number that corresponds to the most truthful answer. Do not spend too much time contemplating each response. Instead, respond as quickly as possible, describing how you feel at this moment. For the 5 physical assessments of Alpha Architecture, fill in the blank with the appropriate information. Consult your physician regarding any preexisting injuries or illnesses, and to make sure you are healthy enough to take this test.

Ready? Pick up your pencil; there's no turning back now and remember, be honest!

The MaleScale

10 MEASURES OF ALPHA ATTITUDE (Circle corresponding number)

Over the past week, I set concrete and specific goals for myself to get where I want to be:

1	2	3	4	5	6	7	8	9	10
Not true		Somewhat true			Mostly true			Absolutely true	

I can resist eating my favorite junk food even when others are eating it in front of me.

1	2	3	4	5	6	7	8	9	10
Never		Rarely			Mostly			Always	

I am satisfied with my current physique.

1	2	3	4	5	6	7	8	9	10
Not satisfied		Somewhat satisfied			Mostly satisfied			Absolutely satisfied	

I am able to handle whatever obstacles life throws in my way.

1	2	3	4	5	6	7	8	9	10
Never		Rarely			Mostly			Always	

I am ready right now to stand up and take charge of a group that needs a leader.

1	2	3	4	5	6	7	8	9	10
No		Unlikely			Likely			Absolutely	

When I'm faced with a tough yet safe challenge that's within my physical capabilities, I face my fear and do it.

1	2	3	4	5	6	7	8	9	10
No way		Unlikely			Likely			Absolutely	

I am very good at looking at things from the viewpoint of other people.

1	2	3	4	5	6	7	8	9	10
No		Somewhat			Mostly			Absolutely	

I tried my hardest over the past week to help people in need, without being rewarded or expecting anything in return.

1	2	3	4	5	6	7	8	9	10
No		Somewhat			Mostly			Absolutely	

I bounce back from hardship by learning from my mistakes.

1	2	3	4	5	6	7	8	9	10
No		Somewhat			Mostly			Absolutely	

If I roll with the punches, everything will work out.

1	2	3	4	5	6	7	8	9	10
No way		Unlikely			Likely			Absolutely	

5 ASSESSMENTS OF ALPHA ARCHITECTURE

Before you begin, enter your current body weight in pounds here _____ .

1) Flexed Biceps Circumference

HOW TO DO IT: Using a cloth or vinyl tape measure, make a muscle and measure your flexed upper arm. The tape should go in a relatively straight vertical line around the largest part of the biceps and triceps, not at an extreme angle. Measure three times for best accuracy, making sure that the tape measure is taut, but not too tight. (You don't want to pinch the skin.) Use the same tape measure for follow-up measurements, to ensure reliability. Do it before you work out—this is a "cold" measurement, not one taken after you pump up!

WHY WE DO IT: "Make a muscle!" For as long as we can remember, the benchmark of male muscularity has been the upper arm. In a poll of *Cosmopolitan* readers, one out of five women confessed that nice, large biceps on a man makes them "absolutely melt." Bodybuilding champions have long boasted of their flexed biceps measurements; Arnold Schwarzenegger was reported to have a 22-inch arm at the peak of his bodybuilding career. Don't worry that circumference doesn't reflect how much fat may be on the arm; we're looking for sheer size here and will deal with body composition later. We assure you, our philosophy calls for a totally balanced body, but a flexed biceps measurement is the perfect way to start the assessment.

My flexed biceps circumference is _____ inches.

2) Chest-to-Waist Differential

HOW TO DO IT: Using a cloth or vinyl tape measure, take a deep breath, expand your chest, spread your upper back muscles (lats), and measure your chest around the largest part. To get an accurate chest measurement, start with your arms slightly raised at your sides. Wrap the tape measure just under your armpits, being sure to keep the measuring tape parallel to the floor. Bring your arms down toward your sides enough to allow proper chest expansion. Then measure your waist at the thinnest part, breathing in deeply and allowing the tape to be tight but not pinching the skin.

WHY WE DO IT: The Chest-to-Waist Differential is a great way to assess your body composition without calipers. The V-taper has been the recognized hallmark of a great physique since the days of Muscle Beach, and it probably dates back to prehistoric times. A study published in the *Journal of Social Psychology* showed that even across cultural settings, the bigger the difference between a guy's chest and his waist, the more likely he was to be found attractive by potential romantic partners. In other words, having a big chest isn't enough; you need a lean midsection to go with it.

My expanded chest circumference is _____ inches.

My waist circumference is _____ inches.

3) Vertical Jump

HOW TO DO IT: Rub a bit of chalk (or dirt, if you don't have any chalk) on the tip of the middle finger of your dominant hand. Stand about 6 inches from the wall, facing sideways, with your dominant hand side near the wall. With both feet flat on the ground, reach as high as possible with your dominant hand. Mark your highest reach on the wall with your chalked fingertip. Put a little more chalk on your finger, resume the same position, and jump up as high as you can. Bring your arms backward, flex your knees and hips, and bring your trunk forward and downward. Then explode upward and reach your dominant hand up to get the maximum height in your jump. At the peak of your jump, tap the wall with your chalked finger. Use a tape measure to measure the vertical distance in inches between the chalk marks. Record the best of three attempts.

Performance Note: Try to be as natural as possible when reaching. You only need a little tap—the chalk will show. Avoid slapping the wall hard or using excessive arm "waving" action, because that will reduce your score.

WHY WE DO IT: The Vertical Jump was first created and used by Dr. Dudley Sargent (1849–1924) to assess physical function. Some years later it was determined that the test could assess physical *power,* and by the mid-1960s the Russians were using this training application to improve power in their athletes. The Vertical Jump has been adapted by many sports (including football) because it indicates not only the rate at which work is performed (power = work/time), but because it also has a high correlation with on-field performance, athleticism, and speed measures. The "Vert" has become a standard for predicting athletic ability and a staple for measuring human performance. It's perfect to bring an element of power, catlike reflexes, and quick-burst speed to round out the Alpha Factor. By improving Vertical Jump scores, you improve overall body power (especially from the hips and legs). This translates into quicker, tighter movements, improved skill, and the ability to quickly develop force needed for everything from jumping and kicking to hitting and punching. All power in human movement comes from the ground, through the hips, and out to the limbs. So improving hip power, as demonstrated in both research and practical application, has profound effects on all performance activities.

My vertical jump height is _____ inches.

4) Maximum Bench-Press to Body-Weight Ratio

HOW TO DO IT: Rather than risk injury by attempting a single repetition to find your maximum bench-press weight, we're going to use a slightly lighter weight and apply a formula to accurately estimate your 1 rep max. *Warning: Recruit the assistance of a spotter throughout the process.* Warm up with 5 to 10 repetitions of a light-to-moderate weight. Rest for 2 minutes. Perform two heavier warmup sets of 2 to 5 reps, with a 2-minute rest between sets. These sets will help you estimate how much weight to load on the bar for the actual test. You should select a weight with which you can perform no more than 6 to 8 repetitions. After a rest of 2 to 4 minutes, perform the set with proper technique. (If you are uncertain how to execute the bench press, see page 193.) Do as many reps as you can until you cannot perform another full repetition. Leave "nothing on the table"—go until you cannot perform another rep without the spotter's assistance. If you perform 10 or fewer repetitions, you have completed the test. If you reach 10 repetitions and still have additional energy to complete more, stop at 10. Increase the load to reflect a better estimate of a weight you can perform for 6 to 8 repetitions. Rest for 4 to 5 minutes, then repeat the test.

WHY WE DO IT: Let's face it: There is no greater measure of male superiority in the gym than the bench press, even though it only measures the strength of your pecs, triceps, and anterior deltoids. Because a heavier man will generally be able to bench-press substantially more weight than a lighter guy, relative strength really tells the story. Relative strength is based on your ability to produce strength per pound of body weight. This measure works well in *most* cases because it assumes that the heavier individual has more muscle tissue. More muscle can produce more force, greater weight can be lifted by heavier individuals. As with all tests, it would be impossible for an easy-to-use measurement system to include the extremes of the weight spectrum. So very light guys and very heavy guys may find themselves fighting for a fair score. But for the average-weight male, pound for pound measurement of your 1 rep max is the way to go. To help guide our Male-Scale scoring system, we used data from combined sources, including the Cooper Institute, research papers, and testing results from both sports and general fitness trainers and coaches.

The number of repetitions (10 or fewer) performed is _____ reps.

The weight on the barbell is _____ pounds.

(The weight of a standard Olympic barbell is 45 pounds. If you are uncertain as to the weight of the bar itself, ask gym personnel.)

5) The 300 Run

HOW TO DO IT: This is a test of your speed, agility, and muscular endurance. Recruit the assistance of a partner to time your run with a watch or stopwatch. Measure out a distance of 25 yards. (You can use your feet, touching heel to toe, 75 times.) You will run back and forth across this 25-yard distance 12 times, for a total run of 300 yards. You must use the 25-yard distance; altering the distance will throw off your numbers. You must have 11 abrupt changes of direction. Warm up properly before the run to avoid injury. Run the distance as quickly as you can, but be mindful of your current physical condition. If you need to jog or even walk part of it, do so. Be careful not to slip or fall each time you switch direction. If you have been sedentary, don't push yourself beyond safe limits.

WHY WE DO IT: Improving cardiovascular health, shedding a few pounds, and becoming quicker and more agile will be a lifelong asset. There are many ways to assess endurance, but only one that can factor in a level of skill and agility that makes the all-around athlete. The Shuttle Run or 300 Run has widely become one of the standards for assessing "usable sport endurance." Due to its distance, it has an endurance component. But due to its short distance switchbacks, agility and speed also become factors. "Watching TV while going for a long endurance walk/run training routine," says David Sandler, a world-renowned strength coach, "is not very manly and certainly won't help improve your ability to run around on the court with your buddies or hang with your kids for a few hours of play. Improving your 300 Run time means you will have improved both your endurance and your speed. Undoubtedly your heart rate profile will improve, meaning that your overall cardiovascular health improves. Your ability to climb a flight of stairs without becoming breathless, or throw out a quick burst of speed here and there without needing to catch your breath, will be the most notable difference of all."

My 300 Run time is _____ seconds.

SCORING:

DETERMINING YOUR ALPHA FACTOR

ALPHA ATTITUDE ASSESSMENTS

1: Goal setting is integral to commitment to exercise and healthy eating. Write your score (1 to 10): _____.

2: Willpower is essential to a true Alpha Male lifestyle. Your ability to resist unhealthy temptations is crucial to success. Your score (1 to 10): _____.

3: Confident and commanding presence increases when you are comfortable with your physicality. Your score (1 to 10): _____.

4: Feeling competent to handle life's curves is key to overall confidence. Your score (1 to 10): _____.

5: The courage to assert your leadership within social groups is quintessential to Alpha Attitude. Your score (1 to 10): _____.

6: Physical courage is at the heart of "manliness." Your score (1 to 10): _____.

7: Strong leaders aren't just the bravest warriors. Empathy for others is truly Alpha. Your score (1 to 10): _____.

8: Altruism is a heroic characteristic of the true Alpha Male. Your score (1 to 10): _____.

9: Resiliency requires the ability to learn from failure. Your score (1 to 10): _____.

10: Maintaining a positive mental outlook about change is a key to resiliency. Your score (1 to 10): _____.

SUBTOTAL (between 10 and 100) _____

Divide by 2 and Round to Nearest Whole Number = _____ (between 5 and 50)

ALPHA ARCHITECTURE ASSESSMENTS

Flexed Biceps Circumference

> 17 inches	10 points
16.5 to 17 inches	9 points
16 to 16.4 inches	8 points
15.5 to 15.9 inches	7 points
15 to 15.4 inches	6 points
14.5 to 14.9 inches	5 points
14 to 14.4 inches	4 points
13.5 to 13.9 inches	3 points
13 to 13.4 inches	2 points
< 13 inches	1 point

Write your score (1 to 10) here _____.

Chest-to-Waist Differential

Subtract your waist measurement from your chest measurement. Write the difference here _____.

> 15 inches	10 points
13 to 15 inches	9 points
11 to 13 inches	8 points
9 to 11 inches	7 points
7 to 9 inches	6 points
5 to 7 inches	5 points
3 to 5 inches	4 points
1 to 3 inches	3 points
-3 to 1 inches	2 points
< -3 inches	1 point

Write your score (1 to 10) here _____.

Vertical Jump

> 27.5 inches	10 points
26 up to 27.5 inches	9 points
24.5 up to 26 inches	8 points
23 up to 24.5 inches	7 points
21.5 up to 23 inches	6 points
20 up to 21.5 inches	5 points
18.5 up to 20 inches	4 points
16.5 up to 18.5 inches	3 points
14.5 up to 16.5 inches	2 points
< 14.5 inches	1 point

Write your score (1 to 10) here _____.

Maximum Bench-Press to Body-Weight Ratio

To find your score, you'll need to use a calculator. Find the percentage associated with the number of reps you performed from the table below.

1 Repetition Maximum Percentages

Reps	% 1 RM
1	100
2	95
3	90
4	88
5	86
6	83
7	80
8	78
9	76
10	75

Now divide the weight you used by that percentage using decimals (83 percent equals 0.83) to get an approximation of your 1-RM. For example, if you can perform 10 reps with 175 pounds in the bench press, that means that 175 pounds is 75 percent (0.75) of your 1-RM. So, 175 divided by 0.75 = 233 pounds.

Having determined your estimated 1-RM bench press, divide it by your body weight in pounds. For example, if your 1-RM bench press is 300 pounds and you weigh 200 pounds, divide 300 by 200 to get 1.5.

My 1-RM bench press divided by my body weight is _____.

> 1.5	10 points
1.4 up to 1.5	9 points
1.3 up to 1.4	8 points

1.2 up to 1.3	7 points
1.1 up to 1.2	6 points
1.0 up to 1.1	5 points
0.9 up to 1.0	4 points
0.8 up to 0.9	3 points
0.7 up to 0.8	2 points
< 0.7	1 point

Write your score (1 to 10) here _____.

The 300 Run (in seconds)

< 60	10 points
62	9 points
64	8 points
66	7 points
68	6 points
70	5 points
72	4 points
74	3 points
76	2 points
> 78	1 point

Write your score (1 to 10) here _____.

SUBTOTAL (between 5 and 50) is _____.

Now add up the Alpha Attitude Subtotal and the Alpha Architecture Assessment Subtotal for a sum between 10 and 100.

Write it here _____.

CONGRATULATIONS!

THIS IS YOUR BASELINE ALPHA FACTOR

Yes, that's your Alpha Factor, your baseline for the transformation to come. Remember, this is only where you are now—it's not a blueprint of where you'll be in 10 weeks.

You may be mulling over the scoring numbers and trying to draw some conclusions. If you're worried about how you stack up against other guys, don't sweat it! That isn't the point. Everyone who undertakes this Challenge is on the same journey: the journey from where you are to where

you want to be. We're all in it together.

What *is* important to notice is that your scores are better in some areas than others. You may have a winning attitude, but your V-taper may need work. You may have more strength than power, or big arms but not a great 300 Run. That's okay; your Challenge is to achieve better *balance*. You want to be the complete package, right—a well-rounded warrior, a gladiator? That's our goal for you. By training more comprehensively and fiercely than ever before, you're going to be better in all respects, and that includes both body and mind.

Get ready for combat. For the next 10 weeks, you'll be on a mission to boost your score! If you meet the Challenge, in just 70 days you'll see astounding improvements in your Alpha Factor—and terrific changes in the way you look and feel!

A COMPREHENSIVE PLAN

You're about to embark on a very different kind of fitness program. Your Challenge is broken down into interrelated components: Alpha Attitude, Alpha Architecture, and the Alpha Fuel Solution. The components aren't sequential. You undertake them all at the same time. You're going to focus on physical exercise, your meals, and also on improving your attitude.

Understandably, you have questions. We'll try to answer them so you can move forward with open eyes . . . and unbridled enthusiasm.

Q: Who came up with this program?
A: We did, after successfully applying its various elements for years and recruiting a multidisciplinary team of experts to assist us in integrating and honing its components. We wanted a plan that *works* for the potato who needs to be "uncouched," but also a plan that can make today's

dedicated and experienced top dogs even better. Simply put: This program *rocks!*

Q: Do I need to be an Alpha male to start the program?

A: Absolutely not. This is a plan for every guy at every level. Haven't mowed a lawn or changed your car's oil in a decade? Resurrection is at hand. Never fired a rifle or climbed a mountain? No problem. Welcome aboard! Transformation is your Destination. We, too, are on an expedition of discovery, always challenging ourselves, learning new skills, and seeking to improve every day.

Q: Why so much emphasis on the mind?

A: Life is about choices and taking action. The choices we make and the actions that flow from them control our destinies. These choices start in the mind; failing to first focus there is the biggest mistake, especially for guys looking to un-couch themselves. Our program goes beyond food and exercise. You want to be a true Alpha Male? Research proves that you can develop your mental muscle through systematic exercise, nutrition, and rest, just like the muscles of your body.

Q: Is *Alpha Male Challenge* just for guys?

A: Yes, this book is dedicated to boosting your masculine Alpha Factor. It's also about helping to guide guys to be better *people*—better citizens, better husbands, better friends, or better fathers. However, most of the general exercise and eating principles of this book will benefit anyone. Developing commitment, confidence, courage, and conscience will spell success not just for men, young and old, but for women, as well. They help build stronger, better people.

Q: What about my family's role in this?

A: They should be very involved, especially if you are new to regular exercise and smart food choices. Involving your loved ones will boost your account-

ability; they are the core of your "Alpha Team"— your personal "A-Team." Their support can help keep you on track, especially when it comes to meal planning—the Alpha Fuel Solution is a good plan for the whole family, and it can provide an opportunity to share some quality time. As husbands and fathers ourselves, we created a program with family in mind. In fact, we highly recommend that you offer this book for your family to read. The Challenge is intended to be a shared experience with your A-Team to as great a degree as you'd like it to be.

Q: Should I check with my doctor before starting?

A: You should check with your physician before taking the MaleScale or starting any exercise program, *especially if you have not been physically active recently* or if you have *any* of the following medical conditions:

- a diagnosed heart condition
- chest pain or pain in the neck and/or arm
- shortness of breath
- dizziness
- a current prescription for cardiac and/or blood pressure medications and/or other prescription medications
- joint and/or bone problems

After your medical doctor gives you the green light, start out gradually and sensibly, based on your existing fitness level. Of course, if you experience any of the physical symptoms listed above when you start your exercise program, cease exercise immediately and contact your physician right away. Also, although the fundamentals of the Alpha Fuel Solution have been tested over the last 2.5 million years, anyone with liver or kidney disease, or who may be predisposed to kidney disease or any other disease, should not adopt this food plan without first obtaining clearance from his doctor. Also, talk to your physician before starting any nutritional supplementation program.

Q: How much exercise will I be doing?

A: Maybe more than you're used to, maybe less. If you're a newly un-couched potato, it'll be more. If you're already a highly trained top dog looking to switch things up to get a renewed burst of progress, maybe less. Lifting weights is a critical and essential part of your program. However, we don't believe in endless hours of working out with weights. For these 10 weeks, you'll be lifting weights only 3 days a week, but the workouts are short, intense, and incredibly effective. You'll also take part in our Work Heart/Play Heart aerobic program, which will integrate fitness into your daily life. We think our program is the optimal balance of weight training, aerobic exercise, rest, and everything else that makes up your waking hours. Time is precious. We have jobs and families, too. Our philosophy is to make the best use of your time.

Q: Will I be doing a traditional bodybuilding workout?

A: The problem with traditional bodybuilding theory is its pure superficiality. It's only about appearance. Some of the bulkiest guys who call themselves "athletes" don't have the flexibility and speed to play Frisbee with their kids. In response to this dilemma, "functional training"—workouts that supposedly focus on building strength and power that can be applied to ordinary life—has become the popular alternative of the moment. But many functional training movements are just plain weird and actually have little relevance in the real world. Besides, most functional training enthusiasts look pretty average. We've improved upon the best of both worlds and created an integrated program to progressively achieve both "show" *and* "go."

Q: What kind of diet will I be on?

A: We're as sick of fad diets as you are. You won't be eating birdseed, and you won't be on a low-carb diet with tons of bacon and sausages filled with saturated animal fat. You won't be obsessing over calories. You won't be starving yourself, either. Our core views on nutrition are about 2.5 million years old. Don't worry: You won't be eating raw meat. Our Alpha Fuel Solution is about eating exactly what you're supposed to be eating. And you'll be getting strong and lean. Unlike the proponents of strict "Paleolithic diets," our model recognizes that not everything "new" is bad. The concept that our bodies have wonderful adaptive capacities is integral to our program. We've taken the best of modern foods and supplements and added them into our simple eating plan of the right Fuel Foods in the proper proportions—and tossed out the trash. You can follow the Alpha Fuel Solution for life. We'll also be introducing you to two highly effective variations: the Handshake Diet and the Spartan Diet. These fuel plans are specifically designed to meet the demands and goals of your 10-week Challenge.

Q: Do I need to join a gym?

A: We've provided a blueprint for building a solid work out of Alpha Architecture in your very own home (page 77). We prefer a gym environment because having training partners and being around all that extra motivating energy from other gym-goers is bound to psyche you up! If you prefer beginning Alpha Wave Basic Training at home, just be sure not to sell yourself short. If you can cajole a partner into joining you, so much the better! Or perhaps just do it for a week or so, build up your confidence, and then get your butt to the local health club. If you knew just how nervous even the huge guys in the gym were when they first started out, you'd be surprised.

Q: Why is a training partner important?

A: Training with a partner or two creates fun, support, competition, motivation, and inspiration. It also enhances training safety by providing an available "spotter," rather than leaving you to train without one or ask a stranger at the gym. There will be days when you'll seem to have a great excuse for not working out, but your training partner will get your tired, overworked, or lazy butt in gear. On other days, you'll do the same for him. Commit to mutual inspiration and to safely pushing each other to excel. Your training partner is most definitely a part of your A-Team!

Q: What kind of changes can I expect?
A: If you put in the time and effort, you're virtually guaranteed to look better, feel better, and perform better in all your daily activities! Results will depend in part on how far you are from your Destination, and generally, the more you put into this Challenge, the more you'll get out of it. You'll soon meet some guys in this book who worked hard and saw amazing results. One guy increased his Alpha Factor by 41 points, dropped 7 inches of fat off his waist, and increased his physical confidence by an amazing 350 percent in 10 weeks! Another dropped 9 inches off his waist and improved his Alpha Factor by 32 points during the Challenge. One star pupil increased his Alpha Factor by 33 points, adding more than 4 inches to his vertical jump while also losing more than 10 inches off his waist and a whopping 52 pounds in 10 weeks.

The tools we provide can be put into action the very first day and may make a difference almost immediately. What's most important to realize is that where you are now doesn't dictate where you can be 10 weeks from now, or even 10 days from now. It doesn't matter how long you may have been lying like a potato on your couch. The requirements of the Challenge are not so burdensome that you can't integrate them into the rest of your life. We always intended this plan to be more than just a road map to better abs. It's a road map to a better life.

THE PLEDGE

If you are ready to face the Challenge, take the Pledge, and vow to keep it. You're not contracting to sell your firstborn child or committing to Fight Club. You're just committing to the search for masculine excellence over the next 10 weeks:

> Having decided that I am ready to improve myself physically and psychologically for the benefit of myself and those I love, I pledge to commit myself wholly to the *Alpha Male Challenge*. I understand that my level of commitment is commensurate with the level of benefit to be gained through this program. For at least the next 10 weeks, I pledge to forgo excuses in favor of accountability. I pledge to sacrifice the comfort of old habits in favor of a new style of living that maximizes my inner and outer potential as one of a new breed of true Alpha Males.

We will hold you to it.

JIM LISA, AGE 51

JIM IS AN ATTORNEY whose hectic schedule left him little time for himself. He was a marathon runner who let his weight reach nearly 250 pounds. "I guess I began to question my physicality upon two major events in my life," Jim notes. "The first was being stricken with cancer in 2004 and the second was turning age 50 in 2008. I wanted to do everything and anything that could possibly extend my life so I could be around to enjoy my family. I felt a first step in that direction was getting my body weight under 200 pounds." Jim was ready to take the Challenge.

Original Alpha Factor: 52.

Jim worked with a True Alpha master trainer for several months and lost 43 pounds.

He started the 10-Week Challenge at 206 pounds.

He weighed 183 pounds at Week 10.

Jim lost 23 pounds in only 10 weeks, while improving his muscle to fat ratio by nearly 30 percent.

He dropped 9 inches of fat from his waist and at the same time increased the size of his biceps. He added an inch-and-a-half of muscle on his chest and increased his maximum bench press by over 20 pounds. His speed on the 300-yard shuttle run improved by an amazing 22 seconds—from 87 seconds down to just 65! "Aches and pains I had in my joints and lower back before I started the Challenge—and I was afraid might get worse—are gone," Jim says with amazement. "I do not remember feeling this good since I was 26. I feel as though I can do anything physically with any person of any age and be competitive."

His MaleScale™ score for willpower increased by 25 percent in 10 weeks, as did his positive outlook on change and his resiliency. And his physical confidence *doubled*!

Overall, Jim soared up 32 points on the MaleScale™.

New Alpha Factor: 84.

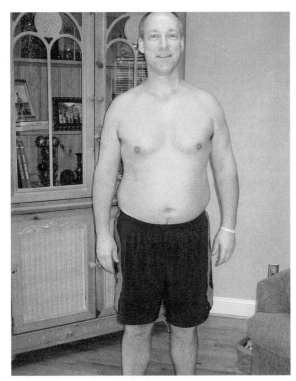

Before

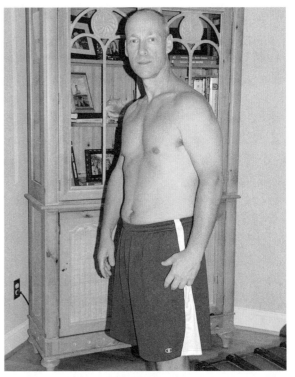

Mid-Challenge

Testimonial:

"The Alpha Male Challenge has changed my body, my attitude and my life beyond any expectations that I had set for myself prior to beginning the Challenge. During the 10-week program I lost 21 pounds, my body now looks muscular, and many of those aches and pains I once had are now gone. I absolutely loved the physical training aspects of the program.

"The physical training concepts under 'Work Heart / Play Heart' and 'Power Boost' plyometric movements were all new to me. What I liked best about these new concepts were the variety and the high intensity levels. I also liked that the duration was generally short for each exercise. The knowledge I gained about nutrition while doing the Alpha Male Challenge was a critical component to my success. As a result of the concepts I learned about food quality and quantity as part of the Alpha Fuel Solution, I now realize how important good nutrition is to be successful.

"I would highly recommend to anyone wanting to make a positive change in their mental and physical well-being that they embrace the concepts laid out in the *Alpha Male Challenge*. The program works and, if you follow it, you will be pleased with the results!"

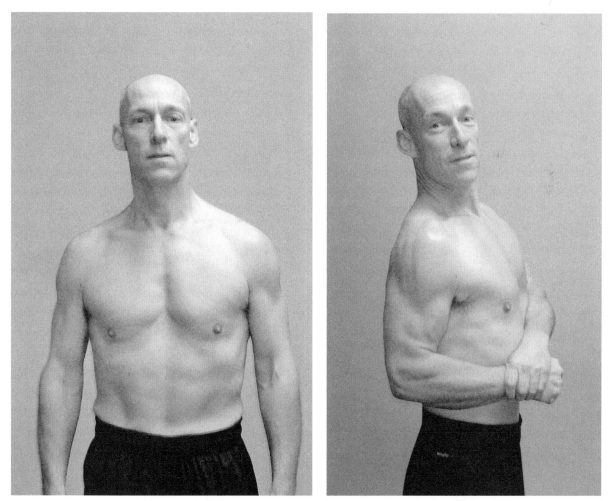

After   After

CHAPTER THREE

TRUE ALPHA ATTITUDE

The bookstore shelves are lined with men's health and fitness books whose authors tell you how to do a barbell curl and why funnel cakes aren't a smart food choice. Do they really think that just providing a food plan or weight-training regimen will catapult readers to the rarefied heights of fitness glory? There are infinitely more of these books on the shelves than six-packs on the men who buy them. Bookstores probably wouldn't need a new one every few months if they worked like they claim.

Unless you're living in a fallout shelter, it's hard to imagine that you haven't gotten the message that eating better and getting more exercise is the way to enhance your health. Yet obesity remains at an all-time high, having reached a new milestone: The population of obese Americans now outweighs the number who are merely overweight. It is clear that knowing that something needs to be changed and even reading a book that tells you how to eat and what exercises to do aren't enough to create true and lasting change.

Floodwaters rise, stock prices fall, traffic snarls on the 4:05. There's a whole world around us, and most of what happens in it is beyond our control.

Our Paleolithic predecessors faced difficult climatic changes and lived a harsh nomadic lifestyle. The dangers they faced were real and life threatening. Today, things such as obligations, illnesses, traffic delays, and spotty cell phone reception have become the stressors for some guys; paying the monthly bills is a stressor for far too many others. Marriages end, jobs are lost. Although you may not see these things as imminently deadly, our bodies react to them that way, and they affect us more than we generally realize.

When you encounter a stressor—for example, a stranger approaching in a dark alley—your brain gets busy. The very same systems that evolved over eons in our prehistoric ancestors as a way to adapt and survive go into action. Our good friend California psychologist Jason Cohen, PsyD, recently described the process like this: Flurries of electrochemical messages unleash a cascade of hormones, causing the sympathetic nervous system reaction sometimes called the "fight or flight" response. This remarkable phenomenon once enabled our spear-wielding ancestors to stay alive in life-or-death situations, such as ice avalanches or saber-toothed tiger attacks. Today, it prepares us for

> "Nothing can stop the man with the right mental attitude from achieving his goal; nothing on earth can help the man with the wrong mental attitude."
>
> ~W.W. ZIEGE~

effective environmental management (aka saving your ass). Your heart rate increases, blood vessels in your skin constrict, your bronchi dilate, your liver releases glucose, you sweat more, your digestion is inhibited, and your pupils dilate. Just imagine that the stranger in the alley is an Ultimate Fighting Champion and he thinks you just messed with his girlfriend. Your brain and body work in harmony to take your best shot at a warrior's defense . . . or a blisteringly hasty retreat. The attacker, the bill collector, the imminent deadline your boss just gave you—all are processed by the same primitive areas of the brain and therefore create similar biological states of readiness.

The fight-or-flight response was explored back in the 1940s by psychologist Hans Selye, who theorized a "General Adaptation Syndrome" (some say he gave us "GAS") that described how our bodies react to stressors. It is marked by three stages. When we are surprised or threatened, we go into a stage characterized by anxiety, called Alarm; a threat is recognized and the body's resources are marshaled to deal with it. In the next stage, Resistance, the body begins to effectively cope with the stressor and the alarm reaction fades. We have the opportunity to successfully adapt to meet the challenge. If the stressor wears us down for too long, we reach the final stage of Exhaustion, in which the body can't keep up with the demands, resulting in fatigue, illness, and, eventually, well, kicking the bucket. But if the threat passes and we have sufficient time to rest before the next hurdle, we will be stronger for having adapted to it.

Our reactions to life's stressors can kill us . . . or make us stronger. How our brains react to the endless variety of environmental factors that surround us can break our bodies down or build our bodies up. This brings us to a preliminary principle, which isn't some New Age mantra but rather a simple fact:

The body and mind are connected.

The connection between mind and body is as obvious as the naked fat guy in the hotel pool. It's a shame that most fitness authors give it such short shrift, or no shrift at all. They plunge—shriftlessly—right into sets and reps, how much protein and carbs to consume, and why nacho chips aren't a food group. But they overlook this initial and most critical connection.

There's no doubt that a successful exercise and eating program will improve your outlook on life and your view of yourself. When your body feels healthier physically, you tend to be in better spirits. When you change yourself on the *outside,* it can change you on the *inside.* When you gain lean muscle, lose belly fat, and get stronger and more powerful, you're going to feel better about yourself. A friend of ours describes how he feels when he's in top shape by gushing, "Dude, when I get to the beach in a T-shirt and board shorts, I just can't wait to tear it all off and show everybody!" Okay, admittedly, he's crazy. But when you like the changes you see in the mirror, you're going to have more inner confidence; you're going to feel more capable and secure. You will, effectively, have "adjusted your attitude" for the better.

But there's a problem. It's Newton's First Law. Huh? Didn't expect that, did you? Well, ol' Sir

"All that we are is the result of what we have thought. The mind is everything. What we think, we become."

~BUDDHA~

"We accept the verdict of the past until the need for change cries out loudly enough to force upon us a choice between the comforts of inertia and the irksomeness of action."

~LEARNED HAND~

Isaac Newton may not have known much about nutrition or resistance training, but he foresaw plenty about modern America's lazy couch potatoes when he created his Law of Inertia:

Objects at rest tend to stay at rest.

And so, a guy on his couch tends to stay on his couch. The human body doesn't rouse itself up to improve unless a force acts upon it, and in most cases it is programmed to fight to stay right where it is. That's called "homeostasis," a set point for the modern-day couch potato. For too many guys, the only force acting on their bodies is the force of gravity, and that isn't going to improve the way you look. So, if you want to improve your body, you're going to need some other force. And if you're seeking a radical or revolutionary transformation, then you are going to need a powerful force to get that ball rolling.

How does your car stay in its lane of traffic when you're driving at night? How does it make all the proper turns to get you home?

Your body may be doing the manual labor, but it's your *mind* that dictates whether your car goes home, or to the gym, or off to a burrito binge at the local fast-food dive. As is all too often the case for so many guys, your mind tells you not to go to the gym at all and to stay home on the comfy couch and eat frozen pizza, instead. What keeps someone on the couch? It's that the perceived cons of going to the gym outweigh the pros, or that the pros of staying on the couch outweigh the cons. So we make conscious decisions to be less than our best.

Take heart, brothers. You've made a commit-ment to us by choosing to pick up this book, and we've made a commitment to you. We feel person-ally invested in your success as a true Alpha Male. And we have a plan to get you to the Destination you want. Science says that the type of transfor-mation we're talking about is best started from the inside, not the outside. Which brings us to another simple principle:

The mind leads; the body follows.

The late Dr. James Dabbs was a psychology researcher and professor at Georgia State Univer-sity. Much of his research focused on gender dif-ferences in social behavior and the relationship between testosterone and behavior in both males and females. In *Heroes, Rogues, and Lovers,* Dr. Dabbs noted something that has been shown in a number of studies over the years: Success or fail-ure in competition affects testosterone levels. Ten-nis players and judo competitors, presumably both exhilarated after winning, experience upward spikes in testosterone levels. But it's more than exhilaration; it is the body's way of preparing for the next challenge, the next competition. Also interesting is the fact that the losers of the match experience drops in testosterone (and increases in stress hormones, including cortisol), which would seem to put them at a disadvantage for the next challenge. And the phenomenon isn't limited to physically active sports; even in an intellectual game like chess video games, gamers' testosterone levels drop when they lose and rise when they win. And even more interesting, our bodies will actu-ally learn to increase testosterone in *anticipation* of competition; when our brain notes a challenge coming, our testosterone levels begin to rise. All in all, it is a pretty complex system. The simple lesson is that our experiences and the way we view them can cause physiological changes, including raising or lowering the levels of the very hormone that makes us men.

Our approach to true Alpha Male fitness starts with the *mind*, which shouldn't really be surprising. We both believe that the mind has an awesome power for controlling the body and achieving "real, lasting, active, revolutionary change."

If your goal were to boost your overall masculine excellence, why would you train only your exterior? Unless your sole goal is professional bodybuilding, why systematically develop only your skeletal muscles—only the façade? When you really think about it, shouldn't every man's goal be not only to look more heroic but also to *be* more heroic? True Alpha Attitude is a quality that resides within. Your most obvious goal in developing your Architecture is to enhance your health, sculpt you into looking like a hard-body hero, and help you build the physical endurance and functional strength to act the part. But we're a little more ambitious than that. After all, does anybody really want a strong and rugged exterior but a weak and soft interior?

Before we tell you how to build awesome arms or blast the fat off your waistline, we're going to retrain the way you *think*. Seems like a tall order for a fitness book, huh? Trust us; we're going to harness the power of your mind to cause as radi-cal a physical metamorphosis as you desire. Your brain is going to start the engine of your fitness goals, and your mind is going to drive the car to your Destination. And if you think that we're just going to give you a little motivational pep talk to stick with your training program and eat better, you're *way* off the mark. We've got something very, very different in mind.

An improved attitude is the kind of powerful force we need to act on the body at rest, and to get it off the comfy couch and into motion. A stronger, more disciplined mind will enhance your commitment to working out and eating right. But those things don't happen just by saying it or because we want them to; they take sustained effort.

Most books in the fitness category take that purely superficial approach. It's all foam and no beer. It's like slapping fresh paint on a Ford Pinto. Our goal is not just to help you build the most magnificent *outer* self you can, but to help you build the most magnificent *inner* self, as well. We want you to *be* more powerfully masculine. And we want you to be able to measure the progress for yourself.

Scientists describe your brain as "plastic," meaning it can be remolded, can be retrained. Experience changes the brain. Decades of research have now shown that substantial changes occur in the lowest neocortical processing areas, and that these changes can profoundly alter the pattern of neuronal activation in response to experience. The more you use your brain, the stronger it becomes and the more efficiently it works. What we're

TOP DOG TIP

Many of the most dedicated weight trainers don't spend much time thinking about developing their mental muscles. Do you? It just isn't part of what guys think about in between rushing to the dry cleaner's and getting to work on time. But there's some truth to the old adage "use it or lose it" when it comes to any muscle. Your mental muscles are being ignored and neglected, like the awkward girl at the high school dance. Those gawky girls sometimes grow up to be gorgeous models, though, and if we pay some attention to our mental muscles we'll find they can transform beautifully, as well.

about to propose is pretty revolutionary. The very idea of it may blow your mind, as it did those we first explained it to. What if you could design a program to exercise and develop your *character* and best *inner* true Alpha Male traits just like a physical training program exercises and develops your skeletal muscles?

The mind is like a muscle.

You're about to embark on a unique program. A progressive regimen to develop the mind along with the body is an unprecedented "cross-training" concept, but it makes perfect sense given the mind-body connection. You will take the same structured approach used in physical training and apply it to attitude training. The components you will target exist naturally within each and every one of us.

Everyone starts with his own individual Alpha Factor. But each and every one of us can build on what nature gave us to be the best *we* can be. That's true of our biceps and triceps, and it's true of our attitude muscles, as well. Like our skeletal muscles, they can and must be *exercised,* and they will respond by adapting. Everyone can develop and strengthen the muscles he was born with. You are truly the architect of the man you will become. Being your own architect gives you the control to overwrite what Mother Nature may have given you.

Sound outrageous? It's not. Accumulating research now suggests that your master "virtue" muscle responds pretty much like any other muscle. After a workout of curls, your biceps will be temporarily depleted of resources. But with adequate rest and recuperation, they can come back to meet a stronger challenge.

Roy F. Baumeister, PhD, and his team of researchers at Florida State University have led the field in research in this area. His studies show that willpower and our ability to resist temptation can be strengthened through exercise. "In addition to the short-term decline in self-control performance after exerting self-control," writes Dr. Baumeister in an article coauthored with Dr. Mark Muraven and published in the APA *Psychological Bulletin,* "the self-control strength model predicts that, like a muscle, repeated practice and rest can improve self-control strength in the long term." It takes energy to exert self-control, and that energy is limited, so using it on one task can make it less likely that we can use it on another—until we have had time to rest. It makes perfect sense. Exercise an ability you want to develop, then give it rest so it can grow, and it will blossom. And that's how we're gonna roll!

Let's use an example: If your desk is next to the snack machine, you might spend the day exerting self-control to avoid buying those salty, fatty chips and instead eating the nuts and raw vegetables that you brought from home. By the time you get home, if there are chips in the cupboard, your self-control resources will be running low and you are more likely to give in. This suggests an important strategy, says psychologist Jack Darkes, PhD, of the University of South Florida: To give your self-control muscles time to rest up from temptation, don't keep tempting foods available at home. You may not be able to control much of our global environment today, but you can control the environment within your own home. Let it help you maintain control while your self-control muscles rest.

WHO DO YOU WANT TO BE?

What qualities are of value to you? We know you want leaner and sharper abs and a stronger and more muscular physique. But what about inner qualities? Most guys have never made any effort to train them at all. But we've talked to guys around the country about the inner traits they prize. When you put them all together, the sum amounts to what most guys think of as traditionally masculine and even, well, "heroic."

Most books about self-improvement speak to their readers as if something were wrong with them. The reader is directed to acknowledge his deficits and failings, and then various recommendations are offered to help "fix" his problems. That's not where we're coming from. This isn't therapy. Rather, we have taken a range of powerful tools and concepts that psychologists have used for years to understand behavior and behavior change, some of which have been used in therapy, and we have reconfigured them to help healthy men like you improve. Behavior change is not always about fixing a problem; it is often about making some things even better.

Let's respectfully push Mother Nature aside. If we were to build the ideal man from the *inside*, what components would we emphasize? What sort of man would we make? We would want to beef up the traits that attract potential mates and also evoke admiration from his masculine peers. We would want to maximally adapt him to survive and succeed in the sometimes-brutal modern world, but also boost the qualities that will help him leave the world a better place than he found it.

What are the inner attributes of the ideal man— the true Alpha Male—a man built on tradition but socially adapted to the modern world? We've identified the Four Cs of Alpha Attitude: commitment, confidence, courage, and conscience. Although they overlap and intertwine, and in some circumstances they may call for a healthy dose of resiliency to go with them (see illustration, left), the Four Cs will help you take a practical approach to developing the inner parts of you that will make you the best man you can be.

Who's in Charge?

We like to think that we consciously choose *every* move we make, but it's really not much like that at all. Sure, we are in control of many of our thoughts and actions, but not all of them—not by a long shot. In general, the human mind operates on (at least) two levels; sometimes we are aware of and actively handle things with what is often called our conscious mind. Most of the time, however, our thoughts, decisions, and actions are controlled automatically by what was traditionally called the unconscious (and we'll avoid scientific jargon and call it that, too).

Our conscious mind plans and sets goals when we say, "I will do this." It is focusing on reading right now; it acts when you tell yourself not to eat your third hot cinnamon bun (although this is where we learn that it is not always in charge). Your conscious mind actively directs thinking and attention and explicitly controls what actions to take (or not to take).

But we also know that such control takes effort, as Dr. Baumeister's research suggests. In fact, because control is valuable and limited, it makes

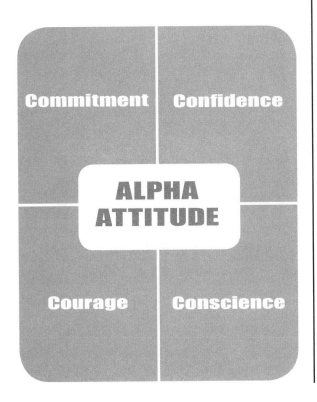

Commitment   Confidence

ALPHA ATTITUDE

Courage   Conscience

sense that we were built to function without it. That is our default condition, although our conscious mind may check in on things every once in a while. If self-control were limitless, then we would never have that all-too-common experience of doing things we did not "want to do." On the other hand, if we consciously decided every move, there'd be little time for doing.

Between the brain's miraculous multitasking functions and the demands of almost unlimited inputs in our hectic lives, we simply can't and don't consciously control all of our mental processes or behaviors. This can lead to lapses; failures to stick to new plans, diets, or fitness regimens (e.g., "failures" of self-control or willpower); or times when we "decide" and try our hardest to do something different but, in the end, go back to the same old (e.g., finding that cinnamon bun or bag of chips half-eaten in your hand).

As our friend Dr. Darkes explains, the unconscious program, once loaded, runs in the background without the operator's attention. That program does not necessarily evaluate the integrity or accuracy of the formula or data with which it works. If there are errors or "cognitive distortions" (e.g., inaccurate memories, negative or unwarranted assumptions), then the output is flawed. Our mind can be like that, as well; once a pattern of automatic beliefs, thoughts, and behaviors becomes programmed, it runs without much consideration of its accuracy or whether it is optimizing our lives or not.

So what does this all mean for the aspiring true Alpha Male? When everything is working well, the system runs along unnoticed. However, when we consciously experience a need for change, decide to learn or do something new, or want to change our thinking or behavior, or when something out of the ordinary grabs our attention, we exert conscious effort. We invest the energy in controlling our thinking and behavior to do something different. But there are no guarantees; over

time, we often end up where we started (e.g., negative thoughts, vegetating on the couch with a bucket o' wings). When we use all our resources and successfully control our thinking and acting in new directions, however, new experiences result and new thoughts and behaviors become part of our life, part of the program, over time. The process becomes effortless again and runs with a hopefully healthier output. So changing thinking and behavior requires a great amount of resources at first, but with planning, time, practice, and persistence, our "good" habits can become as strong as our "bad" ones were.

We've talked about self-control being similar to a muscle, so let's try out one more analogy for this kind of thinking that directly ties together our desire to improve both your physique and your attitude. You may have heard of *myostatin*, a natural growth factor that limits our skeletal muscle tissue growth. Negative automatic thoughts about ourselves and our potential are like "mental myostatin"—a defeatist and negative set of core beliefs that limits the growth and development of true Alpha Attitude and lifestyle. But if you can turn off your mental myostatin, change your behavior (and thus your experiences), and redirect your efforts, then over time your unconscious mind will change, too. You will start to rewrite the program. In so doing, you'll rediscover your life as it was meant to be lived. You'll have more energy, more muscle, less fat, and a better and truer attitude, and you will forever be changed into a better man.

COMMITMENT

We want you to become a master of your own destiny, to set your sights on a goal for your 10-week transformation into a true Alpha Male, and to help you chart the course that will get you there. However, it's important for you to know that we cannot make that commitment for you. You have to want to make the commitment yourself. So we'll start right at the beginning—making a commitment. Not only is commitment central to a winning attitude, but it is also essential to making any change you want to make in life.

You have to want to reach your Destination. You can't do it because you have to. It's much more difficult to build the enthusiasm to engage in something that you feel forced into. Never let goals that others have defined for you or pushed you to aspire to be your guide. Effort is easier to expend when the goals you are pursuing are goals you believe in, goals you want for yourself and have made a commitment to achieve. A study on the relationship between commitment and exercise behavior published in the journal *Psychology of Sport and Exercise* looked at "want to" commitment and "have to" commitment— "want to" meaning goals subjects set for themselves and "have to" meaning goals set forth for subjects by others. The researchers concluded that guys who want to exercise—who make a "want to" commitment—actually follow through with their exercise plan. "Have to" commitment based on a forced obligation or social pressures to get in shape, stop smoking, or slim down just won't cut it. Being cognizant of the idea of "want to" and "have to" commitments is an easy way to pinpoint the triggers that motivate you to act. Choosing aerobic activities that you enjoy and want to do—playing tennis or racquetball, for example—will more effectively keep you exercising than forcing yourself to do something just because you *have to*—such as logging endless, same-pace hours on the treadmill.

The way to develop this ability to commit is through regular practice, and taking the mental and physical steps—no matter how big or small—toward your goal each and every day. Remember that the unconscious program will run as it normally does, as it has been trained to do, if you don't exert your mental force to change it. So you've got to consciously define your goals and your willpower to stick to them.

GOAL SETTING

Your goals are the benchmarks you set on the journey to your Destination. The goals have to be goals you want for yourself, not things that others want for you or you want for others. Setting goals will give you a jump start on your journey to achieving what you want—whether it's professional success, a stronger relationship with your wife or girlfriend, replacing the muffin top above your belt with an abdominal washboard, or bench-pressing 50 pounds more than you can now.

Like most guys reading this book, you probably want to build muscle, burn fat, and reclaim your mental toughness and winning edge. Setting goals involves at least two things—an accurate image of where you are now and a detailed picture of where you want to be. The goals you set must lead to your unique Destination. Start by evaluating your resources; what are your strengths, the skills, abilities, and traits you can use to your advantage? In what areas do you need to improve? If you stick with this program for 10 weeks, what do you want to see in the mirror when you are done? If you do the things you *want* to do, what will you be like a year from now? How will that man be perceived by those around him, and how will they describe him to others? Be detailed, be specific; this is the future you are building.

"There are only two options regarding commitment. You're either in or out. There's no such thing as a life in-between."

~PAT RILEY~

An effective strategy to meet your goals is to set up short-term, midterm, and long-term benchmarks that you can work toward in the next 10 weeks. Monitoring your progress using benchmarks will help you stay committed and increase your chances for the greatest results possible. According to a study published in *Health Education Research,* frequent goal setting is more likely to keep you committed and on track toward your goals. And here again, the power of specific goals was shown; the associations were stronger for goals and strategies related specifically to diet and exercise than for those related to weight loss in general. If your outcome goals (your Destination) are realistic and you evaluate them frequently, then when you set and meet your performance goals (the actions needed to get there), your outcome goals will most often take care of themselves. Create long-term, midterm, and short-term benchmarks for both performance and outcome. Although each of these three goal phases is separate, they all have to do with the very same outcome: reaching your Destination and detailing what it takes to get there.

You'll set your long-term goals first. For our 10-week plan, these will be monthly goals that evolve as you move along in the program, evaluating your progress at monthly intervals. Setting these goals will help you better reach your Destination. Then set your midterm goals, which will be weekly. Lastly, set short-term goals, which will be daily. Short-term goals are actions. They are the little steps—a hard workout tonight, a healthy lunch tomorrow—that lead the way, step by step, to your Destination. Every day, create a new goal for tomorrow. It can be a relatively small feat, but it will still have a powerful effect on your life. You should be setting your daily short-term goals first thing in the morning or the night before. It's simply a matter of identifying what will keep you committed and on track to your Destination. It should only take a minute or two!

Be positive when setting your goals, and look ahead, not back. We learn from our experiences how best to move forward. Research published in the *Journal of Consumer Research* found that sticking to your fitness goals is more driven by where you want to get to than by how far you've come.

Research published in the *Journal of Applied Behavior Analysis* has shown that public goal setting is more effective in changing behavior than private goal setting. A study at Michigan State University found that people who bet $40 that they could stick with their program had a 97 percent success rate, while exercisers who didn't make a bet had a success rate of less than 20 percent. That's why your very first Alpha Attitude drill in Week 1 of the Challenge entails making an "Alpha Bet" with a co-worker or loved one (see page 126). Base the bet on *performance,* not outcome. In other words, bet on what your behavior will be rather than on what the results will be. For example, bet that "I will not eat at any fast food dives for the next 21 days" or "I will work out three times weekly without missing a workout for the next month."

And remember, no man is an island. The help and support of your family and friends can be important for keeping you on track. Wherever you can include and integrate them into the Challenge, you should. They're an invaluable support system. Finding novel and unique ways to involve them from the beginning of your true Alpha Male journey will help create a safety net of enhanced accountability and commitment to the goals you've set.

WILLPOWER

Call it willpower, discipline, or self-control, but whatever the name it goes by, it's a crucial component to success in fitness, in diet, and in life. Willpower gets your butt into the gym on a dark, frosty morning when every fiber of your being says "stay in bed." Willpower keeps your hand from tossing the box of frosted doughnuts into your supermarket cart. For most people, willpower and discipline are what being a warrior is all about.

Take, for example, Stew Smith, former Navy SEAL, popular fitness author, and Certified Strength and Conditioning Specialist (CSCS). After his appearance on the National Geographic Channel's *Fight Science* television episode on Special Ops, he received numerous e-mails from guys wanting to know his trick for handling the death-defying cold water conditions. It wasn't a trick; it was a matter of conditioning. After years of training in tough environments and under stressful conditions during his years in the Navy SEAL Teams, his mind and body simply got used to these encounters and became stronger as a result. "The human body is built for survival and will adapt to better handle cold, heat, stress, pain, and just about anything you can throw at it," Stew told us recently. "How about those days when you feel like crap, but know you need to train? These days occur for every man. It is up to you to will yourself to work out."

Most of the time, when people start the process of changing their lives, whether it is changing themselves physically or the way they think and approach life, the word *willpower* is mentioned. When psychologists talk about this idea, they prefer the term *self-control*, and there has been quite a bit of research looking into this ability and how it works.

One of the really illuminating findings in Dr. Baumeister's research into self-control as a muscle has been that exerting self-control leads to a depletion of resources. (They call it *ego depletion*, because the part of us that exerts control over our actions is often called the ego.) When this happens, our willpower is diminished for a period of time or in subsequent situations. For example, a sensitive conversation of racial politics with a person of another race might require conscious self-control

to such a degree that performance suffers on a subsequent psychological test of directed attention. This effect occurs in physical tasks, as well. For example, people stifling (controlling) their emotions while watching a tearjerker movie gave up more quickly on a subsequent hand-grip stamina test. (Remember that ol' mind-body connection?) So much for watching *Terms of Endearment* before going to the gym! But our point here is simple; you can't constantly be exerting self-control. Just like we have to allow our muscles time to recover their strength after working out, so too do we have to plan for our self-control resources to recover from periods in which we are depleting them. One of the reasons you may have failed in the past was that you did not plan for those times when your ego resources were depleted.

Why does exercising self-control temporarily sap our strength? Your body typically runs on glucose (blood sugar), and so does your brain. Dr. Baumeister found that self-control tasks deplete blood glucose levels. If your body is using glucose as its energy source, the less glucose you have, the less willpower you are able to muster. According to Dr. Baumeister, you can restore your self-control capacity with proper rest (sleep), with positive emotional experiences, and with self-regulatory exercises that are used for managing our emotions.

Remember: While self-control resources can be depleted and restored, they can also be conditioned and, thus, strengthened. Just like your chest muscles will be temporarily exhausted following a set of heavy bench presses, your willpower muscle will also be sapped after it has been exercised. In the short term, that means you have to "pace" yourself and be aware of your limits. But in the longer term, with rest and recovery, both your chest and your willpower will come back bigger and stronger. Systematic exercise of your willpower muscle can start with something as simple as delaying a poor food choice for 5 minutes. Forcing yourself to delay the reward will tax your willpower and strengthen it over time. You'll likely find that once you make it for the 5 minutes, going another 5 will be even easier.

Research shows that regular, targeted willpower efforts in one area (e.g., exercise/working out) lead to improvement not only in willpower in that area but also in many other areas of life. Concentrating on good posture can lead to improvements in study habits and work performance, for example. A study published in the *British Journal of Health Psychology* found that starting and staying on a regular exercise program not only led to the subjects going to the gym more frequently and for a longer duration each visit, but it also improved results on an unrelated lab task of willpower. Remarkably, the subjects also showed decreases in perceived stress, emotional distress, smoking, and alcohol and caffeine consumption while seeing an increase in healthy eating, emotional control, maintenance of household chores, attendance to commitments, monitoring of spending, and regular study habits.

By Week 6 of the Challenge, you'll be strong enough to dare sticking your head in the proverbial lion's mouth. So, your Alpha Attitude drill that week will test your willpower (see page 154). Just like your muscles, your willpower can be strengthened, and it's time to pack some power into yours!

CONFIDENCE

What makes a man "manly"? It's not the amount or thickness of his back hair, his prowess in a burping contest, or the length of time he can wear a T-shirt without washing it. It's also not merely the width of his shoulders or the broadness of his chest. Harvard professor Harvey C. Mansfield, PhD, who wrote the book *Manliness*, observes:

> John Wayne is still every American's idea of manliness. That tells you something about the standing of manliness because John Wayne is not of our generation; in fact, he's dead. He is so far from gender-neutral that one's imagination balks at picturing him as a him/her. How could his manliness be abstracted from his easy male swagger? . . . We are attracted to the manly man because he imparts some of his confidence to everyone else.

That's absolutely right. Confidence is certainly a defining characteristic of the true Alpha Male. Confidence is a dose of testosterone without the injections. But confidence isn't conceit. "Conceit is bragging about yourself," said the late former MVP quarterback Johnny Unitas, widely considered the greatest quarterback of all time. "Confidence means you believe you can get the job done."

Bragging is generally a way to cover a *lack* of confidence. Even in the group context, boasting and "hubristic, pompous displays of group pride" may be a mask for insecurity, suggests new research led by University of California, Davis, psychologists. Truly confident people act with humility. Seven-time Mr. Olympia and California Governor Arnold Schwarzenegger reportedly once explained that if you own a luxury sports car, you don't need to race to show off. Everyone knows how fast it goes. Similarly, the late martial artist Bruce Lee said that the pinnacle of karate skill was never to use it.

Some guys have the gift of natural self-confidence. Others weren't so fortunate. But luckily, confidence can be developed. One way to develop it is to build a more powerful and muscular exterior. Whether it's climbing into a boxing ring, making a speech, or just walking into a room full of strangers, the inner boost you get from the awareness that others perceive you as a physically capable guy who is comfortable in his own skin is a huge advantage. Supreme confidence can inspire respect and admiration.

Looking like pro-wrestler and actor Dwayne "The Rock" Johnson helps when it comes to exuding supreme confidence. The greater level of self-assuredness created by a strong and healthy body boosts your literal and figurative presence among others, both in how you perceive yourself and in how others perceive you, and can provide you with a feeling of physical competence, the assurance that you have the abilities to handle yourself in any rough situation that might come your way. How would *your* current level of endurance, strength, and power hold up if those closest to you really needed your help? Are you confident that you'd have enough stamina and physical and mental prowess to help them?

You don't have to wait until you have 18-inch biceps or a third-degree black belt to start building your confidence levels. What are the two ingredients of supreme confidence? One is a sense of commanding *presence*. The other is a sense of supreme *competence*.

COMMANDING PRESENCE

In his book, *Heroes, Rogues and Lovers*, the late psychologist and testosterone researcher James M. Dabbs, PhD, suggested John Wayne was the epitome of presence—a "quality that suggests physical, moral, or intellectual power." Without a doubt, John Wayne fit that bill; his true Alpha Male presence was larger than life. "People who have presence convey the force of their personalities immediately and effectively," wrote Dr. Dabbs. He and his colleagues at Georgia State University investigated the relationship between presence and testosterone levels by comparing high- and low-testosterone subjects on the qualities associated with the way we carry ourselves—things like speed of movement, patterns of gaze, and general demeanor. Guess what? The high-testosterone subjects seemed more purposeful and confident. They entered a room less hesitantly, looked around less, and focused more directly on the task

assigned to them. Dabbs concluded that they seemed to have more presence. We'll never know what the Duke's testosterone levels were at the peak of his film career, but we might speculate that they weren't too shabby.

How satisfied are you with your physique as it is today? If you like the way you look, and if you believe that you are physically ready to meet your life's demands, then you will have a more confident and commanding presence. If not, you're going to find that your sense of physical presence—of being solid, of having significant muscular mass—rapidly increases when the results of the physical training and nutrition parts of this book kick in. Our physical presence may be further enhanced by good posture and positive body language. How we walk, stand, and hold our heads communicates a lot to others about who we are, how we see ourselves, and how we expect others to see us. Research has shown that, even before competition begins, athletes will use their opponent's appearance and body language to predict their chance of winning. Becoming aware of the visual image we project to others is crucial in the development of a commanding presence. How we perceive ourselves changes how others see us, and how others see us changes how we come to see ourselves. In fact, consciously changing your exterior reality—such as standing to speak while on the telephone—can change how you perceive yourself in that moment and allow you to be more decisive. Poor posture can bring your mood down, and people with hunched-over posture report greater stress. Slouching decreases lung capacity, which makes for a weaker voice.

You can develop a more commanding presence by honestly assessing your current habits. How do you enter a room? Do you walk too fast or too slow? How do you typically stand or sit? Do you look others in the eye or tend to avert your gaze? Here's what we advise to develop a commanding presence.

- **Walk:** You don't have to feign the Duke's swagger. Find a pace that's unrushed but purposeful. Pay attention to the natural movements of your arms as you walk; they should move fluidly and effortlessly. Keep your chest up and your head high and back. No stooping allowed. Better posture will not only make you appear taller and fitter, but it may also save you a few chiropractic visits.

- **Stand:** Are you a sloucher or a leaner? Don't be either one. Pulling your shoulders back and down will allow your chest to move slightly forward so it appears broader—an attribute that contributes to confidence. Envision pushing the top of your head toward the ceiling above you. This will prevent you from slouching or rolling your head down toward your chest. Your weight should be evenly distributed on both sides, feet firmly planted.

- **Sit:** Your feet are best kept flat on the floor, shoulder-width apart. Sit up in the chair with your butt back as far as it will go, your lower back against the chair back, and your shoulders square. Don't slouch forward. If you have to cross your legs, cross at the ankles. If you find your legs crossed with one knee atop the other, smack yourself across the face!

- **Handshake:** Don't overcompensate by trying to crush metacarpals. Similarly, you're not shaking a bottle of salad dressing. We've all shaken hands that felt like dead fish and some of us have suffered the indignity of the tip-gripper—the guy who grasps only the ends of your fingers and makes it impossible to truly shake his hand. Just grip firmly and give two or three subtle shakes.

- **Eye Contact:** Some shy people find it hard to look someone in the eye. On the other hand, it feels weird when someone gives you the blinkless eye-lock in an effort to prove his sincere interest in you. You can usually find the right amount of eye contact by focusing keenly on the conversation and looking for reactions in the other person's eyes.

Body language should look natural. We think it's important to point out that *too much* posturing should also be avoided. We know lots of professional bodybuilders with doorway-wide backs who walk with their massive arms relaxed at their sides. They don't have to walk as if their lats are too big for their arms to hang naturally. Neither does anybody else. Those who walk around with flared lats are *not* confident and not true Alpha Males. This sort of "caricature conduct" is a compensation for insecurities.

If you've developed some bad body language habits over the years—whether strangers are laughing at your silly flared lat swagger or they're mistaking you and your your slump for Quasimodo—it's important to *consciously* focus on changing them. It may initially feel forced, but if you stick with it you will find that you will adapt to your new habits and they will become second nature.

Research published in the journal of *Cognition and Emotion* looked at the relationship between body posture and emotions. Basically, our mothers were right. Whatever you do with your body, you feel and think accordingly. Although smiling when you're heartbroken might not completely dispel the blues, it will help. The researchers found that facial expressions work best, followed very closely by posture. So putting on an angry face and leaning forward with your fists clenched makes you feel angry or aggressive. The same holds true for happiness, sadness, and fear. Muscular feedback triggers systems that are designed to match actions of muscles to emotions—that is, the system works both ways.

Studies show that extroverts are happier than introverts, although the reason is still unknown. One way to have a happier life is to become more extroverted. Researchers at Wake Forest University found that acting extroverted is as good as being extroverted for the positive mood effects. Try the "Walk Tall" drill (page 132) during Week 2 of the Challenge and strive to be outgoing! You'll be amazed at how this simple exercise can enhance your physical presence, overall confidence, and Alpha Factor!

SUPREME COMPETENCE

Being able to "do the job" has always been part of the manly man's traditional job description. Regrettably, many basic skills will soon be lost to the ages. "At about the time that men started to get in touch with their feminine sides, hammer sales around the world began to drop off," observes Sam Martin in *The Lost Art of Being a Man: How to Mow the Lawn.* "Men, it seems, have lost the art of swinging a hammer. . . . Fixing a leaky faucet, these days, means calling a plumber. Knowing how to make oil and vinegar dressing has supplanted any knowledge of basic car maintenance." The complexity and breadth of today's technology doesn't help the cause, nor do the stressful time demands most of us are under. We have often left behind doing for ourselves behind in favor of having others do for us.

Learning the skills of changing a tire, unclogging a sink, or banging nails into a 2 x 4 isn't recommended simply for the sake of building a façade of manliness. They're good things to know how to do so that you can become more self-sufficient and, in turn, more competent. We call things like being able to fix things "manly" because it was our fathers and grandfathers who would always be the ones to fix things back in the day. Back then, they might not have had the luxury of being able to call the local plumber at 2:00 a.m. We're not suggesting that a phone book full of emergency numbers shouldn't be in the kitchen drawer—we're simply saying that if you have a chance to brush up on some of these lost skills, you may very well find a time when they'll come to the rescue.

A large part of what makes us feel, think, and act competently is a sense of task mastery, the belief that we can do things based on our actions. The things we do to gain this sense do not always have to be risky or extreme; they can often be those mundane daily things that take a time-honored and manly skill set.

It isn't too late to reclaim a sense of mastery of basic "guy" things. For many of you, though, time demands will require you to carefully pick and choose which skills to work on.

There are two pieces to competence. One involves knowing what action to take to achieve success, kind of like being given a list of exercises to do and believing that they are effective. We call this an *outcome expectation*, because we think an action will lead to what we want. But psychology research has also looked in another area in relation to competence: "self-efficacy." Albert Bandura, PhD, renowned expert on social learning theory, defined self-efficacy as "beliefs in one's capabilities to mobilize the motivation, cognitive resources, and courses of action needed to meet given situational demands." So it is not just important that we know what action will lead to success. We also need to believe that we have the necessary skills to take that action. We call this *self-efficacy expectation*. Competence then involves knowing what action to take and knowing that *we* can "do it."

Here's the multitasker's way to master a sense of competence *and* enhance your body's appearance and overall health: Tackle new challenges to master new skills. The more physical, the better! You can do it right in the gym. Push your limits, and not with the "same old." If you're pretty much a weight lifter who walks the treadmill for cardio, try something new. Try something competitive, such as tennis, racquetball, or basketball. Not only are they great cardiovascular exercises, but they can also fuel your self-confidence as you progress along the learning curve. If you usually play racquetball, try playing basketball. Even better, take a kickboxing class or try martial arts or any of the other activities suggested on page 80. Step outside your comfort zone! By doing this you learn new skills and learn to believe in your ability to master them. Your sense of competence is founded on the belief that you can master what comes at you.

What challenges do you face daily? Often we meet many challenges throughout our day and don't even notice; we simply accept this as what we do. Stop, take a minute, and note your mastery of those everyday challenges; even look for new ones to master. Then carry those experiences and thoughts with you as you meet life's other, less-expected challenges.

Research on self-efficacy tells us that it is all about believing that you are competent, and thus expecting yourself to succeed. By doing new things, you will see that they are not as uncomfortable as you may think, and are likely fun and rewarding. As you do more and more of this, your belief in yourself as a competent person will grow, encouraging further forays outside your comfort zone. Positive behaviors are self-perpetuating, just as negative ones are. So go out and *be* the taskmaster! In Week 7, you'll have the opportunity to get off the couch, get some physical exercise, and build your sense of competence all at once.

COURAGE

In 480 B.C., the Persian Empire marched its massive armies onto Greek soil, repeating an earlier attempt at invasion and conquest. Standing between them and their goals were 300 Spartans and assorted other Greeks in the narrow pass of Thermopylae in central Greece. For 3 days, Spartan King Leonidas and his small group of Greek warriors kept the Persian armies at bay, killing thousands upon thousands against overwhelming odds. They sacrificed their lives to defend their homelands and their way of life, and their fierce resistance and unparalleled courage ultimately paved the way for the defeat of the Persians.

According to *300*, the movie version of the Battle of Thermopylae, it would appear that extreme courage and a mind-blowing set of abs go together—and that the Spartans trained hard to develop both. In our off-screen world today, courage is just like a razor-sharp six-pack; that is, every guy wants it, many claim to have it, but all too rarely do you see somebody actually throw down and prove it.

If you want true Alpha Male status, you better have courage. "If you want the no-nonsense definition of a man, skip the claim that we are *Homo sapiens* and go directly to 'fearless' and its synonyms—undaunted, bold, intrepid, audacious, brave, courageous, valiant, valorous, doughty, daring, adventurous, heroic, gallant, plucky, gritty," notes Sam Keen in *Fire in the Belly: On Being a Man*. In fact, looking back over history and cultures, it's hard to imagine a quality more coveted by any man than courage. Courage was respected as a virtue by Greek philosopher Aristotle and his works on ethics. It was also one of Roman Catholicism's Four Cardinal Virtues. No wonder courage is one of the Four Cs of Alpha Attitude! It was also highly regarded by the Bushido, the Japanese warrior code of conduct, and by the medieval Knights. "Courage is the one incontrovertible virtue associated with masculinity," writes Willard Gaylin, MD, in *The Male Ego*. "In the history of Western culture and from the data evident in current tribal cultures, courage has

"Courage is fear holding on a minute longer."

~GEORGE S. PATTON~

always been the substance of masculinity." When we think of the great men in history—from military heroes to activists for social change and justice—it is often their courage that stands out as their defining characteristic. It's a primary yardstick by which we measure ourselves.

So what fueled King Leonidas and his 299 Spartan soldiers to stand their ground against the hundreds of thousands of Persian invaders? It went well beyond commitment and confidence to a characteristic that relies on both of those capacities, but reflects how such strengths are put to use. Courage is putting our skills and abilities to the test in the face of fear, when our first thought might be uncertainty about our ability to prevail. Mark Twain said it in *Pudd'nhead Wilson*: "Courage is resistance to fear, mastery of fear—not absence of fear." Or as John Wayne once said, "Courage is being scared to death—but saddling up anyway." You gotta love the Duke.

Recognize, though, that courage is not recklessness. The difference between courage and recklessness is *worthiness*. Courage means picking your battles and knowing when the challenge is worth it. It is not always about taking action; sometimes our fears can be in the form of, "If I do not respond to this challenge, everyone will think I am a coward," and courage may take the form of walking away when it is the wiser choice. Courage is not just charging the hill, asserting one's authority, or steadfastly clinging to a culture of honor; sometimes courage asserts itself against fear in a calm and retiring fashion. Sometimes standing up means being willing to sit down, too. Often the most courageous among us is also the most humble.

Aristotle's advice on courage was that you have to train yourself to be ready when you're put to the test. Courage is like a muscle; flexing it regularly will build it to a higher and higher peak, whether it's the assertive courage that made King Leonidas the leader he was, or the mental toughness that made all 300 Spartans stand their ground for freedom. True courage comprises both.

> ## "Courage is grace under pressure."
> ### ~ERNEST HEMINGWAY~

ASSERTIVE COURAGE

Why do some people come on strong and stand their ground when conflicts arise, and others yield and surrender? When obstacles or the wants of others stand between you and your needs or wants, having the courage to stick up for yourself without bullying others can make the difference between getting what you want and going home empty-handed. How badly do you want it? How strongly do you believe in it? Sometimes called "social courage" and sometimes "assertiveness," this type of courage builds on two of the other Four Cs: commitment and confidence.

The true Alpha Male stands his ground and sticks up for himself and what he believes in. Dominance and leadership are built on the bedrock of assertiveness. But assertiveness requires balance. Too little assertiveness makes you passive—a human doormat. Too much of it is just as bad, making you confrontational, overly aggressive, and not very likable at all. Learning to be assertive without being aggressive will help you get what you want without being a bully. Of course, differing situations will call for different levels of vigor, tenacity, and force of assertiveness. We call the perfect balance of assertiveness for a given situation *assertive courage*.

Assertive courage is what makes a good leader. Research at Columbia University, using an anonymous online survey to obtain comments from graduate students about specific former colleagues' strengths and weaknesses as leaders, found that a significant weakness is having either too much or too little assertiveness.

Every day presents situations where assertive courage can mean the difference between the satisfaction of getting what you want and disappointment. It can be something as minor as getting a retail clerk to accept a return on broken merchandise. Or it can be one of life's defining moments: getting the job, getting the promotion, or getting the girl. Sometimes it's about haggling in a business or legal negotiation to get a better deal than what's being offered. Sometimes it's not about *getting* something, but about saying *no*, such as when you must forcefully ward off the pushy salesman or telemarketer or refuse to accept an unfair work schedule. Sometimes it's about keeping something you already have, such as the sales territory your boss is now trying to give to your co-worker. All too often the interests of another person stand in the way of your needs and desires. You can surrender and retreat, or you can muster the fortitude to push forward and get your due.

Stew Smith, the former Navy SEAL and fitness author mentioned earlier, is a prime example of a true Alpha Male who effectively asserts himself without ever seeming pushy or abrasive. Stew told us that assertive courage is both a personal skill and a tool of good leadership:

> I equate the term "true Alpha Male" to "leader," and leaders are people who command respect and admiration through their achievements and the effectiveness by which they assert their convictions. As a former Navy leadership instructor at the United States Naval Academy, I saw classrooms filled with above-average men and women, all with leadership potential. Just as a person can be a natural athlete, there are natural leaders or natural Alpha Males. At the Naval Academy, we took natural leaders and less than natural leaders and made better leaders for the Navy and Marine Corps. The best leaders combine assertiveness, charisma, physical presence, and intelligence. Of these characteristics, assertiveness is less of a trait and more of a skill. Assertiveness makes leaders clear about what they want and direct about communicating it. Asser-

tiveness *can* be learned, so that a good leader can become an even better leader.

Look, there's almost no guy who, when pressed, can't think back to a particular place and time when he wished he'd done a better job of standing up for himself or a position he believed in. Can you recall incidents in which you wish you had faced up to a challenge or risked more than you did? What was the consequence? If you identify common elements that existed when you fell short on assertive courage, you're on to something.

How could you have handled yourself more effectively in the situations you've looked at? To change the consequence, you have to change your beliefs about things or yourself. One way to challenge those beliefs is to behave in assertively courageous ways to test whether they are true or not. If you are automatically telling yourself you cannot handle it, and then you do, you have evidence that your belief about yourself is not true.

When you exercise assertive courage, keep four things in mind:

1. *Honesty.* If you don't believe it, neither will anyone else.
2. *Clarity.* There should be no guesswork about where you stand and what you want.
3. *Respect.* Recite the facts, what you want, and, if appropriate, your feelings about the situation. Do not vent, belittle, or name-call.
4. *Appropriateness.* The vigor and duration of your effort should be calibrated to each situation.

Check out Week 3 (page 137) for a simple drill we call "Straight Talk," designed to help improve your ability to effectively exercise assertive courage.

MENTAL TOUGHNESS

Bravery in the face of physical danger is often called "physical courage." But courage isn't physical. It's mental. You can't be heroic without the mental toughness to step outside your comfort zone and take a physical risk, maybe even an extreme one. A tough and rugged physical exterior may, in some situations, lend confidence and competence, but it's just a façade unless you have the mental toughness to go with it. As Karl Kuehl, John Kuehl, and Casey Tefertiller say in their book *Mental Toughness,* mental toughness "is not about what gifts we may be granted, physically or intellectually; it is about what we do with them." It's a skill to be learned and nurtured and, the authors state, "is, simply, the most effective approach to virtually all arenas of competition. Mental toughness is a quality that has been exhibited by virtually all leading athletes, by military leaders from Hannibal to Colin Powell, and by exemplary titans of business."

It takes mental toughness to act in the face of danger. But remember: no fear, no courage. To build your courage, you need to fully acknowledge your fears. What scares you? Heights? Snakes? Tight spaces? Find what you fear, find out what unconscious thoughts relate to those fears, and face them down. We're not suggesting that you go out and get into a fist fight—it's generally more courageous to walk away from unnecessary conflict. Face your fear intelligently and conquer it by dealing with it and learning from it. You'll often find that what you thought you'd be fearful about really wasn't that scary at all!

An effective technique to enhance your mental toughness uses graded or gradual exposure to things that may scare you. Just as your physical training routine uses resistance or obstacles, such as barbells and machines, so too does a courage-training routine use resistance or obstacles, such as your fears and hesitations. Here's a simple technique:

- If the object of your courage shortcomings is a specific thing or situation, try systematically desensitizing yourself to it in your imagination. This takes advantage of our ability to visualize and works great with traditional psychother-

apy in dealing with phobias, such as fear of heights, snakes, and the like. By progressively building up your exposure to the object in your imagination, either in nearness or duration of exposure, while working to remain calm and resolute, you'll gradually lose your fear of it. Close your eyes and imagine a relaxing scene for yourself. It could be lying on the beach in a favorite vacation spot, for example. Now imagine the threat object. Every time you feel your courage ebb below a 3 on a scale of 1 to 5, 1 being fearful and 5 being courageous, focus on the relaxing scene. This distracting technique will help your mind adapt and foster progressive achievement of enhanced courage.

- Now, apply the desensitization technique to the real world. If you are afraid of heights, begin by simply standing on the ground and looking up at a tall building. Then, while remaining calm and resolute, begin to gradually expose yourself to greater heights. Our lack of courage in the face of such fears is most often a result of having either run away from them or avoided them altogether. The reduction in anxiety that we feel by escaping or avoiding our fears makes our fears even stronger. So the best way to overcome these fears can be to face them gradually, not allowing ourselves to run from them or escape them until our anxiety levels have gone down.

Research published in the *Journal of Humanistic Psychology* examined what could be learned about courage and humility from extreme sports—such as BASE (building, antenna, span, earth) jumping, big wave surfing, extreme skiing, waterfall kayaking, extreme mountaineering, and solo rope-free climbing. Participants are often considered crazy thrill-seekers with a death wish or an absence of any fear. But interviews with extreme sports participants revealed that it's not the absence of fear, but the balancing of it with a sense of personal capability and technical expertise that propels extreme sports participants. Their death-defying experiences both humble and empower them.

A word of warning: If you try to change things too drastically, you may find that you don't achieve your goal. This can become destructive, because it could reinforce your "fearful" perceptions about yourself (i.e., mental myostatin). These are very likely the things that have inhibited your growth all along. The last thing you want to do is set yourself up to fail. Choose *reasonable* tests of your mental toughness, just like you set reasonable goals for yourself in committing to the Challenge. Start small and work slowly. Looking at it all as a process of gradual and progressive achievement is the key to lasting change.

Boosting your Alpha Factor means boosting your mental toughness. You don't necessarily have to climb the Matterhorn or run with the bulls at Pamplona, but you should look for opportunities to exercise your true Alpha Male mental toughness throughout the Challenge. When you get to Week 8, you'll be ready for a bigger test, one we call the "Alpha Extreme Triumph" (see page 164).

CONSCIENCE

We've spent a lot of time extolling the benefits of true Alpha Male manliness. In an age in which testosterone is dwindling and manliness is mostly something to apologize for, we've dared to suggest that if we reintroduce masculinity into modern society, good things can happen. Enhanced commitment, confidence, and courage all equip today's urban/suburban/rural warrior to compete and succeed on the various testing grounds of life. They give you the very best chance of mining gold from all areas of your life, including sticking with and succeeding at an exercise and nutrition plan. However, there's another piece to the puzzle that has to be put in place. Still, without it, no man is whole; it is at the core of who we are and the rea-

son the other attributes exist. It, too, must be nurtured and developed if those other attributes are to have meaning for us and the people around us.

The timeworn stereotype of the alpha male often evokes a rather nasty image. In the animal world, the alpha male is assumed to always be the strongest, meanest, hairiest beast in the group, dominating the others by threat or force. But science shows otherwise. Researchers studied 10 years of alpha male chimpanzee behavioral data collected in Gombe National Park, Tanzania. Their findings, reported in the *American Journal of Primatology*, show that being attentive and kindly to others appears to be one factor by which to obtain and maintain alpha male status in chimpanzee society. There's a lot more to the true Alpha Male than chest-thumping, even among the beasts.

Historically, human alpha males have not always been viewed as the most socially conscientious people. The authors of *Alpha Male Syndrome* begin their book with:

> Human history is the story of alphas, those indispensable powerhouses who take charge, conquer new worlds, and move heaven and earth to make things happen. Whether heading a band of warriors, bringing a vital new product to market, guiding a team to glory, or steering a giant conglomerate, alphas are hardwired for achievement and eager to tackle challenges that others find intimidating. Along the way, they inspire awe and admiration—and sometimes fear and trembling.

This seems to suggest that the alpha male has his place, but often people want that place to be somewhere else. In fact, "too much testosterone" is blamed for all sorts of selfish and brutish male behavior. Back in the 1970s, *Ms. Magazine* published an article, "What Every Woman Should Know about Men," written by former *M*A*S*H* actor Alan Alda. The piece accused men of having such a high "overdose" of testosterone that their "abnormal" behavior supports the hypothesis that almost all men are suffering from the ailment of testosterone poisoning. Alda's idea was later referenced in the 1985 book, *A Feminist Dictionary*.

"If ever there were a human hormone to achieve 'rock star' status, no doubt it would be our old friend testosterone," notes Brian O'Neill, in *The Testosterone Edge*.

> It's become a code word for virility, manliness, and attractiveness. It's also become a code word for lunk-headedness. Certain behaviors and personality qualities commonly considered exclusively male, including competitiveness, stoicism, aggressiveness, ambitiousness, egotism, thrill-seeking, and assertiveness, are routinely traced back to testosterone in the court of public opinion. . . . Highway speeding, libidinous barroom antics, corporate backstabbing—testosterone was there without an excuse, the potion that turns Jekyll into Hyde.

In some circles today, the testosterone-fueled alpha male has the rep of being pushy, selfish, uncaring, or even psychopathic! The problem is that the "poster children" for the alpha male archetype have been the ones who misbehaved. The most aggressive and the least evolved ones who've perpetrated all manner of brutality—from battles to bar fights—over a few thousand years are the ones by whom all others are judged. The negative stereotype leaves out all the other characteristics of the true Alpha Male and simplifies his relationships with others. That kind of posturing "faux" alpha male isn't what this book is about, and you no doubt know this by now. Nope, *Alpha Male Challenge* isn't just about being more manly or even being a better man solely for your own gratification, but about putting all the right qualities in place to be a better person and a better citizen, a better father and a better husband, a better co-worker or a better boss, a better caretaker of yourself and those around you.

Sure, testosterone is part of the discussion when we speak of behaviors such as assertiveness and dominance. But research shows that it also correlates with leadership and heroism. Being dominant or a good leader within a group is about a lot more than being the strongest or bravest of warriors; it serves a social function, too.

The virtues of respect, compassion, and tolerance that are so integral to being a true Alpha Male aren't really new. The Japanese Bushido and samurai codes stressed not only fighting skills but also loyalty and honor. These values appear in many various styles of martial arts from around the world.

The ancient Roman soldiers fought for the ideals of "strength and honor." In the film *Gladiator*, the Roman soldiers often use the phrase as a motto. And with good reason. Without honor, strength lacks meaningfulness. Without respect for others, and mercy and tolerance, courage and confidence may approach brutality. Without a higher purpose, we all are but "shadows and dust."

The medieval knights adopted the code of chivalry to construct a set of rules that men of great honor should live by. These men were warriors, without question, but yet honor, mercy, and tolerance were always a part of their value system. If, as we believe, ideal manliness involves balance, then there must be something to balance out the ruggedness of the true Alpha Male.

Many have asked, "Is chivalry dead?" in the modern world now that men and women are equals. Some folks of both genders are uncomfortable with modern displays of chivalry. Some women have been brought up to believe that any such displays are sexist or condescending, and that submitting to them is a sign of weakness. So many men are uncertain as to how to act, even wondering whether "gentle" displays may be seen as "unmanly." We see them as essential to being a complete man. It has nothing to do with gender politics, or who is stronger or better. It is that the complete man is committed to the welfare of both himself and all around him, confident in his abilities, and empathic and courageous in his interactions with others. However imperfect, he strives to be heroic.

The true Alpha Male is a balanced breed—strength and muscle, but with heart and humanity. Conscience is our term for a critical matrix of virtues and values, emphasizing the respect, empathy, and tolerance so needed to be a better man in an oftentimes brutal world. It includes the "emotional intelligence" and "social intelligence"—which we call "Alpha empathy"—that facilitate a more benevolent relationship with the world and those around us. And it incorporates the concept of "heroic altruism," a selflessness expressed by helping others despite there being no benefit—or even some risk—to yourself. These attributes are essential components of success.

ALPHA EMPATHY

Many men might tune out when the word *emotion* rears its flowery head in a discussion of manliness. And "emotional intelligence" might seem to be an oxymoron. But the term appears to have originated with none other than Charles Darwin, who used it to refer to an ability crucial for survival and adaptation in humans. As social animals, it wasn't just physical prowess and fitness that ensured our survival; it was also the ability to recognize and appropriately respond to social cues. Our primal ancestors did not survive solely on brute strength and intestinal fortitude; they also adapted complex social routines that ensured mutual support in the many tasks needed to survive.

The term "emotional intelligence" was popularized in the 1990s by Dr. Daniel Goleman, whose book of the same title made the *New York Times* bestseller list. The current meaning of the term concerns the ability to understand and manage your own emotions and those of others. In 2006, Goleman followed up with a book called *Social Intelligence,* focusing more on the interactions between people than on their individual emotions. The notion addresses the functional need for social expertise and a connectedness. It is in this context—person to person—that empathy is best understood.

Confidence and courage are hallmarks of heroic leaders. But the very best leaders are empathic. A growing body of research suggests that the people we look up to as leaders are those who make us feel understood and valued as individuals through displays of empathy. Several studies published in the *Leadership Quarterly* suggest that true Alpha Male leaders demonstrate greater consideration of and sensitivity to the needs of their followers. Empathy is the ability to put yourself in somebody else's shoes. Nationwide surveys published in the *Leadership Quarterly* suggest that empathy is the bedrock for the thoughts and behaviors that determine who rises to positions of leadership within a group.

If the true Alpha Male is the ideal man for contemporary times, he must relate on a social level in ways that transcend the ordinary. He must be better at relationships with superiors, subordinates, co-workers, and loved ones. Building a more enjoyable and successful career and improving who you are and the way you're perceived in the world are what we're talking about. It's about learning to connect with people more fully, to create deep levels of rapport. And, believe it or not, connecting with people and maintaining and nurturing our relationships takes commitment, confidence, and courage, and when things don't go our way, a good dose of resilience.

Here's a good example of nurturing our relationships: Have you ever heard two people talking to each other—or should we say, *at* each other, as is too often the case? A typical conversation usually includes each person having a chance to voice his thoughts while the other, in a true conversation, actively listens. Unfortunately, what typically occurs is that neither of them is really listening to the other very much. Each person is immersed in his own thoughts, serving his own personal agenda. While one person talks, the other listens only enough to know when to jump in and express his own views. This ultimately gets them nowhere and leads to pent-up frustration on both sides because nothing gets solved. They are not communicating; that takes listening as well as talking, something called "active listening."

Adding a little emotional/social intelligence to this dynamic would work wonders for the two of them. They would each attentively listen to what each other is really saying, process it well, ask for clarification if something were not clear, and even restate what they heard as part of their response—a powerful method of validation called mirroring. Together, these two would then know what the other was thinking. Sometimes one person's views might make sense, sometimes the other's might, but in the end, by listening actively and expressing themselves clearly, they will best understand each other's views.

Empathy is the ability to put yourself into someone else's shoes, understand how he may be feeling, and really grasp what it's like for that person. Empathic people make the best leaders and managers; they often command the love and respect of their troops. They make the best boyfriends, husbands, fathers, and friends. They also make the best training partners. Being empathic does not mean that you always do what others feel is right, but that you take others' feelings, thoughts, and concerns into account, you attend to them, you consider them important, you try to understand them, and you consider them when you plan your own actions. You'll have an opportunity to flex your empathy muscles—and try to get a sense of what it's like to be in the other person's shoes—during Week 4 in a drill we call "The Moccasin Mile" (see page 144).

HEROIC ALTRUISM

Are humans capable of truly nonselfish actions? Wouldn't Darwin's theory of natural selection predict that each of us is solely out for Numero Uno, to take everything and give nothing? Isn't that what Survival of the Fittest is all about? Why would somebody act, as Richard Dawkins describes altruism in *The Selfish Gene,* "in such a way as to increase another entity's welfare at the expense of his own"?

The late Dr. Dabbs hit the nail on the head when he discussed the concept as "heroic altruism" in his book on testosterone and behavior. When Dr. Dabbs first began researching testosterone, he expected to find selfishness and violence; however, he also found generosity and altruism. Altruism encompasses a wide range of behavior, from little acts of kindness to the ultimate sacrifice that combat soldiers sometimes make to spare the lives of their comrades. It can be soft and gentle or bold and heroic. Any selfless act that puts the interests of others above your own, if only for a moment, is altruistic.

In the rocket-speed world we live in, time is a precious commodity. How does all the rushing we do affect our altruism? The famous "Good Samaritan study" conducted at Princeton in the early '70s and published in the *Journal of Personality and Social Psychology* found that the biggest factor in whether we help our fellow man is whether or not we are in a hurry. John Ray, a doctoral student in the Department of Clinical Psychology at the University of South Florida, puts it this way:

> Altruism and empathy are about more than just being a good guy. A landmark study on altruistic behavior showed that it is important to maintain a steady focus on actually *doing* the right thing. Darley and Batson, of Princeton University, conducted an experiment using future ministers from the Princeton Theological Seminary as their subjects; it is hard to imagine a group of people more likely to be altruistic in nature. The seminary students were told they were to give a talk to an incoming group of freshmen. Half were told they'd be speaking on seminary job opportunities, while the other half were told they'd be delivering the parable of the Good Samaritan, a biblical story about people who professed to live their lives helping others in the name of God, but then

ignored a beaten robbery victim they encountered in their travels. The person who did help the injured man was a Samaritan, hence the name of the parable. The students were told they would have to walk across campus to the lecture site. Finally, in equal numbers, some students were told they were already late and would need to hurry, some were told they were right on time, and some were told they had several minutes to spare and could take their time.

What the students didn't know was that on their way to the talk, just as in the parable, they would encounter an ostensibly sick or injured man, who was actually in on the experiment. When he saw a student coming, the "sick" guy, already sitting on the ground and slumped against a wall, would groan and cough pitifully, making it readily apparent that he was sick or injured, or maybe drunk, though the student couldn't have known which.

You might think that, because these guys were religious students, they each would have stopped to help the sick man. Or, alternatively, that even if some didn't, surely the ones who were going to talk about being altruistic and empathetic would. It turns out that only about 40 percent of the students offered any help at all. More surprising (though the researchers expected this), planning to give the Good Samaritan talk, and thus actively thinking about "doing good," didn't make a difference. Some people even stepped over the poor guy on the way to the talk! It was their degree of *hurriedness* that made the real difference in who helped the man. Sixty-three percent of those who were not in a hurry helped, 45 percent of those who were in a mild hurry helped, and of those in a major hurry, only 10 percent helped. Can you think of a more appropriate lesson

in the context of today's super fast-paced multitasking lifestyle?

It isn't enough to be well-intentioned. After all, these guys were studying to do God's work. The true Alpha Male is a guy who recognizes that his opportunities to help others in need won't fit neatly into his schedule between dinner and *Family Guy,* when demands on him are low. He realizes that an altruistic and empathetic man is a "doer" of good deeds, always on the lookout for someone who may need help, and ready to *act.*

We need to make time for selfless acts. Failing to do so is failing to achieve your true Alpha Male potential. Being a true Alpha Male means balancing self-interest with selflessness. Donating to a worthy cause is a selfless act we endorse. Giving a donation of blood can save a life—you can check with your local house of worship or blood bank service to arrange a donation.

Donating blood and giving money to bona fide charities is a way of helping the less fortunate around you, but they aren't the same as volunteering your time and effort when it comes to the rewards to *you.* Researchers at the London School of Economics used U.S. data to examine whether people who do volunteer work report better health and happiness than those who don't. But the high association isn't seen in those who simply donate money or blood. Their findings, published in *Social Science and Medicine,* suggest that volunteer work might stimulate the development of empathic emotions. People engaged in helping behavior generally report feeling good about themselves, and studies using biological markers show immune-enhancing biological changes in subjects after engaging in altruistic moods and behaviors. Moderate amounts of volunteerism have been shown to be associated with less depression, more happiness, and a lowered risk of death. You don't have to do too much volunteer work to receive benefits; too much volunteering to the point of strain can overwhelm you and offset the benefits. Approximately 44 percent of American adults engage in formal voluntary activities each year. Isn't it time you joined them?

In 2000, Catherine Ryan Hyde's novel *Pay It Forward* was published. It was an action plan within a work of fiction. Adapted into a Warner Brothers film, the concept of the book and movie is that for each good deed received you must do three good deeds for others. In other words, instead of paying the debt back, you pay it forward to others. The spontaneous acts of kindness should be things that the recipients couldn't do on their own. The intended effect is that altruism would spread exponentially and launch a social movement with the goal of making the world a better place. You can exercise heroic altruism through the Pay It Forward Foundation (www.payitforwardfoundation.org), which was established to inspire students to change the world "one favor at a time." It's a real-world social movement popularized in public schools and on college campuses. In 2006, Oprah Winfrey promoted it on her television show, and we think it's a great idea for the true Alpha Male, too.

However, you don't necessarily need to join a foundation to work heroic altruism into your life. And you don't have to limit your good deeds to three, or wait until you receive a good deed to start. There can never be enough random acts of kindness. Caring about others is truly Alpha Male.

In Week 9, you'll have the chance to put your own heroic altruism to the test. Don't miss the opportunity to be a hero to someone.

WITH GREAT POWER . . .

You bought this book and you've read this far for a reason. You could have opted for a simple "idiot's guide" about which exercises to do and what not to eat. But you chose a more comprehensive and revolutionary program to not only look better and feel better, but also to *be* better. You want more endurance, strength, and power, and more lean, hard muscle; you want less unsightly, ab-obscuring body fat, too. Well, 10 weeks from now, you'll have achieved all those things and be wanting even more. In picking up this book, you decided to build up your true Alpha Attitude as well. You'll have those gains, too, but what do you plan to *do* with them?

In the first *Spiderman* film, Uncle Ben warns Peter Parker that just because you can beat someone up doesn't give you the right to. In fact, with great power so too comes great responsibility. Your increased commitment, confidence, and courage are performance-enhancing tools that give you a distinct "Alpha advantage" over those around you. Unchecked, these tools are a volatile weapon. Alpha dominance and power must be balanced, and that's where conscience comes in. Commitment can't be allowed to become stubbornness and rigidity. Confidence can't become egomania and conceit. Courage can't become recklessness or bullying. You will have powerful tools to do well for yourself in the arena of today, to take control of what you can in a world in which so much is beyond your control. But it is not just about doing well. It is about doing *good*. Make time to do good. And just because your objective is not to be rewarded for these self-less acts doesn't mean that people, especially the emotionally intelligent ones, won't notice your goodwill. More than ever, this world needs a heroic new breed of leaders and role models that others, especially the young or misguided, can look up to and learn from. It was Mahatma Gandhi who said, "You must be the change you wish to see in the world." A better world starts with you.

We hope we've given you a new appreciation for the vital role mental attitude plays in true Alpha Male status—including a pivotal role in the *physical* part of your transformation. You started your journey standing in your underwear taking a long hard look in the mirror, so let's now turn to directly training those physical muscles, burning any excess body fat you may have hanging around, and creating a whole new reflection of yourself.

ALPHA MALE CHALLENGE CLIENT:
MATT BAXTER, AGE 37

MATT OWNS AND OPERATES a tire and auto repair store. "My physical activity dropped at about 25 years old, due to marriage, career, and the birth of my first child," he observes. His weight reached 212 with a 38-inch waist.

Original Alpha Factor: 45.

Matt took the Alpha Male Challenge and put in 10 weeks of effort.

He started the Challenge at 212 pounds.

He weighed 182 at Week 10.

Matt lost 30 pounds in only 10 weeks, with an improvement in his chest to waist ratio of nearly 22 percent.

He dropped 5 inches of fat from his waist and at the same time gained 2 inches of muscle on his chest. His vertical jump increased by a whopping 4 inches.

His maximum bench-press-to-body-weight ratio soared by 20 percent and his time on the 300-yard shuttle run decreased from 71 to a lightning fast 59 seconds! "I'm lighter now than when I got married," he says. "I can see muscle tone I've never seen before. My stamina is increased. I'm proud of my body and more confident when speaking." He's also both stronger and quicker when playing hoops, and his kids don't have to wait for him to catch up. The kids say they really like "healthy Daddy."

Matt's MaleScale™ score for overall courage improved by over 54 percent. His willpower improved by over 66 percent, and his physical confidence increased by over 166 percent!

Matt achieved an increase of 28 points on the MaleScale™ in 10 weeks.

New Alpha Factor: 73.

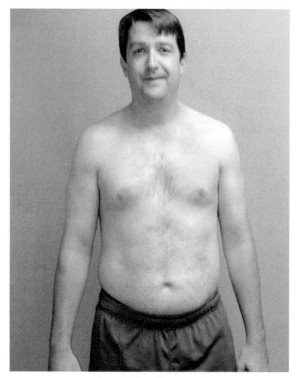
Before

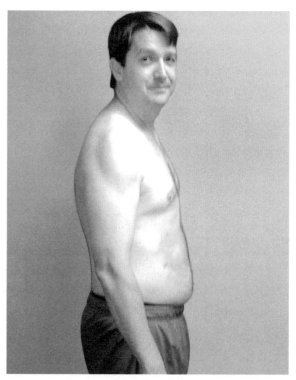
Before

Testimonial:

"The Alpha Male Challenge brought out the best in me. At 37 years old, I still enjoy playing basketball; I have played with the same group of guys for years. After the Challenge, I'm considerably quicker and my stamina has gone way up. As other guys are gasping for air, I'm still running full speed. Though I dropped considerable weight during the Challenge, my strength increased so I'm still able to hold my own pushing guys around in the post.

"Many guys have complimented my transformation. My confidence has grown as well. Recently I committed to play in a league where most of the players are under 30 years old. Thanks again for a phenomenal program!"

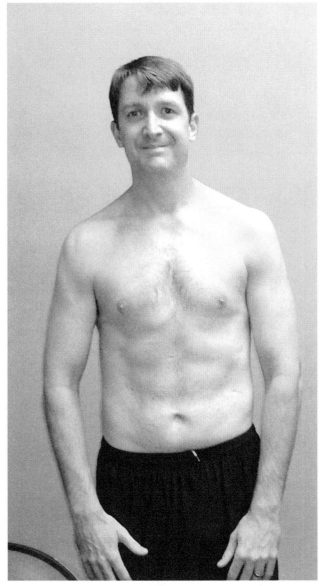

After

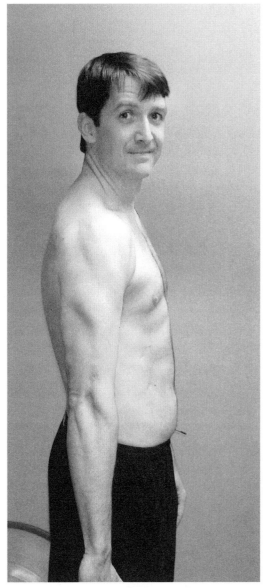

After

CHAPTER FOUR
ALPHA ARCHI-TECTURE

In the animal kingdom, the alpha male must be large and strong enough to hold his own among his jungle or grassland peers. While thumping your chest and baring your teeth like a silverback is generally frowned upon around the water cooler, physicality is nonetheless one universal measure by which human males are judged. Size and strength have helped separate the leaders from the followers since we were nomadic hunter-gatherers traversing the ancient grasslands. Back then, the fittest men survived; the others, not so much. Today, physical stature still affects the impression others have of us. What does your body say about you? Do you exude confidence? Strength? Dominance? Do you appear ordinary . . . or heroic? A winner . . . or a loser? A top dog . . . or a victim, ripe for a mugging?

ALPHA WAVE BASIC TRAINING

We're betting you'd like the rugged and chiseled muscularity of a Roman gladiator or a Spartan warrior. And we aim to get you into that kind of shape as quickly as possible. Although many gladiators were slaves, our philosophy is not about making you a slave to the gym. We designed a system for maximum results in minimum time. None

of us wants to spend all of our time working out. We know you have limited time and a tangle of responsibilities too numerous to mention. You may work crazy hours. You may spend your life living out of a suitcase. You may have a family to support. We understand. We've been there. This program will not ask you to neglect your family, your job, or your friends. It won't make you spend 3 hours a day or 7 days a week in the gym. We don't have time for that, and neither do you.

ONLY 27 WORKOUTS TO AN AWESOME NEW BODY

Our mission is to teach you the most cutting-edge, scientific training techniques so you can get *better* results with *less* time training. Our program consists of 27 resistance training sessions—no more, no less. From the perspective of the full 10-week Challenge, that's just three workouts per week for the first 9 weeks. That's all. A pretty modest investment of time in the weight room, don't you think? But that's all the weight training you need to build a muscular masterpiece of Alpha Architecture and to establish a new lifestyle that will take you far into the future.

EVERY ALPHA WAVE BASIC TRAINING WORKOUT IS DIFFERENT!

We wanted to create an exhilarating experience, so we made sure to add as much variety and as many tests and surprises as possible over the next 10 weeks. These aren't boring gym workouts. We wanted to tap into your "want to" commitment, not your old "have to" thinking. We wanted you to be excited about your next workout! So, you'll never do the same workout twice during the Challenge. You'll likely train harder than you've ever trained in your life, but you'll have fun doing it. You'll get stronger, faster, and more powerful. And when you take off your shirt in front of a mirror, you'll be amazed at the results you'll see. We fully understand that you're anxious to change the way you look and feel, and we've done everything necessary to help you do just that.

We pledge to provide you with everything you need to know to get into the very best physical shape of your life. Our exercise system is challenging. It's *supposed* to be challenging. As the 10 weeks roll along, you'll push yourself harder and harder, dig deeper and deeper, to soldier past your previous bests and reach new heights. We call that *progressive achievement*, and it's what the Alpha Male Challenge is all about.

RESISTANCE TRAINING: BE A BELIEVER!

Years ago, many athletes were afraid that weight training would make them muscle-bound and hinder their functional performance. Yeah, right, tell that to Tiger Woods today. The fact is, athletes from virtually all areas of sports now use regular resistance training to increase their competitive advantage. It'll work for you, too.

Hitting the weights should be your first step when forging a better body. Resistance training boosts your muscle-building hormones and raises your fat-incinerating metabolic rate so that you reap the benefits during workouts and even afterward, at rest. The "underappreciated role of muscle" was detailed in the *American Journal of Clinical Nutrition*. Among the benefits: Every pound of muscle on your body effortlessly burns approximately six calories per day. If you have 75 pounds of lean muscle mass on your frame, you're talking an additional 450 calories burned without any physical effort, each and every day.

We've talked about testosterone already. It's certainly a marker of manliness. Well, guess what resistance training does? It increases your body's circulating concentrations of testosterone! Many studies show that large-muscle-group, multi-joint movements, such as relatively heavy squats, deadlifts, and squat jumps (all of which are incorporated into the Alpha Wave Basic Training program),

MALE ANATOMY: WHAT WOMEN WANT

Research suggests that women are evolutionarily predisposed to prefer muscularity in men. A study conducted at the University of California, Los Angeles, found that women rated muscular men nearly twice as sexy as non-muscular men. Other research, published in *Current Research in Social Psychology*, offers relevant insight: "A problem women faced in their evolutionary past was finding a mate who was able to (a) protect her and her children from predators, and (b) provide resources for her and her children." Strength—especially upper-body strength—dominance, and overall muscle mass were noted as good predictors of a man's ability to provide.

force your body to open the spigot of manly testosterone. As training expert Steven J. Fleck, PhD, a distinguished scientist and recognized authority in physical training and human performance, points out in *Designing Resistance Training Programs,* other variables recommended to boost serum testosterone concentrations include a moderate to high volume of exercise and short rest intervals. So a properly designed training system can actually boost your testosterone—the hormone most correlated with your Alpha Factor and your score on the MaleScale. If that isn't a compelling reason to get off the couch and into the gym, we don't know what is. And a nice little bonus: Resistance training also boosts your circulating levels of growth hormone, another natural muscle-building hormone that'll help speed your progress toward an awesome new body. Growth hormone is prized by Hollywood celebrities in its high-priced injectable form. But the right training can maximize your own body's production . . . for free.

Everybody knows that aerobic exercise can improve circulation and lower blood pressure. But what about resistance training? According to a study by the American Heart Association, hitting the weights just two or three times a week is enough to lower resting blood pressure.

Need still more motivation to exercise? How about turning back the aging clock? Startling data released by molecular gerontologist Dr.

Simon Melov of the Buck Institute for Age Research demonstrates that a strength-training regimen can replenish aging muscle tissue and reverse impairments. After 6 months of exercise, the muscle tissue of subjects over age 65 looked remarkably more like the muscle tissue of young adults. Nice, huh?

Maybe you're concerned about one of the big problem areas for most guys over 30: the ol' joints. Well, here's a tip from Victor R. Prisk, MD, assistant professor, Department of Orthopedic Surgery, University of Pittsburgh Medical Center:

As we age, we experience more aches and pains in the joints. Your knees and hips can experience forces of up to seven times your body weight when you run up a flight of stairs. So, every pound you gain adds 5 to 7 pounds of pressure on your joints. You can spend all the money you want on glucosamine and chondroitin supplements and you may or may not get relief. Or you can take the Challenge and lose the excess adipose baggage. With regular exercise, the lining of your joints begin to produce healthier joint fluid that lubricates and soothes pain. You joints will thank you for it!

Not convinced yet? How about keeping your bones strong and healthy? Again, resistance train-

ALPHA FORM/ALPHA FUNCTION

We think you want it all just like we do. We want to look strong and conditioned, and we want to be strong and conditioned. So, our exercise approach for you is to take the best of *both* worlds—form and function, appearance and performance—for a complete physical journey from ordinary to extraordinary. And guess what? That's pretty much what the gladiators did. Obviously, functional strength and skill were essential for their survival. But did you know that gladiators had to *look* buff, too? Historians point out that a gladiator's popularity and crowd appeal—and, consequently, his income—was based on a combination of performance and appearance.

It's obvious that some things never change. According to research studies published in the *Journal of Applied Social Psychology,* people who look good are more likely to get hired and more successfully pitch ideas and products. Maybe when you look good, you just feel a whole lot better about yourself. And when the people around you respond to that, success follows.

ing is the way to go, and again our approach gets the thumbs-up from Dr. Prisk:

> The only time in our lives men acquire bone mineral density is during our youth and adolescent years. As we settle down in our thirties, our bone mineral (calcium) slowly leaks out. Osteopenia, when your bone mineral density is lower than normal, is a precursor to the dreaded osteoporosis, and the incidence of osteopenia in men in this country is increasing. Weight training, such as the Alpha Wave Basic Training regimen, prevents the loss of bone mineral density.

What about the brain? Research shows that men who exercise perform better on memory tests. A Columbia University Medical Center study found that exercise targets a region of the brain that underlies the memory decline that begins around age 30 for most adults. Research at the University of Edinburgh showed that subjects who took cognitive tests at age 11 and again nearly 70 years later showed better cognitive function if they were in good physical shape. As researchers continue to explore how exercise can reverse aging, we figure the time to start turning back the clock is right now. Don't you?

How about just plain living longer? A new long-term study of more than 10,000 men conducted at the Cooper Clinic in Dallas found that stronger muscles reduced the risk of cancer and heart attack. We know you're ready to make that commitment to a stronger, leaner body right *now*!

THE POWER OF COMMITMENT REVISITED

So hitting the weights can make you stronger, healthier, more attractive, more youthful, and smarter, and might even extend your life. What's

not to like? Well, even with all those motivators, if you look at weight training as the endless lifting and lowering of gray metal discs, you probably won't enjoy it much. And when you don't enjoy something, it's hard to stick with it despite your best intentions. Our job is to put you on the fun and challenging path to success—both in and out of the workout room.

We designed our Alpha Wave Basic Training system to get you excited about and psychologically invested in your workouts. At any given time during each workout, you'll know your primary objective for that workout and the reasons behind it. This attention to detail brings more focus to the game and keeps your eye on the prize. Our innovative and exciting exercise protocols will bring out your competitive warrior nature. No other exercise regimen brings this kind of fun fitness to the table. Don't get us wrong, you're going to be busting your butt, but you'll enjoy the innovative style of all the workouts.

These workouts are also short and intense. Studies show that resistance training sessions lasting much longer than 1 hour will result in *lower* testosterone and growth hormone levels. Long, drawn-out workouts lasting several hours will put the body into a "catabolic" state in which you can actually burn some of that valuable muscle you've worked so hard to build. Our training methods demand brutal intensity during your workouts; the harder you work, the better your gains. The higher your intensity, the less time you can spend exerting yourself at that level. There will be times during your 10-week program when some workouts will take a bit longer than others, but if your Alpha Wave Basic Training workouts last longer than 60 to 90 minutes, you're not working out intensely enough or you're resting too long between sets.

Our program requires a commitment to train your major muscle groups with a variety of the most effective compound exercise movements. It requires investing the necessary time—but the least amount of time possible—to bring about the metabolic changes you expect. You might be new to the whole weight-training arena, and that's all right. This is precisely why we developed a program that took a guy's current fitness level into account. You begin where *you're* fit to begin. If you follow the program, you will naturally and quickly progress to more advanced levels of training. The climb from one level to the next will be natural, as your body adapts to the multiple facets of this awesome training program. Yes, the workouts will take some time and they will be intense, but in only 10 weeks' time, you will witness the dramatic results of your commitment and hard work.

BEYOND THE POWER OF ONE

Many guys train alone, either because they prefer the flexibility or because they work odd shifts and can't find anyone with a similar schedule. If that's you, fine. You can fit Alpha Wave Basic Training into your schedule, odd or irregular as it may be. As long as you hold yourself to the timing schedule of each session, you're golden. A portable music player and headphones are key to solo training—music keeps you focused and discourages you from being distracted by conversation. A watch with a second hand—or preferably a stopwatch—is essential. We've valued your time enough to create a system that economizes it. All you have to do is adhere to it.

Of course, if you can find somebody to partner up with on your Alpha Wave Basic Training, it can be a tremendous plus. A motivated gym partner is one of the most effective insurance policies to keep you on your fitness track. We all have days when we'd prefer to do something other than go to the gym. The role of a training partner is to be strong when you're weak. Neither of you should want to let down the other. A sworn commitment to training together makes it harder to simply "blow off" a workout. Over the long run, you'll both exercise a lot more if you hang tough for each other. A good training partner brings accountability, motivation, inspiration, and assistance to your training.

In the 2000 film *Gladiator*, Maximus, the title character played by Russell Crowe, finds himself on the floor of the Roman Colosseum, standing among a small group of unfortunates facing probable death at the hands of unknown adversaries. "Anyone here been in the army?" he asks. An unknown gladiator responds affirmatively. "You can help me," says Maximus. "Whatever comes out of these gates, we've got a better chance of survival if we work together. Do you understand? If we stay together we survive." As it was then with survival in the Colosseum, so it is today with success in the gym. Working together for a common goal maximizes success. Alpha Wave Basic Training with a buddy not only ratchets up adherence, but also solves issues of safety: You've always got a spot when you need one.

Best of all, training with a partner adds rugged but supportive competition to each and every workout. Our good friend, top fitness expert, and Delaware personal trainer, Jud Dean, regularly organizes group training sessions for his clients. He believes there's nothing like going mano a mano in fierce gym competition to boost testosterone both physiologically and psychologically. For example, instead of standing alone doing stationary barbell lunges, try doing "cross the river lunges" with a partner. Instead of counting repetitions, you take turns getting to a fixed point across the gym floor and back while doing walking lunges with dumbbells. Innovative and competitive exercises like this are "outside the box" of traditional training but are remarkably effective and fun.

DESIGNING THE ULTIMATE TRAINING PLAN

In designing the Alpha Wave Basic Training regimen, we started out with a list of program requirements. We wanted a plan that was based on science, not guesswork. For us, that meant a program with three distinct but integrated phases, or "waves," each one designed primarily to build lean muscularity, maximum strength, and explosive power. The program needed multiple levels of intensity, so as to be challenging enough for hardcore top dogs but also something that couch potatoes could handle. It needed to be for a definite, 10-week duration—long enough to see dramatic change but brief enough that it wouldn't be overwhelming. It needed a version of the program for training at home. Its workout sessions needed to be short enough that even the busiest execs would have no excuses. And the program needed to provide startling results.

We reached out to some of the top names in the fields of exercise physiology and resistance training to help create a masterpiece—the ultimate male training program. We wanted an expert with not only mastery of theory but also years of real-world experience. David Sandler, MS, CSCS*D, CCS, HFD, fit the bill to perfection. A doctoral candidate at the University of Miami, David is the president and cofounder of StrengthPro, Inc., and a former competitive powerlifter with regional, national, and world records. A strength and conditioning consultant for more than 18 years, David

has authored or coauthored 5 books, published more than 20 scientific abstracts and articles, written more than 75 articles on power and strength training for various magazines and pieces of literature, and is a consultant and member of the advisory board for *Muscle and Fitness Magazine*. He's the chairman of The Arnold Strength Training Summit at the Arnold Classic, the country's largest fitness symposium, and is currently the state director of Nevada for the National Strength and Conditioning Association.

David was excited about becoming part of the team to design the next evolutionary step in resistance training.

> When the Alpha Wave Basic Training concept was presented to me, I immediately saw two other guys who have that same passion to look at what people really want and figure out how to make it happen. . . . To get a chance to work on a revolutionary program that integrates old-school lifting with the latest science was an offer only a fool would pass up. The resulting training system is going to shake things up big time.

Our goal is to help you build effortless endurance, brute strength, Herculean power, and a body that grabs attention, all without giving up your day job to become a slave to the gym. Our revolutionary program is designed to raise your Alpha Factor.

Each of your physical assessments on the MaleScale will be improved during Alpha Wave Basic Training. You'll burn more calories, build more foundational functional muscle, and improve coordination and skill. And you'll look better than ever on the beach.

Resistance Training 101

There are very few guys today who have never been in a weight room. But for those of you who haven't been there since high school, we're happy to provide a refresher course on the basics.

A **repetition,** or rep, is one complete movement of an exercise, typically raising and lowering a weight. **Concentric contraction** is the shortening of the muscle to lift the weight during a repetition. **Eccentric contraction** is the lengthening of the muscle to lower the weight during a repetition.

A series of repetitions without a break is a **set.**

The total number of sets and reps in a workout is the **volume** of that workout.

There are different kinds of sets. We will be using a variety of both traditional and innovative training protocols. The traditional **straight set** is one in which you perform one exercise for a sequence of reps and then rest for a recommended period of time before performing the next set of the exercise. A **superset** is two exercises performed back to back with no rest between them. A modified compound superset, which we call a **circuit set,** is a set of three exercises performed in a consecutive sequence with 1 minute of rest between the first two movements. A **drop set** is one in which you begin a set, lifting a weight for as many repetitions as you can do. When you reach momentary muscular failure, you pick up a lighter weight and continue lifting for as many repetitions as you can do. A drop set will continue in this fashion until you've reached a target weight or repetition range. Our drop set protocols involve three descending levels of resistance, or steps.

The **Punisher** is a grueling 100-rep giant set, during which you must try to reach the 100-rep mark in as few sets as possible. You may get 40 reps on the first set, 20 on the second, 15 on the third, 15 on the fourth, and 10 on the fifth. It would be both more time-efficient and more intense if you got 60 reps on the first set, 30 on the second, and 10 on the last. If you choose the proper weight—often about half of your strength-training weights—you may come out somewhere in between. Either way,

you want to reach 100 reps with as few sets as possible. Remember to perform 50 reps on each leg for all single-leg movements. It's more than tough and we're sure that you'll be cursing us when you're smack in the middle of this bad boy.

The **pushup challenge,** inspired by the martial arts and sometimes used as a training test for black belt status, requires you to perform as many consecutive full repetitions as you can without stopping. You'll bring your chest to about 2 inches off the floor on each rep. Levels A and B will do two sets, separated by a 1-minute rest interval. To pass a black belt test, the minimum required is 75 repetitions.

The duration of the **rest intervals** between sets plays an important role in the training equation. Rest periods are vital for strength recovery, but you must stay focused. It's very easy to become distracted and taken out of your "zone" during rest intervals. Use this time to dynamically stretch out, walk off the muscle burn from the last set, or step outside for a quick breath of air. Not only will keeping tabs on your rest time between sets help you cruise through your workouts more efficiently, but it will also stimulate a metabolic effect to add muscle, build power and strength, and torch those waist-bulging calories! Short rest periods provoke a release of growth hormone and maximize muscle growth and endurance. Longer rest periods are best for boosting strength and power. Our system is designed to maximize your progress on multiple levels—that's why you'll notice a variety of rest periods in the workouts, depending on which of the three training goals (see page 62) is being targeted.

- Movements to build muscle size and endurance will have you resting either 1 or 2 minutes between sets.

- Movements to target strength will have you resting between 2 or 3 minutes between sets.

- Movements to increase explosive power will have you resting 1½ or 2 minutes between sets.

Keeping to the prescribed rest periods is vital to Alpha Wave Basic Training, so it would be wise to purchase an inexpensive stopwatch.

The **training tempo** of a repetition is the speed at which you perform the repetition. For example, for a bench press, the training tempo is the time during which the weight is lowered, how long it's held at the bottom of the movement, how fast it's lifted, and how long it's held at the top before being lowered again. Each of the four phases of the rep is measured in seconds. Varying the training tempo will vary the stimulation to the muscles being worked and elicit different responses. It's also a terrific way to keep your training fresh! Let's use the bench press example again. For a training tempo of 2-0-1-0, you should:

- Lower the bar to your chest over a span of 2 seconds.
- Begin lifting the bar without a discernable pause at the bottom.
- Lift the bar over a 1-second span.
- Begin lowering the bar again without a discernable pause at the top.

Recognize that some exercises start by lowering a weight (squats, leg press, bench press, flies) and some start by raising it (leg curls, shoulder press, biceps curl, pec deck). The first number *always* corresponds to the eccentric contraction in any movement, regardless of which phase typically starts that exercise.

Time under tension (TUT) refers to the total time a muscle is contracted and under stress in response to resistance. It can refer to the total time a muscle is under tension in a whole workout (all your sets combined), or during just one set, or during each rep. The training tempo of a repetition will determine the muscle's TUT for that rep.

For example, if you do a dumbbell squat with a training tempo of 3-0-1-0 (3 seconds to lower the weight, no discernable pause at the bottom, 1 second to return to the standing position, and no discernable pause at the top before descending again), the TUT for that rep would be 4 seconds. Performing 10 reps at this tempo would take a total of 40 seconds. Therefore, the TUT for that set is 40 seconds. If you elongated the tempo of the concentric phase of the reps to 3 seconds as well (3-0-3-0), it would take you 60 seconds to complete a 10-rep set. Slowing the repetitions and extending the duration of sets can dramatically increase intensity and pack on the muscle mass quickly, provided the resistance is heavy enough to challenge your muscles.

One way to intensify a training program and enhance results is to work hard to reach momentary **muscular failure** during a set. This is simply a matter of lifting a weight until your muscles can no longer lift that weight using good form and proper exercise technique. Reaching momentary muscular failure is a great training strategy to recruit the maximum number of muscle fibers in the muscle you're working. However, don't use this strategy all of the time, because too much of it can lead to overuse injuries such as tendonitis. Since the intensity required to reach momentary muscular failure is so extreme, it's much wiser to select only one or two movements per workout and then go for only a couple sets of momentary muscular failure on them. Other high-intensity training techniques should be used prudently as well. The drop set, for example, is extremely effective, but if you used this training protocol all the time, you'd overtax your body and hinder your results, or even get injured. We strategically placed drop sets into your Alpha Wave Basic Training program to an extent that balances intensity with prudence. Don't try to do more than the program advocates!

Every modern muscle-building exercise plan utilizes a training protocol called **progressive overload** or **progressive resistance**. This means incrementally increasing the training stimulus to trigger your body's adaptive response. Progressive resistance yields progressive achievement! Your body will adapt to the demands placed on it—or, as Nietzsche said, "That which does not kill us makes us stronger." Continuously going through the same motions of the same tired workout routine week after week, month after month, and year after year, will reap few rewards. If you want bigger, fuller, harder muscles, you've got to ratchet up the demands on your body. That means regularly adding more weight to your workouts or otherwise increasing training variables to force your body to meet the challenge by packing on new muscle. It's the only way to shake your body out of its comfort zone and allow you to make improvements.

Which brings us to the question of **resistance**: How much weight should you be lifting? Obviously, there are too many variables to give an answer that would apply to everyone. The only viable answer is this: as much as you can with good form and without hurting yourself. More weight is only one of many factors (such as number of sets, number of reps, and rep tempo) that can be manipulated to add intensity to your training. But as surely as lifting weights that are too heavy for you will subject you to the risk of injury, lifting weights that are too light for you will mostly waste your time. Although movements to build power are meant to be performed quickly and with somewhat lighter weight, both the lean muscle mass/endurance and the strength-building exercises work best when you are using poundages that allow you to finish each set with very little gas left in the tank, so to speak. Be mindful that slower rep tempos (e.g., 3-0-3-0) will be much harder than more traditional tempos (e.g., 1-0-1-0) using the same weights. There will be some trial and error at first to find the poundages that make you struggle to finish each set of your workout while maintaining good form and

remaining injury-free. But the results will speak for themselves.

ALPHA WAVE BASIC TRAINING: THE NUTS AND BOLTS

Alpha Wave Basic Training has three distinct goals, addressed over three rolling training Waves, and offers three training levels. These components interact and work beautifully together, creating a simple training system that's fresh, exciting, and incredibly effective!

The Three Basic Goals

- Build muscular, lean (fat-free) body mass and muscle endurance
- Maximize brute strength
- Boost explosive power

The overall objective is to dramatically improve in all three areas over the 10 weeks of the Challenge. Each and every one of the 27 Alpha Wave Basic Training workouts incorporates specific exercise protocols—varying repetition ranges, strategic rest intervals, and prescribed training tempos—to optimally meet all three basic goals. However, specifically trying to target all three basic goals equally, in every workout, would require marathon workout sessions that would stall your gains and lead to overtraining. Our system is designed so that each individual workout predominantly targets only *one* of the three training objectives. An Alpha Wave Basic Training workout targets a basic goal when roughly 60 percent of its protocols address that goal. In a given workout, each of the other two basic goals receives 20 percent of the focus.

- Muscle Up resistance training exercises that are performed to target the goal of building lean body mass and muscle endurance.

- Strength Max exercises are executed to target increased brute strength.
- Power Boost movements are performed to target enhanced explosive power.

In practice, the 60-20-20 system amounts to six exercise movements for the targeted basic goal and two movements for each of the other two. That's 10 exercises, every workout, along with a couple of bonus movements for a strong core and rock-hard abdominals.

We've provided you with a lot of exercises within the Alpha Wave Basic Training program. You will notice that there are multiple exercises for each major muscle group. At first glance, some of you may find the broad variety a bit overwhelming, but it is truly of great benefit—it will keep your muscles consistently challenged and will help you stay mentally motivated throughout the Challenge. The variation of the exercises extends beyond just the type of machine or training apparatus that you'll be using. You will also be instructed to put your body in various positions that will allow you to isolate specific muscle groups. For example, when you do a chest press on an incline bench, you are engaging the upper chest (pectoral) muscles. If you move to a flat bench and perform a chest press, you will move the primary muscle concentration to the center of the chest. These slight changes in body positioning, or "training angles," will allow you to hone in on specific areas of each muscle group. These training angles apply to all of your major muscle groups. Just follow the plan and you'll be hitting all of the areas of each muscle group to ensure total development.

Another one of the training variations that you'll notice in our program is how certain exercises can be performed using various alternative pieces of equipment. For example, you can perform the incline chest press using a barbell, dumbbells, machines, or even a Smith Machine. The same variation applies for all your major muscle groups. The quadriceps muscles located on your frontal thigh can be stimulated by a variety of different exercises. You'll engage the quadriceps during the barbell squat, any lunge movement, the leg extension exercise, and many more. The biceps muscles can be stimulated during the barbell curl, the incline dumbbell curl, the chinup, and more. Variety will add a refreshing component to your workouts. You will perform specific exercises for certain muscle groups in one workout and then use different exercises to hit that same muscle group during that next muscle group's workout. This variation is what will keep your body guessing, and it's what will keep you motivated to keep going strong. When you get used to doing the same exercises and workouts all the time, it gets pretty boring and your progress stagnates.

Remember Alpha Wave Basic Training requires you to carefully track your rest periods between sets and between exercises. This is crucial if you're looking to make your workout time most efficient. However, in the real world you may not be the only person in the gym. There may very well be someone already using the machine you need, or even other people waiting for their turn. The last thing you want to do is waste time waiting for a machine to become available. You should, of course, feel comfortable enough to ask the person on a "manned" machine how many sets he has left. If it turns out that he still has more than one set to go or if there are other people waiting to use it, don't wait. It will throw off your workout! Instead, substitute an alternative exercise and keep the workout moving along. Check out the substitutes exercise list located in the "Alpha Wave Home Body/Substitutes" section (see page 77). We've carefully selected each exercise and its replacement for you!

The Three Rolling Waves

Alpha Wave Basic Training comprises three independent training Waves, followed by a fourth 1-week "Breaking Wave" of active rest and recovery.

The three training Waves are broken down into a weekly countdown, as follows:

- 1st Wave: 4 weeks
- 2nd Wave: 3 weeks
- 3rd Wave: 2 weeks

The 1st Wave focuses on building muscular lean body mass and muscle endurance; the 2nd Wave on maximizing strength; and the 3rd Wave on boosting explosive power. They follow each other just as each ocean wave follows another to the shore. As you can see, each of the first three training Waves specifically targets one of the three basic goals. However, each Wave also incorporates elements from the other two training Waves. This is where the true power of the program exists! In each and every one of the 27 workouts, you will devote 60 percent of your efforts to one of the three basic goals—Muscle Up, Strength Max, or Power Boost—and 20 percent each to the other two goals. Over the course of the 10 weeks of your Challenge, this ratio has the incredible effect of helping you get the most out of the present Wave's primary training target, while maintaining the results you've already earned and laying the foundation for the work yet to come. You see, most "periodized" training programs will have you train for a specific goal but will eventually move on to a different training goal without devoting any maintenance training to those hard-earned results you've already achieved. True progress is often futile, as you are bound to lose what you don't maintain. (You've heard of the "use it or lose it" principle, haven't you?) To achieve optimum fitness results, during each workout you will dedicate a majority (60 percent) of your training to one basic goal, and another portion (20 percent and 20 percent) of your training to each of the other basic goals to maintain results already achieved from prior training. This is what you call smart training, guys, and it's the future of fitness.

The Rolling Wave approach helps you achieve new results, maintain them, and optimally prepare your body for each of the upcoming Waves.

If you skip a specific Wave, you will have left out a vital ingredient in the recipe for an extraordinarily better-looking physique. By the end of the 10-week training cycle, you will have increased every factor and not compromised any factor. In a nutshell, to experience the greatest results from the Alpha Wave Basic Training regimen, you must follow the program as directed!

Three Training Levels

Alpha Wave Basic Training offers three training levels of volume and intensity to account for differences in initial strength and fitness levels:

- Level A
- Level B
- Level C

Research shows that the hormonal response to exercise differs between untrained guys and guys with years of strength training under their belts. Experienced lifters need a higher level of training than the newly un-couched. A study of adult men (mean age, 40.6 years, ± 4 years) published in the *Journal of Strength and Conditioning Research* suggests that a high volume of training is best for maximizing testosterone release in long-term lifters, but too much volume for untrained men leads to a greater release of the muscle-diminishing stress hormone cortisol. Our program is designed to offer just the right training stimulus for *you*.

If you've never lifted weights before or haven't in many years, you start at training level C. Otherwise, just refer to the results of your physical assessments on the MaleScale (see page 15). Add up your scores. If your total is between 5 and 20, start at level C. If it's between 20 and 35, start at level B. If your score is above 35, start at level A, which is the most advanced training level. It's this simple:

Physical MaleScale Results Training Level

Greater than 35	A
20 to 35	B
Less than 20	C

A very small minority of guys may find after beginning Alpha Wave Basic Training that the training provided by the level is either too easy or too difficult. If so, you may adjust by switching one level up or down.

The total number of sets you will complete in any given workout (excluding four to six sets of core and abdominal movements) will depend on your training level.

- Level C trainers should complete 12 to 18 total sets in a workout session.
- Level B trainers should complete 20 to 26 total sets in a workout session.
- Level A trainers should complete 24 to 30 total sets in a workout session.

Get the idea? If you are at level C, you will perform the lowest number of sets of each exercise. You can always work up later. Level B will perform more sets than C, and level A even more.

How many sets of each movement should you do to reach the total sets for a session? It will depend on your level. For level C, most movements will call for one or two sets. For level B, you'll do two or three sets of most of the 10 movements. For level A, you'll do either two or three sets of all exercises. When you review your workouts and refer to your particular training level, everything is already mapped out for you. Just follow the guidelines and add intensity—it's a guaranteed recipe for success!

FIRST THINGS FIRST: THE DYNAMIC WARMUP

You've learned how each of our Alpha Wave Basic Training workouts includes three training objectives: building muscular mass and endurance (Muscle Up), maximizing strength (Strength Max), and boosting raw power (Power Boost). You will want to thoroughly prepare or warm up your muscles immediately prior to each training session. To do this most effectively, you need warmup movements that sufficiently ready your body as whole and each of your muscles for the work ahead.

Let's talk about proper warmup. A warmup is a sequence of movements that prepares your body for the demands of an upcoming workout. The Dynamic Warmup was designed to limber you up enough to avoid injury and maximize your performance. Yeah, yeah, we all know self-professed tough guys who say warmups are for "sissies," but we're betting you're more mature than that. The benefits of a proper warmup are that you:

- Prevent injury through an increase in your respiratory rate and the flow of blood to your muscles
- Make your muscles more flexible through muscle elasticity
- Improve your focus on the exercise that follows

So don't blow off this important step. Just do the warmups, okay?

The Alpha Male Challenge Dynamic Warmup uses both dynamic activity and static stretching. Note that preworkout stretching shouldn't be done "cold"—the best research suggests that to avoid the risk of injury you shouldn't stretch until after you've warmed up the muscles you intend to stretch.

Power Boost movements start every Alpha Wave Basic Training session. That's because the explosive actions of power training require skill, coordination, and precise execution that are not yet diminished by fatigue. Our Dynamic Warmup is the perfect lead-in to your Power Boost movements, taking you in a gradual progression from a "cold," slower-moving body to a faster, warmer body that is prepared for the impending battle with the iron. Additionally, because the Strength Max movements and Muscle Up movements also require warm muscles and a full range of motion, the Dynamic Warmup provides a thorough body stretch to promote flexibility and help reduce the possibility of injury.

Our exclusive Dynamic Warmup should precede every single one of the 27 Alpha Wave Basic Training workouts. Perform the Dynamic Warmup exactly as it's laid out here:

- 5-minute treadmill walk (grade 1.5, speed 3.0)

Now perform the sequence below for one circuit. Begin the circuit with a slower and more deliberate pace, then accelerate the pace as you continue.

- 10 bodyweight Good Mornings
- Walking Lunges (Cross the River) (8 lunges on each leg)
- Rotational Hamstring Stretch (8 stretches on each side)
- Trunk Rotations (10 to each side)
- 10 Deep Squats
- Static Quad Stretch (hold for 15 seconds on each leg)
- Static Lunge Hip Flexor Stretch (hold for 15 seconds on each leg)
- Static Chest Stretch (hold for 15 seconds on each side)
- Static Lat Stretch (hold for 15 seconds on each side)
- 10 Pushups (full range of motion)
- Stationary Inchworm (8 reps)
- 10 Jumping Jacks
- Butt-Kickers (20 total—10 on each leg)
- Lateral Shuffle (10 total—5 to each side)

Check out Appendix A, page 299 for movement descriptions. Now let's catch those Waves!

1ST WAVE— WEEKS 1 THROUGH 4

Target: Muscle Up

This 1st Wave is the one responsible for opening the spigots of testosterone and growth hormone production. Research conducted at the University of Nebraska on male subjects who had some experience in weight training but had not been involved in recent consistent training concluded that during a 10-week resistance training program, shorter between-set rest intervals elicited a greater hormonal response—testosterone and growth hormone—than longer rest intervals. But the greatest differences were seen during the first 4 weeks. (By Week 10, the differences had disappeared.)

This Wave—consisting of 4 weeks—targets the higher repetitions and shorter rest intervals of Muscle Up to rapidly spike your muscle-building hormone levels, increase your lean muscle mass (bigger, better-looking muscles), and dramatically improve your muscular endurance (the ability to repeatedly perform a movement using a specific muscle or group of muscles). Improving your muscular endurance, or staying power, will have great practical benefits for your life. The next time you're late for an appointment on the 10th floor and the elevator's broken, you'll scale the 10 flights of stairs in a sweat-free minute, while the Beta males wait for the technician.

Beginning lifters can expect to quickly gain not only muscular size and endurance but also improved coordination.

To build bigger muscles, 1st Wave workouts maximize the length of time that your muscles are forced to endure a load. The two most common methods for accomplishing this are increasing the number of reps and taking shorter rests between sets. Other ways include using slower, deliberate movements, where single reps may take several seconds, and dropping or stripping weight and continuing sets maximizing the total time a group of muscles is exposed to the same stresses.

The 1st Wave will include predominantly Muscle Up movements, designed to stimulate the growth of lean body mass by lifting moderately heavy weights, taking rest periods of 1 to 2 minutes, and keeping the reps moderately high. In the first week, reps are up to 20 per set, providing an opportunity for top dogs and gym rats to boost endurance, shock their neural systems, and flush those muscles will nutrient-rich blood, while also resting and repairing tendons and ligaments. (Most seasoned lifters will have mainly been training with heavy weights and low repetitions.) For new lifters, this is a time to condition the muscles, tendons, ligaments, and joints for the intense journey ahead. Then the reps drop down to 15, and then 12, and then 10 reps for Muscle Up movements in the weeks that follow.

2ND WAVE— WEEKS 5 THROUGH 7

Target: Strength Max

This 2nd Wave is designed to increase your overall maximum strength. Only in competitive body building are muscle size, shape, and definition the judging criteria for actual strength—without regard for actual strength. Being strong, in addition to looking great, is a top priority for men who want practical fitness they can use in everyday life. The 2nd Wave will help you to gain the kind of upper and lower body strength that is needed to lift or carry a load. Most guys train using the wrong criteria for increasing strength. During 2nd Wave workouts, you will develop strength by using relatively heavy resistance in lower repetition sets—4 to 6 reps—and taking longer timed rest intervals—between 2 and 3 minutes. The longer rest intervals will allow for you to properly recover. More time between Strength Max sets will enable you to push and pull the heavy iron needed to build truly impressive strength.

Lifting a heavy weight for lower reps, while performing multi-joint or compound exercises, such as squats, deadlifts, and lunges, will continue to force your body to release muscle-building testosterone. The muscularity and endurance gains made during your 4 weeks of 1st Wave training and the raw strength gains yielded over the 3 weeks of 2nd Wave training will result in a body that looks strong and is strong.

INJURY PREVENTION

As you prepare for your new training program, a few words about injury prevention are in order. We don't expect you to become injured, but from having been in the strength and fitness world for a combined 50 years, we know that guys can hurt themselves from time to time. This is often a consequence of lifting beyond their means, not practicing proper form, or simply pushing their recuperative capacities beyond the natural limits.

One of the finest physical therapists in the country, our friend Dr. Michael Camp, DPT, CSCS, PES, has helped countless people, from famous athletes to average Joes, by rehabilitating their injuries and by teaching them his proprietary pre-habilitation strengthening protocols to prevent recurrences. Mike points out that "a very large piece of my practice is dedicated toward treating the 'weekend warrior' types of injuries. If you are suffering from a shoulder or low back injury, it is absolutely essential that you first seek medical advice before beginning any physical protocol within the Challenge. Remember, even what you may now consider to be a small problem, in time, will often become a bigger one." To read Mike's pre-hab routine online, check out www. alphamalechallenge.com.

We want you to push as hard as you can on all Alpha Wave Basic Training workouts, but be mindful that neither Rome nor a gladiator's physique was built in a day. Never try to lift more weight than you can handle in good form. You can always increase the poundages on the next workout.

3RD WAVE— WEEKS 8 AND 9

Target: Power Boost

In the 2 weeks of your 3rd Wave training, you'll target developing explosive power, fueled by the testosterone and growth hormone production that first began in the 1st Wave. Developing muscular power will challenge your central nervous system by teaching your muscles to react and fire faster. Challenging your muscles with explosive movements—"plyometrics" (see opposite)—will ultimately teach you to control your muscles much more efficiently. This has obvious advantages not just for sports athletes, but for the average guy, as well. Power is the combination of speed and strength; explosive power training improves both. You'll get quicker and more agile, with better balance and overall coordination.

There is an important distinction between strength and power. Power is the maximum rate at which a load is lifted. Most people believe that using very heavy weight will help develop power; however, the opposite is true. In power training, the objective is to lift a manageable weight as fast as possible. (Remember our friend gravity.) Essentially, it's strength with a time factor added. To develop true explosive power, both the concentric and the eccentric phases should be performed as explosively as possible.

Numerous studies show the benefits of explosive lifting, including its efficacy in improving not only power but also everyday life function—things you do with your kids, for example, such as running, jumping, and throwing. In fact, several studies show that power training even improves functionality in both active and frail senior citizens. For example, if a person were about to fall down, increased power could help break or prevent the fall through a quicker and more explosive response—a potential lifesaver for older folks.

We have selected Power Boost movements that are generally regarded as both safe and effective by experts. Explosive lifting requires attention to proper form to maximize safety while minimizing time spent learning specific skills. When using resistance (such as a barbell or dumbbell) during explosive movements, you must take care to avoid injury. Your most effective means to avoid injury here will be your undivided attention to the movement you're performing. Your training partner can also assist by letting you know how your form looks and how to adjust it if it's lacking.

After the Dynamic Warmup, each and every Alpha Wave Basic Training workout begins with a Power Boost (plyo) movement. If you are over 200 pounds and not used to jumping or doing upper body plyos such as power pushups, we advise that you perform these movements using either a modified form or a limited range of motion. For a jump, this will simply mean not squatting as deeply both during the jump and on landing. Just always be sure to jump from and back to soft knees (a bend in the knees so that they act as shock absorbers). As for the power pushup, you may simply modify the movement by doing it from your knees. Do not feel inadequate about the need to take it easier at first. If you stick to the program and you are free from any preexisting injuries or congenital medical issues, you will eventually become conditioned enough to perform all the movements as they were meant to be performed.

In 3rd Wave Power Boost training, your rest intervals will be 1½ minutes between each set of power movements. Your repetition range is still low, with 5 reps total in each set. Your repetition tempo is super-fast and explosive. Think about it: To be faster and more explosive, you need to specifically train for it. All of your power movements will be executed as explosively as possible after the first rep. Use the first rep to learn technique and control, and then hit it hard for 4 more reps. Power training, including plyometric movements, is heavily taxing. Note that if your muscles are sore or your joints (knees, ankles, lower back, etc.) are bothering you, you should completely avoid these movements until you have recovered. Performing power exercises at anything less than explosive speed is a waste of time.

By using all of the Alpha Wave Basic Training methods, you will focus on all of the physical training it takes to be a true Alpha Male. You'll have the muscle size and endurance, the maximal strength, and the extreme power, speed, and agility. Who among us wouldn't want all of that?

WHAT ARE PLYOMETRICS AND DO I NEED TO DO THEM?

Plyometrics, or "plyos," are a method of training that enhances the muscle's natural ability to contract more forcefully and rapidly. Plyometric movements are performed very differently from traditional weight-training exercises. They are performed as rapid movements—typically as jumps or explosive pushes—for low repetition ranges (typically 3 to 6). The tempo is best represented as 0-0-0-0, meaning as fast as you can do them. This explosive style of training leads to an improved ability to generate greater force more rapidly. Another benefit of plyometric training is that the higher intensity demands they place on the body place greater demands on the metabolism, resulting in more calories burned.

Think of stretching a rubber band, then releasing it at one end. The release will produce extreme force, all generated from that stretch. Now imagine your muscles reacting in the same way during a plyo movement. An example of one plyometric movement that we will be utilizing in and throughout the Challenge is the squat jump. The squat jump movement consists of quickly squatting down from a standing position, then explosively jumping up as high as you possibly can. After landing back in a squat position and without resting, you then explode back into a jump (and repeat for the required repetitions). This fast action movement will excite your muscle fibers and nervous system and ultimately improve your ability to jump higher at a faster rate. When your muscle becomes stretched, such as in the landing of a squat jump, the landing triggers a stretch within your muscles/tendons and will generate pent-up energy forces that will actually help you jump more explosively as you jump back up. This process is known as the "stretch shortening cycle."

Plyometric activity utilizes the muscle's inherent stretch-contract mechanism and, over time, improves the rate at which force is developed. Even endurance athletes, general fitness enthusiasts, and senior citizens should perform some plyometric training. Can you think of how this would benefit you in your life, right now? How about in a situation where you need to quickly jump to safety, saving yourself or a loved one? Building up power will also help you perform better at the things you love doing. If you love sports, more power means being quicker and more agile. If you love playing with your kids, which guy would you rather be: the one chasing your kids as they laugh at your embarrassingly futile attempt to catch them, or the one who has your kids chase you, as you quickly break away with ease and enjoyment?

We have purposely added a Wave dedicated to boosting your power through the use of plyometric movements. Professional athletes have been using similar movements in their training for as long as sports have existed. If you question whether they should be part of a program like this, the answer is an unequivocal yes, they should. It's one thing to look great; it's another to perform and feel great. Adding plyos to your program will have you moving quicker with less effort than you're used to exerting. You'll be conditioning your body to move in ways you're not used to, and probably haven't since you were a kid. These movements will actually lead to fewer aches and pains, because many aches and pains that men experience are a result of moving in ways they are not used to. You will be training and conditioning your body and muscles to move so that when you need to—or, better yet, choose to—move more quickly and explosively, you'll be able to do so with little effort.

THE BREAKING WAVE—WEEK 10

Target: Active Rest and Recovery

We call the final Wave of the 10-week plan the Breaking Wave. Unlike the three training Waves, it lasts only 1 week. The main objective is to allow your body to actively rest and recover from the previous 9 brutally productive weeks of training. We suggest only Work Heart and Play Heart activities (see page 73), and at most 2 days of circuit training (usually a line of weight stack equipment specifically set up at most gyms) with light to moderate weight and higher repetitions. We promise that you won't sacrifice gains by taking it easy during the Breaking Wave. Your body will have been pushed hard and will absolutely need the rest. So yes—this Wave is mandatory.

The Breaking Wave should be made up of activities that get you moving without overtaxing your muscles, connective tissue, or aerobic system. There are a few schools of thought as to which activities are best for an active rest week. Is it weight training with less volume and intensity, or is it getting out of the weight room and engaging in some Play Heart activities (see page 79)? According to renowned exercise gurus Bill Kraemer and Steve Fleck, active rest should involve activities outside of the weight room. They suggest that games, hiking, and swimming can provide recovery for the neuromuscular system.

We're up for a couple of less-intense weight-training sessions if you like, but we believe that you'll actually gain more from your Play Heart time. You've worked diligently and intensely for 9 weeks, and your body will soak up a new form of activity. During your Breaking Wave week, dedicate some time to doing something different. Try something exciting and novel: a new sport or an adventure trip with friends or the family (you'll know when you're scheduled for your Breaking Wave week, so plan ahead for some fun). Do something challenging and enjoyable. It will reenergize your body, your dedication, and your drive. Recuperative low-intensity, low-volume activities don't have to lack excitement. Live it up!

After 9 weeks of rugged training, reward yourself with a therapeutic massage. This is an ideal time to allow a licensed massage therapist to dig deep into those tight and taxed muscles. It will help you recover more quickly, stimulate your circulation, and even help bring about better training results after all your hard work. It's also great for preparing muscles for upcoming physical activities. In fact, if you can afford it, it's a great way of recovering and preparing for all your weekly workouts over the 10-week program. Or try visiting a chiropractor or even a physical therapist; because he may be able to show you how to more effectively recover from intense training. Try some acupuncture, tai chi, yoga, or any other modality that's ever intrigued you. The new activity, like a new exercise or exercise variation, can spark new results.

Your week-by-week Alpha Wave Basic Training regimen—all 27 workouts—is set forth in the 10-week Challenge, beginning on page 126. For now, let's turn to the unique system of heart-pumping, fat-burning aerobic exercise we have got in store for you!

BUILDING A BRAVE HEART

During the Stone Age, daily aerobic exertion was a necessity to secure food and water and to escape predators with huge fangs and claws. "Our remote ancestors participated in various physical activities daily," notes research published in *Mayo Clinic Proceedings*. "They walked and ran 5 to 10 miles daily as they foraged and hunted for their food sources. They also lifted, carried, climbed, stretched, leaped, and did whatever else was necessary to secure their sustenance and protection. Days of heavy exertion were followed by recovery days. In modern terms, these people cross-trained with aerobic, resistance, and flexibility exercises." Although technology has made physical activity mostly optional, it's still important to exercise as though our lives depended on it. For in fact they do depend on it, given the current state of our gender described.

A healthy heart and lungs play an important part in overall health. Cardiovascular or aerobic exercise—"cardio" as it's commonly called—will deliver oxygen and nutrients to the tissues of your body. You will powerfully increase the circulation of blood to and through your heart and blood vessels, strengthening your heart and its ability to pump blood more effortlessly to all areas of your body. When you exert yourself during the aerobic exercises and activities of the Challenge, your heart and lungs will begin to work more efficiently. You'll soon feel the benefits of having more energy to do all those things you love doing. And it will play a key part in getting you lean.

MAKING "CARDIO" COUNT!

Nobody will dispute the fact that aerobic exercise should be part of any conditioning program. Aer-

obic exercise is anything that involves or improves your body's consumption of oxygen. The intensity level can vary. A question many guys ask is, "How hard should I be working to get the best results?" The answer depends on the activity. For walking, bicycling, and other low- or moderate-intensity activities, try using a "conversational pace." If you can walk and talk at the same time, you aren't overdoing it. If you're so short of breath that you can't, scale it back. On the other hand, if you can sing "Stairway to Heaven" while you're exercising, you should step it up. Training at low or moderate intensity is terrific for torching excess body fat. That's why we've incorporated these types of activities into our program.

If you want to track your aerobic intensity during more strenuous exercise, we advocate a simple method called the "Rating of Perceived Exertion." It uses a 20-point scale called the Borg scale to communicate your level of exertion during your aerobic workout. The scale begins at the number 6, which is no exertion at all, and goes up to 20, which is maximal exertion (see "Borg Scale" below).

The object is to assess what you're feeling in the way of exertion at a specific point in your exercise. Choose the expression/number that best describes what you're feeling at that moment. A number 9, expressed as "very light" exercise, is often chosen when a person is walking slowly at a constant pace. A number 13 is expressed as

BORG SCALE

6 No exertion at all	13 Somewhat hard
7 Extremely light	14
(7.5)	15 Hard (heavy)
8	16
9 Very light	17 Very hard
10	18
11 Light	19 Extremely hard
12	20 Maximal exertion

"somewhat hard" exertion, but you're managing your exertion well.

A 17, expressed as "very hard," is considered strenuous exertion. This level of exertion is still okay to push through, but it will take extreme intensity and laser focus to maintain. A 19 on the scale is expressed as "extremely hard." This is considered an intensely strenuous exercise level and calls for caution, because you may be nearly at the brink of exhaustion. Always stay focused and listen to your body. Ignoring your current fitness capabilities and pushing excessively hard can subject you to more harm than good.

This 20-point Borg scale is a great way of assessing how hard you're working during activities of higher intensity. It can provide a great indicator as to whether you're working as hard as you should be in order to improve your cardiovascular conditioning.

Monitoring Your Heart Rate

One long-accepted benchmark for cardiovascular intensity is your heart rate. Your heart beats approximately 70 beats per minute (give or take, depending on your fitness level) when you're sitting and haven't exerted yourself for a while. That's your *resting heart rate*. Your *maximal heart rate* is the fastest rate at which your heart can beat and is generally estimated to decline with age.

You can use your heart rate as a guide to determine the proper intensity for your aerobic intensity. The standard formula to use as a guideline is subtracting your age from the number 220 to estimate your maximal heart rate (e.g., a 40-year-old guy would have an estimated maximal heart rate of 180; of course, this is a very rough estimate, and his actual maximal heart rate may be much higher or lower depending on his individual fitness level). Somewhere in the zone between your resting heart rate and your maximal heart rate is the optimal heart rate for cardiovascular exercise. This is called your *training heart rate*.

Your training heart rate should be between 50 and 85 percent of your maximal heart rate (e.g., if you're 40, your training heart rate should be between 90 and 153 beats per minute). You can check to see whether you're within that range during exercise by placing your index and middle fingers on the side of your neck (carotid artery). Count the beats in a 10-second interval, then multiply by 6 to get the number of beats per minute. Of course, most treadmills will monitor your heart rate if you simply squeeze and hold the handle.

A more accurate way to estimate your optimal training heart rate is the Karvonen method, a mathematical formula that factors in your individual resting heart rate to find your "target heart rate" for aerobic exercise. The formula is:

Target Heart Rate = [(Maximal Heart Rate – Resting Heart Rate) × % Intensity)] + Resting Heart Rate

Let's say you're 40 years old (maximal heart rate: 180) and your actual resting heart rate is 70 beats per minute. If you want to find your target heart rate for training (either 50 or 85 percent intensity), you'd use the formula:

At 50% intensity: [(180 – 70) × 0.50] + 70 = 125 beats per minute
At 85% intensity: [(180 – 70) × 0.85] + 70 = 163 beats per minute

Exactly what *your* actual training heart rate should be depends on many factors, including your age, fitness level, and training goals. Getting your heart rate closer to maximal levels can be a great way to improve your cardiovascular efficiency and burn lots of calories, but lower heart rates within the zone can more effectively use body fat as a fuel source. The bottom line: Using a variety of training heart rates within the zone is a terrific way to condition your heart and lungs *and* melt that excess body fat!

TRUE ALPHA MALES DON'T JOG

We're not fans of endless slow-pace jogging sessions. For one thing, it's painfully boring. For another, our species doesn't seem to be adapted for it. We think there are better choices. Besides, prehistoric man didn't run unless he had to. This was often a means of surviving an attack from a nasty predator, or of being a predator himself to hunt for his next meal. Cavemen sprinted in intermittent bursts. They didn't jog, and they didn't "jazzercise." It would have served little purpose. Maybe the reason that today's runners tend to experience so many sports injuries, including fallen arches, shin splints, strained Achilles tendons, bruised heels, and various knee and back ailments, is that the human body just isn't evolved for it. If you're predisposed to degenerative arthritis, running has been shown to induce the onset and exacerbate the damage. According to exercise scientists at the University of Amsterdam, the average recreational runner who trains steadily and regularly participates in long-distance runs is subjecting himself to otherwise avoidable injuries.

If you love running, we ask you to consider is swapping out some running sessions for some other types of aerobic activities. As you'll soon see, there are plenty of them. And don't think jogging alone will get you into amazing shape. It won't. Do the math yourself. A 200-pound man jogging for a half hour burns fewer than 320 calories. But that's less than what's in just one Grande Java Chip Frappuccino—even minus the whipped cream! Focusing on calorie burning as your main fat-loss strategy is a fool's errand. From a pure net calorie perspective, you'd almost be better off skipping the treadmill and simply eating a McDonald's Double Cheeseburger instead of a Double Quarter Pounder with Cheese—you'd save a full 300 calories in the swap! Of course, we're not discouraging daily aerobic activity. On the contrary, we think it's an important part of overall conditioning, and it's an essential component of the Challenge. We're just saying that you also need to control your weight on the front end—by watching what you eat and drink, and by increasing your lean body mass through resistance exercise. And we're also saying that choosing a variety of activities that are *fun* to do will be more effective at getting you in shape and keeping you committed to exercise.

TRUE ALPHA MALES DO WORK HEART AND PLAY HEART

Our revolutionary approach to cardiovascular fitness not only improves your health but also enhances your maleness. Our plan purposely minimizes or avoids those long and boring bouts of sustained endurance activities such as jogging. We focus on cardiovascular activities that will certainly improve your endurance, but will also allow you to simultaneously build muscle, burn fat, and save your joints from the repetitive stress injuries often associated with jogging and long-distance running. The Challenge incorporates two categories of mandatory aerobic activity: 1) the Work Heart system and 2) Play Heart activities.

Our Work Heart/Play Heart model is based on a combination of functional aerobic efforts (Work Heart) and enjoyable recreational aerobic activities (Play Heart). Work Heart allows you to make better use of or add to activities that you're already doing anyway, such as walking from your car to work and back, or taking the stairs to get to your floor at the office. Play Heart options include both standard gym-based cardio machine training (i.e., treadmills, stationary bicycles, and steppers) with creative cardiovascular activities performed both in and outside the gym.

Note that as the 10-week Challenge progresses, the requirements for both Work Heart and Play

Heart generally increase. That's because the longer you've been invested in the Challenge, the more dividends you've received. You can see the Challenge is paying off! So, by increasing your weekly investments of time—without any excessive demands on your hectic schedule—you'll get even more back!

The Work Heart System

Our Work Heart system is a completely unique program that simply yet powerfully makes the best use of your daily activities and time. This point-based system will have you looking at your daily grind in a whole new way. It not only will improve your overall conditioning, it also will regularly and repeatedly strengthen your mental commitment and pledge to this Challenge.

We know how easy it is to forget about health and fitness as soon as you leave the gym. Even the most dedicated men who already train conscientiously tend to leave their fitness commitment at the gym when they leave. You can just motor through a day without even thinking about it. Our Work Heart system enables you to recommit to the Challenge and your fitness goals not just in the gym and during meals, but throughout the day, every day. Exercising your commitment through Work Heart will only strengthen it.

Why does the elevator trump the stairs for most men every time? With too much pressure and too little time, most guys favor the shortest distance between two points. Speed and convenience beat out healthier choices. So you drive rather than walk. You circle the lot endlessly to park close by your destination. Each moment of decision (e.g., stairs or elevator?) stands alone—random and disconnected. Immediately you make the choice, and you never look back on it. Each is a solitary choice in a series of isolated choices, meaningless "dots" unconnected and soon forgotten, so that at the end of the day, you might shrug and figure, who really cares whether you took the stairs or not?

Clearly, the solution to integrating healthy cardiovascular activity into each and every day is to connect the dots! You can do this by *quantifying* your daily aerobic activity with the Work Heart system. Just as the MaleScale quantifies your Alpha Factor, the Work Heart system quantifies your aerobic exercise with a daily point system. Your objective is to collect a specific number of points by the end of each day. Let's use 20 points daily as an example. Each point is equal to 1 minute's worth of activity, give or take. Your focus should not be so much on exact time as on making the best use of each activity. In other words, we've given you a point system based on time, but what we'd like most for you to think about is getting in a purposeful activity each day that roughly corresponds to 20 minutes. If you fail to collect 20 points, you lose all credit for that day. In our example, at the end of the 5-day workweek, you would need to have collected 100 points.

Work Heart is simply taking the roads less traveled (but keeping your Destination always in mind). Let's say you consciously choose to park your car at the far end of the parking lot and briskly walk 5 minutes to your building, plus 5 minutes back later in the day. You accumulate 10 points (5 points each way) toward your total of 100 points in our example. If in addition to parking farther away you take the stairs instead of the elevator and it takes you 2 minutes, you get 2 points more. A minute to come back down, you get 1 point. Get the picture?

Rather than looking at these extra steps as inconveniences, see them as opportunities. That's Alpha Attitude, right? Five flights of stairs might, at first, take you 2 minutes to climb, but rest assured that after a week or so, those minutes will turn into seconds. Recent research suggests that the benefits of intermittent exercise throughout the day can approach that of a continued block of low-intensity exercise such as treadmill walking. Why waste a half hour treading to nowhere when you can integrate functional Work Heart into your daily routine?

It's all about making each moment really count. If you're walking, put some oomph in your step. If you're climbing stairs, step a little faster or try taking two steps at a time. We really want you to get into it! According to the folks at *Runner's World* magazine, walking briskly at 3.5 mph burns more calories than slowly running at 3.5 mph, because the body's mechanics are designed to walk slow and run fast. Walking fast creates stride inefficiencies that force your body to work harder, and the harder you work, the more calories you burn—and the more benefits you'll reap.

Every time you consciously think about choices such as taking the stairs instead of the escalator, you'll strengthen your commitment muscle. When you become aware of your heart-healthy activity choices throughout the day, you become more sensitized to all aspects of your fitness lifestyle. Your overall outlook on life becomes positively energized. Your muscle endurance, strength, and power begin to improve. Even the smarter dietary choices you make will become an empowering factor. In other words, you'll get better and faster results in all areas of your life! Think of it this way: Every step brings you closer to your destination.

Of course, if you ever feel like you're overdoing it (in any aspect of the Challenge), scale it back a bit. Start out slowly, especially if you've been largely sedentary for years, but try to improve each and every day.

The majority of your Work Heart points will come from two activities: walking and climbing stairs. These are the most common activities most of us will do throughout the day.

One of the best Work Heart opportunities for most guys involves getting to and from work.

- If you drive to work, park far enough away to add a brisk 5-minute walk. Walking this extra distance from your car and back to it at the day's end will add 10 minutes of Work Heart effort to your day. But remember: It's not so much the exact time that matters, but the effort you put into it; that is, 8 minutes of higher intensity brisk walking is better than 10 minutes of a lazy stride.
- If you work in a high-rise office building, choose the stairs over the elevator. You'll only be doing 5 minutes at a time, so you won't even work up a sweat. If your building is extremely tall, walk up for 5 minutes and then take the elevator up for the balance. If you carry a briefcase, even better! Just switch hands halfway through to balance out the effort.

We also want you to get creative here; don't be afraid to add some spice and intensity to the mix. Instead of pulling your suitcases on wheels at the airport, pick them up and carry them to increase the demands on your body. If you see an opportunity to lend someone else a hand, help him or her. Let's say you see someone who needs help pushing her car into the gas station lot. Will you be an onlooker or a doer? Why not push that car and reap all the benefits: good feelings from lending support and the awesome exercise. How about if you see a person who'll have a difficult

WORK HEART SMART

If you need fresh ideas on how to best fit the Work Heart system into your day, check out www.alphamalechallenge.com. Some guys like to bookend each workday with some Work Heart effort, with a few additional minutes during lunch or a break. That certainly doesn't seem like much extra effort, does it? If you already have a co-worker committed to Work Heart efforts with you, by all means continue, even if it means a solid block of time during the workday. Recognize that by getting all your weekly minutes, you'll be cumulatively adding a whole lot of fat-burning Work Heart effort to your week.

time getting a carry-on into the overhead compartment of a plane? Ask if you can help! You're not only collecting Work Heart points but also exercising some heroic altruism (see page 50).

Play Heart Activities

This is where the fun comes in. Fitness should be fun. Play Heart consists of fun activities that amuse and stimulate the human body and spirit. We look at it as rugged, manly playtime. Remember the benefits of "want to" over "have to" commitment? Your Play Heart choices should be things you *want to* do, things you enjoy and look forward to. Play Heart is your chance to really challenge yourself with new and exhilarating physical activities. There are countless options for Play Heart choices at all levels of difficulty and intensity. Some can be done alone, but most of the best ones are *competitive*, such as tennis, basketball, squash, and racquetball. And contact activities such as boxing and martial arts are even better. Not only do they provide great cardio training, but they can also help boost testosterone levels! They also offer the opportunity to develop Alpha Attitude. That's right. If you find the idea of a martial arts class intimidating, then you're *exactly* the guy who should sign up for one today. Talk your training partner into it, also. As you learned from the start, the only way to develop Alpha Attitude is to challenge yourself. Regularly test your confidence and courage, accepting that both are works in progress and knowing that just by doing so you are scaling rarified heights among your peers.

How much Play Heart activity should you do? It depends on your goals. If burning excess body fat fast is paramount to you, you should aim for three

WHITE COLLAR BOXING: THE BOARDROOM BRAWL

John Oden is typical of many career-oriented people in America today. As an executive in a global money management and research firm, he faces all of the pressures one might expect to accompany such a position. He travels constantly and spends his spare time in various cultural and community activities and philanthropic initiatives. Yet despite his remarkably busy schedule, John still manages to find time to stay physically fit via his favorite recreational sport: white collar boxing. Having taken up the sport more than 15 years ago when he was in his early 40s, John now has 20 competitive white collar boxing matches under his belt and claims to be in the best shape of his life. Here's his primer for anyone looking for a healthy and challenging new way to get fit.

"The terms 'white collar boxing' and 'white collar sparring' are used interchangeably to refer to this particular subset of nonprofessional, nonamateur boxing. Contests are staged in local gyms and clubs around the world, and consist of three 2-minute rounds, with 1 minute between rounds. Sixteen-ounce gloves are used. In many gyms, both participants normally receive an identical trophy at the end of the match. White collar boxing was conceived and implemented by Gleason's Gym in Brooklyn beginning in 1988, by the owner of the gym, Bruce Silverglade.

"Participants, as a general rule, are not out to kill each other. Rather, they are involved in the sport to get a good workout, meet new people interested in the sport, and enjoy good camaraderie as they acquire new skills and make new friends. It is a most congenial sport, fostered by mutual respect and common goals. Yet it is a most challenging sport, and all who participate quickly recognize this as well and try to help each other.

"I would rather be a white collar boxer than anything else, as far as athletics and physical fitness are concerned. In my opinion, there is simply nothing like the exhilaration of a boxing workout, which has terrific cardiovascular and aerobic benefits. Boxing has not only helped me stay in great physical shape, but it has also made my life more interesting and unique. It has helped me in innumerable ways to become a stronger human being and more successful businessman. It has strengthened my constitution and helped me focus better on my work. It has sharpened my time-management skills, allowing me to set and achieve my goals in both athletics and business."

sessions per week. Two can be performed in the gym, right after your Alpha Wave Basic Training session. If you're already in the gym for your resistance training, this economizes your valuable time—a key to adhering to any exercise regimen. The third should be on one of your days off. We make this suggestion for two reasons. First, the prospect of new and exciting activities gives you something to look forward to during the workweek. Second, we don't want you to burn out. The overall Alpha Architecture program requires a lot of balanced conditioning. You don't want to overdo it and overtrain with too much exercise in a 5-day span.

The idea is to choose just one Play Heart activity per weekend. It shouldn't take you more than an hour or two, at most, to complete many of the activities we recommend, although some options—such as surfing or skiing—may take up a good part of the day. (And keep in mind that the great majority will take less time than 18 holes of golf, but offer far better fitness benefits.)

Your approach to the Play Heart system will vary with your current fitness condition as reflected with your level on the MaleScale. For level C trainers and/or those who have been "on hiatus" from exercise in general, this will be a new and exciting challenge for you. For level A or B trainers, and/or those who are already involved in a regularly scheduled competitive Play Heart activity, such as tennis or racquetball, this will seem more standard practice at first.

Those are just a few of our favorites, to get your creative and competitive cardio juices flowing. Remember, always take precautions when trying any new and challenging sports, exercises, or activities. The Challenge is all about becoming the man you want to be, but that doesn't mean showing off and being reckless. Whichever activity you decide to engage in, please be careful to choose facilities and instructors whose first priority is making sure that you are safe and properly prepared. Don't be afraid to ask staff for client referrals. It's better to be safe than sorry.

Check out the list of Play Heart suggestions on page 79. Pick the first one that makes you nervously twitch. (You will soon enough, in the Alpha Extreme Triumph!) Seriously, choose an activity that seems fun and challenging. Better yet, review the list with your training partner or gym buddies and arrange a group session. Or go over it with your family or friends and make a go of it for some quality together time. If you don't see anything on the list that you think you'll like, by all means, get creative. You might have a new idea that we didn't think of. If you do, be sure to visit our Web page at www.alphamalechallenge.com and let your true Alpha Male brothers know about it, too.

You will notice that some of the activities listed are seasonal and some may require at least half a day, with anticipated travel time and setup. With this in mind, construct your Play Heart time to be quality interactive time with friends or family members. Remember, most of us work hard, so Play Heart, too!

ALPHA WAVE HOME BODY/ SUBSTITUTES

We realize that not every guy can or will want to leave the comfort of his cave, lair, or fallout shelter to train in a communal gym or health club. If you live on an ice floe above the Arctic Circle or in a bunker in the Mojave, getting to a gym facility may require impossible expenditures of time and effort. It may be that you simply enjoy working out at home or require more convenience that a home gym can provide. Training at home can fit into even the tightest schedule, and it's also one way to economize during especially tough financial times. We've made things very simple for you, by creating a list of alternative exercises to accommodate your Home Body.

James initially built his own physique while training exclusively at home. So he can attest that it's great to have access to your training equipment in mere seconds whenever you choose. Rick also began his training in his parents' basement before joining the local gym. There are, however, some drawbacks to training only at home. (You didn't think we were going to let you off that easy, did you?) Unless you're planning to turn your basement into a state-of-the-art training facility, which could cost you literally thousands of dollars, a home gym may limit your exercise options. You're also unlikely to meet a new training partner in a corner of your garage. Plus, at home you'll be in an atmosphere where it can be hard to avoid distractions, such as a ringing phone or little Junior deciding that the weight bench is a great place to arrange a display of his action figure collection.

If you choose the home gym set up, you'll need to take a little time to plan ahead and figure out how to go about setting up your home gym. Here are some key questions that you'll need to answer:

How much space do you have available?

What is your budget for home gym equipment?

If you set up in a garage, will you be warm enough in colder climates or cool enough in warm ones?

Will you have more potential distractions at home; and if so, can you set some ground rules to help avoid them?

Do you have enough room to set up a mirror or two? (This is a great way to monitor your form.)

Although we're giving you a solid list of substitute at-home exercises and ways to get the most from a home gym, your greatest long-term results will most likely be achieved in a commercial gym setting. You may choose to set up a smaller home gym (a multi-bench and a set of dumbbells) in addition to your commercial gym membership, as it will give you the best of both worlds.

The home-based program should be treated no differently than the gym-based version of Alpha Wave Basic Training. The only major difference is the modification or substitution of exercises to better fit home equipment. Your intensity, set, rep, tempo, and rest protocols should remain identical, or at least as similar as possible. It may be difficult to do some of the "advanced techniques" such as drop sets unless you have more than one set of dumbbells or

use Power Blocks (see below). You should have more than enough weight plates to do drop sets using your barbell and leg extension/leg curl apparatus.

For your home-based program to be successful, you will obviously need to turn a part of your home into a gym area. There are a few companies that specifically design equipment that will really help you get a great workout. Even some of the popular television infomercial systems can provide an excellent workout.

The simplest solution for many exercises is a few sets of adjustable dumbbells. For example, a bench press using a barbell can be easily modified to a dumbbell bench press. Keeping the dumbbells preset to a few different weights will keep them ready for action on a variety of exercises and minimize adjustments within a workout.

An extremely convenient option is investing in a set of Power Blocks. This multi-weight quick-change dumbbell system happens to be one of the most effective pieces of home exercise equipment available. Power Blocks provide just as many weight choices as a whole commercial gym dumbbell rack, but in one single pair. These little gems have proven to be some of the most versatile equipment that we have ever used to help build our bodies.

A chinup bar adds more options for back (chinups, both wide grip and narrow underhand) and abdominal training (hanging leg raises). Some require that you drill holes into a door frame and others only require placement inside a door frame. These no-drill-required bars use body weight leverage to hold the bar securely in place. You can purchase one of these or a standard chinup bar set at your local sporting goods store or the Web. Most bars will conveniently adjust to fit a doorway—just make sure it's completely secure before using it!

In addition to dumbbells and a chin-up bar, resistance tubing will give you even more options. Tubing is an amazing training tool that you can easily adapt to many standard weight-training movements.

Most tubes were originally designed with rehab in mind. But now there are a few specialty equip-

PLAY HEART ACTIVITY MENU

ALPHA ACTIVE	ALPHA ACTION	ALPHA EXTREME: SUPERVISION REQUIRED
Match	**Match**	**Match**
Cross-Country Skiing	Skiing/Snowboarding	Extreme Skiing
Boogie Boarding/Wake Boarding	Surfing	Big Wave Surfing
Touch Football	Tackle Football	Rugby
Kickboxing Class	Mixed Martial Arts Class/Ultimate Fighting Class	Actual Mixed Martial Arts Cage Match
Handball	Racquetball or Squash	Jai Alai
Street Biking (Street Cycling)	Mountain Biking	Rough Terrain Mountain Biking
Snorkeling	Scuba Diving	Free Diving/Cave Diving
Speed Bag/Heavy Bag Training/Shadowboxing	Boxing Class	White Collar Boxing Match
Canoeing	Ocean Kayaking	White-Water Rafting
Lake Kayaking	White-Water Kayaking	Waterfall Kayaking
Parasailing	Tandem Sky Diving	Solo Sky Diving/Paragliding/Hang Gliding
Frisbee	Ultimate Frisbee	Extreme Mountaineering
Swimming Laps	Swim for Speed/Time/Race	Triathlon
Surf Kite Maneuvers	Wind Surfing	Kite Surfing
Street Hockey	Roller Hockey	Ice Hockey
Boat Tow Rafting	Jet Skiing	Water-skiing
Riding ATVs	Snow Mobile	Extreme Snow Mobile Journey
Trail Hiking/Jogging	Indoor Rock Climbing	Mountain Climbing
Cliff Jumping/Diving	Bungee Jumping	Base Jumping
Horseback Riding with Guide	Solo Horseback Riding	Bareback Horseback Riding or Rodeo
Juggling	Weighted Juggling	Power Juggling
Unmatched	**Unmatched**	**Unmatched**
Hill Walking	Hill Sprints/Bleacher Runs	Mountain Boarding
Rollerblading	5K Marathon	Parkour/Free Running
Speed Walking	Inline Skating	Land Yachting
Beach/Sand Running	Big Game Fishing	Snow Kiting
Snow Rafting	Tournament Paintball	Wingsuit Flying
Dodgeball Extreme	Jumping Stilts	Sphering
Skateboarding	Slam Ball	Solo Free Climbing
Rowing	Go-Carting	Sand Boarding
Ping-Pong		Land Luge
Paintball		Ice Climbing
Golf		Sand Kiting
Soccer		Fire Walking
Softball/Baseball		Dog Sledding
Tennis		Adventure Racing
Baseball/Football Catch		Ballooning
Volleyball		Extreme Roller Coaster
Basketball		

ment groups like Power Systems (www.power-systems.com) that make solid, 3-inch wide, ¼-inch thick, 6-foot long (looped like a rubber band) resistance bands that come in several different "weights" designed specifically for endurance and strength training. It's been reported that the heaviest type of this tubing can provide as much as 250 pounds of additional resistance when fully stretched! These bands are used extensively in college and professional athletic programs; they can give you all the resistance you need. As long as it is tough enough, it makes muscles bigger and stronger. Use bands and tubes just like you would use barbells and dumbbells. Follow the set and rep schemes in these workouts; just use a little ingenuity to create the tubing exercise you need. For pictures and descriptions of tubing exercises, along with some innovative ways to turn a home gym into an amazing training facility, visit us at www.AlphaMaleChallenge.com.

If you get a few different tubes, you can easily create more or less resistance and perform drop sets and other methods of training. Keep in mind that resistance bands or tubes function just like a rubber band. The more you stretch it, the greater the resistance created. To make the same tube or band more difficult to stretch, shorten it by looping it around a pole a few times, or stepping on it to shorten its distance. This alone can make a single tube have a variance of nearly 20 to 30 pounds of resistance, according to most professionals. The only major concern you have is to make sure the tube or band is tightly affixed to whatever it is you are using for an anchor. Some popular home "anchors" are: the leg of a chair (if you are sitting on it), a door handle on the opposite side of a closed door, banisters, your car, and solid structures outside your house.

A heavy-duty multi-bench with an adjustable leg extension/leg curl attachment is a necessity for any worthy home gym. They don't always come together, so make sure you ask a store representative to show you some that include these attachments. As a combined unit, these pieces of equipment are priceless, because they will allow you to do most upper and lower body exercises in the convenience of your home.

There are many variations of the exercises presented in the Alpha Wave Basic Training system. We offer substitutes for all of them, most suitable for home trainers. We only name exercise substitutes for exercise machines that are uncommon in a typical home gym setup, and replace them with the use of dumbbells and tubing exercises. Not all substitute exercises are described or shown, as many are performed almost identically to the gym exercise. We also offer these exercises as alternatives for gym trainers, for times when someone will be using the training equipment you need. Rather than wait you should immediately switch to a substitute. The awesome effectiveness of Alpha Wave Basic Training is due in part to strict adherence to the prescribed rest intervals between sets and exercises. Don't get bogged down waiting! Get to it!

Here's a list of gym exercises and their home substitutes using mostly dumbbells and a bit of tubing. If you don't recognize a particular substitute exercise, visit www.alphamalechallenge.com.

Exercise List	Substitute Exercise List
LEGS	**LEGS**
· Leg Press (Narrow Stance)	· DUMBBELL Squat / Tubing Leg Press
· Leg Press (Wide Stance)	· DUMBBELL Lunge / Tubing Leg Press
· Barbell Squat	· DUMBBELL Squat / Tubing Squat
· Barbell Lunge	· DUMBBELL Lunge
· Cross the River	· DUMBBELL Lunge/Barbell Lunge
· All Barbell Deadlifts	· DUMBBELL Deadlifts
· Smith Machine Hack Squat	· DUMBBELL Squat
· Leg Extension Machine	· Leg Extension Attachment

Exercise List	Substitute Exercise List
· Lying Leg Curl Machine	· Leg Curl Attachment / Tubing Leg Curl
· Standing Calf Raise Machine	· Standing Tubing Calf Raise
· Seated Calf Raise Machine	· Seated Tubing Calf Raise
· Donkey Heel Raise Machine	· Donkey Calf Raise Using Weight Belt w/Chain for Added Resistance
· Leg Press Calf Press	· Standing DUMBBELL Calf Raise
CHEST	**CHEST**
· Chest Dip	· DUMBBELL Bench Press
· Incline Barbell Bench Press	· Incline DUMBBELL Bench Press
· Flat Barbell Bench Press	· Flat DUMBBELL Bench Press / Band Bench
· Pec Deck Fly	· Any DUMBBELL Fly
BACK	**BACK**
· Lat Pulldown	· Pullup / One-Arm DUMBBELL Row
· Narrow-Grip Pulldown (neutral grip)	· Narrow-Grip Pullup
· Seated Cable Row (neutral grip)	· DUMBBELL Bent-Over Row
· Machine Row (neutral grip)	· DUMBBELL Bent-Over Underhand Row
· Machine Row	· DUMBBELL Bent-Over Two-Arm Overhand Row
· One-Arm Machine Row	· DUMBBELL Bent-Over One-Arm Row
· Barbell Bent-Over Row	· DUMBBELL Bent-Over Row
· Lat Pulldown	· Pullup
· Narrow-Grip Pulldown	· Narrow-Grip Pullup
· Lat Pulldown	· Pullup
· Chindownp	· Chinupup
· Power Row	· Power Tubing Row
· T-Bar Row	· DUMBBELL Bent-Over Row
SHOULDERS	**SHOULDERS**
· Barbell Shrug	· DUMBBELL Shrug
· Rear Deltoid Machine	· DUMBBELL Bent-Over Lateral Raise
· Shoulder Machine Press	· Tubing Shoulder Press
· Barbell Shoulder Press	· DUMBBELL Shoulder Press
· Barbell Upright Power Row	· DUMBBELL Upright Row
· Cable Lateral Raise	· DUMBBELL Lateral Raise
· Clean and Power Press	· Dumbbell Clean and Power Press
TRICEPS	**TRICEPS**
· Triceps Pushdown (V-Bar & Rope)	· DUMBBELL Skull Crusher
· Triceps X-tension	· Bench Dip / DUMBBELL Skull Crusher
· Triceps Dip	· Bench Dip
· Barbell Close-Grip Bench Press	· DUMBBELL Close-Grip Bench Press
BICEPS	**BICEPS**
· Barbell Curl	· DUMBBELL Curl
· Preacher Machine	· DUMBBELL Preacher Curl Against Incline Bench
· E-Z Bar Preacher Curl	· DUMBBELL Preacher Curl
· 21 Curls using Barbell	· 21 Curls using DUMBBELLS
ABDOMINALS/CORE	**ABDOMINALS/CORE**
· Captain Chair Leg Lift	· Bench Leg Lift
· Swiss Ball Crunch—Alternate Holding Barbell Plate	· Floor Crunch
· Swiss Ball Throw	· Swiss Ball Crunch
· Partner-Assisted Leg Throws—Alternate Twisting	· Bench Leg Lift
· Full Body Resisted Cable Extension	· Full Body Resisted Tubing Extension
· Samurai Swing	· Tubing Samurai Swing
· Grand Slam	· Tubing Grand Slam

Without a doubt, you can boost your Alpha Factor working out at home if you put in the hard work and discipline. As you continue to improve in strength and power, however, you will likely have to invest in heavier dumbbells and more sophisticated equipment or else join a gym. Some people think of joining a gym the same way they think of buying a car: many choices, aggressive salespeople, and when you leave, you feel like you are no better off than before you got there. Frankly, we think exposing yourself to the sights and sounds of a gym—especially a rugged, hard-core gym like the Powerhouse Gym where we train in Syosset, Long Island—is a way to boost your Alpha Factor on a multitude of levels.

Our hope is that the Alpha Male Challenge program will ultimately empower you to get into the

ALPHA MALE CHALLENGE CLIENT:
MEL BROOKS, AGE 56

MEL, A RAILCAR REPAIR AND BILLING EXECUTIVE, was an athlete earlier in his life. But as 30 years came and went, he wasn't happy with his physical condition and knew his eating habits left much to be desired. "Junk food, chips, pizza, and fast food made for a physical look and extra weight that I was not real pleased with." His son Chris encouraged him to take the Challenge. Mel began the Challenge with a waist measurement of 39½ inches.

Original Alpha Factor: 56.

Mel accepted the Challenge at 200 pounds.

He weighed 171 at Week 10.

Mel lost 29 pounds in only 10 weeks!

He dropped 6 inches of fat from his waist and increased his chest size. He shaved 18 seconds off his time on the 300-yard shuttle run and increased the height of his vertical jump. As a nice little bonus, his physician reported that his triglycerides dropped from 164 to 77.

Mel's overall confidence on the MaleScale™ improved by over 23 percent. His positive outlook on life's changes improved by 60 percent.

Mel increased 20 points on the MaleScale™! He now wants to continue training to build yet a little more muscle mass!

His New Alpha Factor: 76.

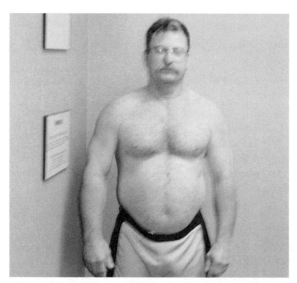

Before

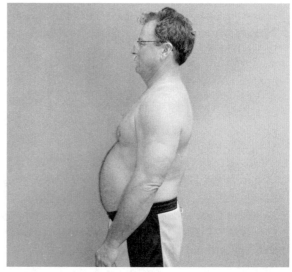

Before

gym no matter what your time constraints or any other reservations you have. This may sound like a long shot for those of you who have never thought about making fitness part of your lifestyle. We understand that it sounds like a big commitment—and you're right: It is a big commitment. But recognize that when you make this program part of your lifestyle, you will improve the overall quality of your life for years to come. Meanwhile, home training can help many guys make an effective transition from the couch to a whole new world of possibilities. It's never too late to take back control over your body and your health. So, now it's time to start your home gym plan of action. Find the best choice of space in your home and plan the setup of your new training bunker.

Testimonial:

"Participating in and completing the Alpha Male Challenge was one of the most rewarding and gratifying things that I have done, not only for myself, but for my family too. Being a middle-aged man, I had basically settled into the daily grind of everyday life at work and at home. I had begun to think of retirement as the next big step towards change in my life. But then along came the Alpha Male Challenge. What a difference it has made! Changes such as weight loss, physical appearance and surprising reductions in certain cholesterols, blood sugar, and body fat levels were all exciting!

"However, the thing I enjoyed most was actually doing the whole Alpha Male Challenge. The 10 weeks of training, were they grueling? Absolutely. The new diet, was it "willpower" testing? Of course. But the overwhelming excitement on that final day with the achievement of goals that you, in the beginning, never thought were within reach—what a confidence and attitude boost! Do something for yourself. Accept the challenge!"

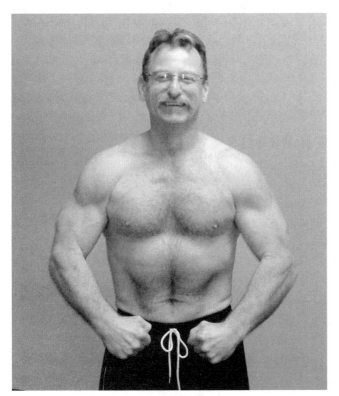

After

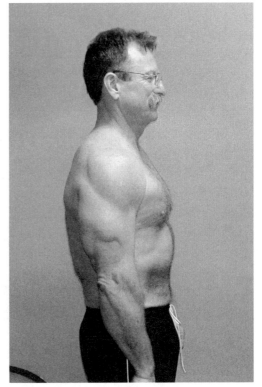

After

CHAPTER FIVE
ALPHA FUEL

THE GREAT AMERICAN DIET DISASTER

It's bad enough that American manliness has dissipated like gun smoke in a Wild West stage show. But men are also getting fatter by the minute—and their health is eroding, to boot. Obesity, which is linked to most chronic diseases, including type 2 diabetes, heart disease, osteoarthritis, high blood pressure, some forms of cancer, and many a lonely night alone, is generally defined as a body mass index (BMI) of 30 or greater. For most people (other than bodybuilders), BMI corresponds to the portion of your weight that is body fat.

Obesity is rising at an unprecedented rate. According to data in the *Chartbook on Trends in the Health of Americans* from the National Center for Health Statistics, the prevalence of obesity

from 1960 to 2004 more than doubled among adults ages 20 to 74, with most of this rise occurring since 1980. For guys only, the picture is even worse: Obesity went from 10.7 percent in 1960 to 33.3 percent in 2005–2006!

Although four states claimed an obesity rate of 15 to 19 percent in 1990, a statewide obesity rate of 20 percent or more was unheard of then. In 1995, still no state had breached the 20 percent obesity mark. Only 5 years later, however, just 28 states maintained obesity rates of less than 20 percent. By 2005, only four states had obesity prevalence rates of less than 20 percent, while 17 states had prevalence rates equal to or greater than 25 percent; the three fattest states (Louisiana, Mississippi, and West Virginia) blasted to an obesity prevalence of 30 percent or more! By 2007, only one state, Colorado, had an obesity prevalence of less than 20 percent! Gentlemen: Unless we spring

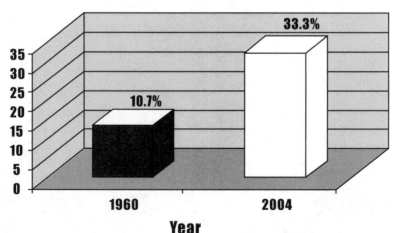

Obesity in American Adults Aged 20-74

Diabetes Prevalence of Americans

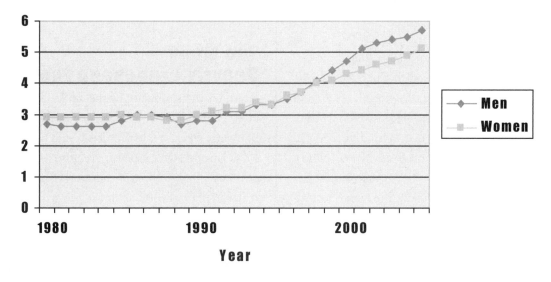

into action now, the outlook for 5 years from now is belt-busting!

The potbellies and muffin tops of our countrymen are expanding at breakneck speeds, that accelerate with each passing year. A study of 9,179 adults published in the *Annals of Internal Medicine* in 2002 found that young adults are getting obese faster. Americans born in 1964 became obese 26 to 28 percent faster than the study subjects born in 1957. Twenty-six percent of men were obese by the time they were 35 to 37 years old. In 2007, researchers at the University of New Hampshire presented their data from a survey of 800 college students at a meeting of the American Physiological Society. The ongoing survey reveals that university students lead generally unhealthy lives, characterized by little physical activity and diets packed with junk food and low in nutrients; nearly half of the male students surveyed were overweight or obese.

Forty million American adults have high cholesterol. According to the CDC, 30 percent of men have high blood pressure. Diabetes rates are rising faster than gas prices. Between 1980 and 1998, the prevalence of confirmed diabetes for men and women was comparable. In 1999, however, men began to outpace women in the race for high sugar levels; from 1980 to 2005, the prevalence of diagnosed diabetes increased 76 percent for women but a whopping 111 percent for men. With all the advancements in pharmacology and technology, coupled with our greater awareness of how to combat illness, how is it that we are a nation of diminishing health?

And guess what else, guys? Obesity has an opposite relationship with your manliness—at least as reflected in your hormones. A host of studies have shown that the fatter you are, the less testosterone you generally have—especially the all-important free testosterone. One study published in the *Journal of Clinical Endocrinology and Metabolism* identified obesity as the *most* important determinant of total testosterone over time; obese men were found to have levels 25 percent lower than non-obese men. Moreover, there is a "revolving door" relationship, or mutual influence, between sex hormones and obesity. In other words, not only does obesity tend to lead to decreased total and free testosterone, but lower testosterone itself can also result in increased abdominal obesity, blood triglycerides, and insulin resistance. What follows is a downward spiral of overall health and wellness, not to mention the way you might look in a Speedo. It's hard to feel confident when you're embarrassed to take off your shirt at the beach.

What a mess. And it's not simply due to the fact that we have become fused to the easy chair—Americans are making *astoundingly* bad food choices. With the dizzying pace of modern life, many men are relying on fast food joints or local greasy spoons for their food fixes. Nearly half of the typical family's food budget goes toward foods prepared and consumed outside the home, according to research published in the *Annual Review of Nutrition*. It's an "eat out" society. Breakfast at the doughnut shop. Lunch at Mickey D's. A massive frozen cappuccino to plug through the midafternoon blood sugar crash. Dinner wolfed down at the pizza joint. This pattern of unrestrained oral indulgence is considered so "normal" that health-conscious men who eat wisely are suspiciously interrogated about their "abnormal" food choices. Meanwhile, the growing population of obese men convince themselves that their "on the go" diets are "not that bad." Yet fully one-third of all vegetables consumed in America come from only three sources: french fries, potato chips, and iceberg lettuce. No wonder guys are getting paunchier with every glance in the mirror.

The supermarket aisles are filled with products touted as "low-fat" or "low-carb" or "all-natural" or "a great-tasting part of a healthy breakfast." The taglines may be literally true, but the product itself could nevertheless be a ridiculously unhealthy addition to the human diet. Despite the multimedia overload of diet and nutrition information, even men who think their nutrition is right on target don't have a clue.

What you're about to read is the result of an analysis of *all* the information—not only interviews with the top experts, but also thorough evaluations of the most up-to-date scientific nutri-

tion literature. It's the science-based, no-holds-barred truth about what's specifically wrong with the modern American male diet.

Too Many Heavily Processed Foods

Consider the simplicity of the apple. Nature created a winner. It requires no processing, has lots of dietary fiber, is nutrient dense, and tastes good. In its natural state, it doesn't require laboratories, chemicals, or people with hairnets. The problem: It doesn't last. Lose one in the hot trunk of your car for a few months, and you won't find it too appealing when it resurfaces.

That's why much of the food industry shoves nature aside. From the outset, pesticides and other toxins are used to maintain fruit orchards, vegetable farms, and even fish farms. Antibiotics and hormones are pumped into livestock. Then the foods are processed to make them last longer. The nutrients are processed right out of them. These "foodlike substances" have the unnatural ability to exist in a humid environment for years without rotting or changing form. Heavy processing extends product shelf life and fattens the corporate books of manufacturers and distributors. Heavy processing is also likely to fatten your waist, diminish your health, and send your Alpha Factor to the basement.

The typical American diet is stacked with eats that are engineered in laboratory-like processing plants. Grab the typical boxed, bagged, or canned product and you'll notice an unpronounceable list of unrecognized ingredients—most of these compounds are chemical flavorings and preservatives. On top of that, piles of sugar, salt, and high-fructose corn syrup are added to most processed foods to make them taste edible again. Dangerous trans fatty acids or "trans fats"—which increase your cholesterol and risk of heart disease—have been substituted for traditional oils in many processed foods. The high-fructose corn syrup and trans fatty acids in highly processed foods deliver a one-two punch to your nutritional health—a "metabolic nightmare" that makes it even easier to shuttle calories toward fat (especially belly fat, or visceral adipose tissue) and away from muscle and lean body mass. The nutrients are processed out; empty calories and chemicals are funneled in. Heavily processed foods contain lots of stuff you might not want or need, but few, if any, ingredients of value. You know the sort—"junk food." And Americans are shoveling it in . . . and paying the price.

Excessive Portion Sizes

According to the CDC, modern Americans are eating more calories on average than our parents and grandparents did. The problem may have started when Americans began "eating out" more than ever before. In the 1970s, U.S. residents spent 34 percent of their food budget on meals away from home; that figure rose to 47 percent by the 1990s. Fast-food joints started offering "supersized" portions to entice customers, and other restaurants followed suit. Today, some fast-food meals may contain over 2,000 calories—all the calories many guys need for a whole day!

Having become accustomed to bigger portions when eating out, Americans have gotten used to eating more food overall. Between 1971 and 2000, the typical guy increased his total weekly food intake by more than 1,175 calories. The Department of Agriculture reports that during the 1990s, total food consumption rose by about 140 pounds per person per year.

You name the food, and today's offered portion size is likely to be more than you ought to be eating. Research published in the *American Journal of Public Health* examined a wide variety of food products and found that the portions were larger—sometimes tremendously larger—than USDA standard portion sizes. Bagels, steaks, muffins, and cooked pasta exceeded USDA standards by 195 percent, 224 percent, 333 percent,

A SUGAR BY ANY OTHER NAME . . .

Added sugars, like a skulking spy, can be disguised on food labels by many names.

All the sugar alcohols: sorbitol, malitol, xylitol, and so on	Honey
Beet sugar	Invert sugar
Brown rice syrup	Lactose
Brown sugar	Maltose
Corn sweetener	Malt syrup
Corn syrup	Molasses
Dextrose	Pure cane sugar
Fructose	Raw sugar
Fruit juice concentrates	Sucrose
Glucose	Sugar
High-fructose corn syrup	Syrup
	Turbinado

and 480 percent, respectively. Some cookie products were 700 percent larger than USDA standards! But research shows that most people will often eat whatever portion is put in front of them, even after they're already full. (See page 36 to refresh your memory on the importance of willpower.)

Too Much of the Wrong Fats

It's time to debunk the simplistic myth that "fats make you fat," once and for all. The problem isn't the fact that there's fat in your diet. Listen carefully: Fats are a crucial and essential part of your diet, and don't listen to anyone who tells you differently! Our problems with fat have only become worse, despite a reduced overall proportion of fat in the American diet. The problem is eating the *wrong* fats, and too much of them. Not all fats are equal!

Beware: When you see a "partially hydrogenated" oil on an ingredient label, you know that you're dealing with a trans fat! Trans fatty acids, also called trans fats, are unsaturated vegetable oils subjected to the industrial process of partial hydrogenation, in which the chemical structure of the fat is changed so the oil becomes more solid. Hydrogenated vegetable oils are generally found in highly processed, packaged foods, because solid fats are more stable for deep-frying and creating baked goods with long shelf lives. You'll find them in ready-made baked and fried foods, salad dressings, crackers, mayonnaise, and many other items. Although some manufacturers have eliminated or reduced the amount of trans fats in products on store shelves, fast-food joints can be bursting with them. Unfortunately, synthetic trans fats promote a host of health problems, including heart disease, gallstones, and obesity.

Saturated fat is found mostly in products of animal origin, but also high in saturated fat are coconut oil, palm oil, and palm kernel oil, which are also regular players in heavily processed edibles. And for you coffee drinkers, be aware that nondairy creamers may also contain high amounts of saturated fats. Diets too high in saturated fat (particularly lauric and myristic acid) are correlated with an increased incidence of atherosclerosis and coronary heart disease based on numerous studies. However, unlike trans fats, a healthy amount of saturated fat is necessary for optimal health. In fact, without enough saturated fat, your testosterone production is hampered—not a helpful push toward a higher Alpha Factor!

Not Enough of the Right Essential Fatty Acids

Essential fatty acids, or EFAs, are necessary fats that the human body can't make. We can only get EFAs through our diet. There are two families of EFAs: omega-3 and omega-6. Men need to take in both kinds from food to support the cardiovascular, endocrine/reproductive, immune, musculoskeletal, and nervous systems. When these organ systems are functioning at peak levels, recovery and adaptation from exercise are optimized. But we need these two kinds of fatty acids to be properly balanced. The typical American male diet is way off the mark. We consume mostly omega-6

SAT FAT!

You need some saturated fat to stay healthy and manly, but Americans eat too much. Is beef the worst offender in this excess? Nope, cheese is (13.1 percent of saturated fat consumed). Fatty beef is in second place (11.7 percent), followed by milk (7.8 percent). So limit your dairy intake to mostly low-fat and fat-free milk, yogurt, and cottage cheese.

fatty acids and not enough omega-3 fatty acids. Some scientists suggest that the ideal intake ratio of omega-6 to omega-3 fatty acids is somewhere between 1:1 and 4:1. The omega-6 to omega-3 ratio in modern Western diets averages about 12:1, and some say it's more like 14:1 or even 20:1. Dr. Artemis Simopoulos of the Center for Genetics, Nutrition, and Health, in Washington, DC, is a leading proponent of *reducing* your intake of omega-6s. She points out that it wasn't until the past 150 years—and mostly just in the past 50— that our species ate a diet so high in omega-6 fatty acids. Research by Dr. Simopoulos and others shows that high dietary omega-6 to omega-3 ratios are associated with increased risks for cardiovascular disease and some types of cancer, and they tend to exacerbate many inflammatory disease responses. It seems we'd all do a whole lot better with more omega-3s in our diet, and might generally do better with fewer omega-6s.

A Lopsided Food Pyramid

The modern American diet relies heavily on grains, such as cereal, bread, and pasta. For most people, starchy carbohydrates form the bulk of their daily food intake. In fact, most of us grew up with the old Food Pyramid of the U.S. Department of Agriculture (USDA), which emphasized bread, cereal, rice, and pasta by their placement at the base of the pyramid. The traditional food pyramid you've been taught says:

1) Meat, Poultry, Fish, Dry Beans, Eggs, and Nuts Group—2 or 3 servings

2) Milk, Yogurt, and Cheese Group—2 or 3 servings

3) Fruit Group—2 to 4 servings

4) Vegetable Group—3 to 5 servings

5) Bread, Cereal, Rice, and Pasta Group—6 to 11 servings

That's right: The USDA advised us to eat 6 to 11 servings of these grains per day—more servings than of any other single group, and even more than the total vegetable and fruit group servings combined! The USDA's new pyramid scheme (www.mypyramid.gov) recommends that a 35-year-old guy, 6 feet tall and 200 pounds, who is physically active 30 to 60 minutes a day, should eat a whopping 10 slices of bread a day, or the equivalent in grains—and up to half of them can be refined grains like plain white bread! Should we rely so heavily on a foodstuff that, as we will see, is a relatively new addition to the human diet, and one that sends our blood glucose and insulin levels soaring? Not only do humans eat a disproportionate amount of grains, but so do most of our cattle. Ranchers feed cattle lots of grains to fatten them up faster. So, most of the beef we buy is heavier in omega-6s and lighter in omega-3s than it would be if the cattle were allowed to graze on their natural diet: grass.

Scientists have begun to link the high proportion of refined grains we eat to health problems. *Diabetes Care* published a study of almost 43,000 men, between the ages of 40 and 75, that showed that a high intake of refined grains significantly increases the risk of type 2 diabetes.

Sky-High Glycemic Carbs

As is the case with fats, it is too simplistic to claim that all carbohydrates are bad for us. Eating a diet containing too much of the *wrong* carbohydrates sets a guy up for a lifetime of disease and a basement MaleScale score. To distinguish the good carbs from the ugly, an "index" was created as a method of ranking carbohydrates based on their effect on the blood sugar (glucose) levels of our bodies. Carbs that break down quickly in the digestive process release glucose quickly into the bloodstream, which results in the highest scores on this "glycemic index," or

GI. Research published in *Diabetes Care* concluded that "5 weeks of [a low glycemic index] diet ameliorates some plasma lipid parameters, decreases total fat mass, and tends to increase lean body mass without changing body weight. . . . Such a diet could be of benefit to healthy, slightly overweight subjects and might play a role in the prevention of metabolic diseases and their cardiovascular complications."

Added Sugars and High-Fructose Corn Syrup

The wonders of modern technology have enabled us to create foodstuffs that didn't even exist in the food chain until the 1970s! High-fructose corn syrup (HFCS) was invented through an enzymatic process by which the fructose content of corn syrup was increased. The resulting product was a sweeter syrup with a longer shelf life and a cheaper cost. Stiff tariffs on foreign sugar importation have made HFCS most attractive to American food and beverage manufacturers. By the mid-1980s, HFCS was replacing sugar in many edible goodies. HFCS lurks in the ingredients list of just about any processed product with a sweet taste. It's the sweetener of choice in American soft drinks today, and it's in many sweetened juices, candy, ice cream, frozen yogurts, and popsicles, too. You'll also find it in sauces and condiments (including ketchup and barbecue sauce). One study found that the average American eats nearly *70 pounds* of HFCS per year.

Look, 70 pounds a year of *any* sugar is hardly a recipe for sustained energy or abdominal glory. But Americans consume nearly 70 pounds of table sugar in addition to HFCS, for a belt-busting annual total of nearly *140 pounds* of refined sugars!

Susan M. Kleiner, PhD, RD, CNS, FACN, author of *Power Eating* and *The Good Mood Diet*, describes HFCS as "the Devil's candy." "It has been understood for several years that fructose is metabolized differently in the body than glucose," explains Dr. Kleiner. "While the body prefers to metabolize glucose into energy or store it as glycogen to fuel muscle cells, fructose is metabolically processed in the liver and preferentially turned into fat, rather than used as energy. Human studies have shown that fructose ingestion increases rates of fat production, but ingesting the same number of calories as glucose does not cause the same response."

A review of the scientific literature on fructose, weight gain, and the insulin resistance syndrome, popularly called Syndrome X, was conducted by researchers from the University of California, the U.S. Department of Agriculture, the Monell Chemical Sense Institute, and the University of Pennsylvania. They suggest that the finger of blame for the epidemic of obesity and abnormalities seen as part of Syndrome X should be pointed primarily at HFCS. "When you mess with the food supply to the degree that has been done with high-fructose corn syrup," warns Dr. Kleiner, "you're making a deal with the devil, and someone's going to pay. The food manufacturers have made the deal, and we've been paying with our health and our lives."

FRUCTOSE EQUALS FAT

"Not only does the fructose that you eat turn into fat, but it shuts down the body's mechanisms that keep it from turning into a fat-making machine. According to numerous animal studies and several human studies, fructose does not stimulate the production of two key hormones, insulin and leptin, which are involved in the long-term regulation of energy balance."

—Susan Kleiner, PhD, RD, CNS, FACN

Too Little Protein

The current recommended daily allowance (RDA) of dietary protein, which in healthy adults is 0.36 gram per pound of body weight per day (80 grams of protein for a 220-pound man). According to the CDC, the typical American gets about 15 percent of daily calories from protein. In a 2,000-calorie diet, that's only about 75 grams of protein a day. Some experts say it's quite enough and that any more than that will ruin your kidneys and cause your body to lose calcium. Others argue that while such low intakes may be enough to keep a couch potato from losing what little muscle mass he may have, it's hardly optimal for masculine excellence. Let's see what the science says.

In 2007, José Antonio, PhD, and a team of researchers on behalf of the International Society of Sports Nutrition (ISSN) conducted a comprehensive review of the scientific literature on protein and exercise. They looked at scores of studies to determine whether people who work out need more protein than the average couch potato. Consistent with the research conducted by Canadian protein research pioneer Dr. Peter Lemon, the team concluded in their published Position Paper that the protein needs of physically active individuals are increased by as much as a 100 percent over those of sedentary individuals. They found that there is a genuine risk in consuming insufficient amounts of protein, especially in the context of exercise; a negative nitrogen balance will likely be created, leading to increased catabolism and impaired recovery from exercise.

The team deduced seven important points regarding protein intake:

1) A "vast" body of research shows that if you're working out regularly, you need *more* dietary protein than the typical couch potato.

2) Consuming 1.4 to 2.0 grams of protein per kilogram of body weight (0.64 to 0.91 grams per pound) each day is not only *safe* for physically active individuals, but may also *improve* your adaptive response to exercise. That's 140 to 200 grams daily for the 220-pound guy.

3) For healthy, active people, the protein intakes stated above are *not* harmful to the kidneys or bone metabolism as part of a balanced, nutrient-dense diet.

4) Although it's *possible* to get enough protein through food, taking supplemental protein is a practical way to ensure adequate and quality protein intake for intense resistance trainers.

5) Although different types and quality of protein can affect amino acid bioavailability, the superiority of one protein supplement type over another hasn't yet been convincingly demonstrated.

6) Timing your protein intake is an important component of an overall exercise training program and is essential for proper recovery, immune function, and the growth and maintenance of lean body mass.

7) Specific amino acid supplements, such as branched-chain amino acids (BCAAs), may improve exercise performance and recovery under some circumstances.

Unless you have preexisting kidney disease, a moderately high-protein diet will not damage your kidneys. In fact, researchers in Belgium put the safe ceiling for protein even higher, at 2.8 grams per kilogram (1.27 grams per pound) daily. That's 280 grams daily for our 220-pound guy.

So where does that leave any guy seeking to boost his rank on the MaleScale? You can forget the typical American protein intake.

Too Much Salt

Your body needs salt to function. The sodium in salt is the main component of the body's extracellular fluids and helps carry nutrients into the cells and regulate other body functions, including blood pressure. But the amount you need is fairly minor. Primitive man was adapted to a low salt intake. When our ancestors switched over from hunting and gathering to cultivating crops and raising animals, their survival depended on stockpiling foods over the winter. One way to preserve food for an extended period is to salt it.

Today, excessive amounts of salt are added to processed foods. Americans today consume 9 to 12 grams of salt daily. Salting most foods at the table is overkill: 75 percent of the American sodium intake is already in processed foods when we bring them home from the supermarket.

According to the National Research Council of the National Academy of Sciences, the recommended safe minimum daily amount is about 500 milligrams of sodium and the upper limit is 2,400 milligrams. However, the council suggests that reducing daily sodium intake to 1,800 milligrams would probably be healthier. Many guys can reduce their chances of developing high blood pressure by consuming less salt.

A study conducted by researchers at the University of California, San Francisco, used a computer simulation model to determine the impact that reducing salt intake could have on reducing heart disease. The researchers found that removing only 1 gram of salt from the diet could result in 250,000 fewer new cases of heart disease and more than 200,000 fewer deaths over a decade.

Insufficient Fiber

Fiber is the indigestible part of plant foods. Current recommendations from the Institute of Medicine of the National Academies suggest that the average male should consume 30 to 38 grams of dietary fiber each day. The odds are that you're not getting it. The average American takes in only 12 to 18 grams of dietary fiber daily. The effects of eating too little fiber may be worse than mere constipation, hemorrhoids, and colon polyps. A Harvard study of more than 40,000 male health professionals found that a low total dietary fiber intake was linked to a 40 percent higher risk of coronary heart disease compared to a high total dietary fiber intake.

REAL SOLUTIONS

What's the best nutrition plan for any man seeking to improve his health, sculpt his body, boost his testosterone, and raise his rank on the MaleScale?

The solution to the Great American Diet Disaster isn't a "diet." The solution is simply a better way of eating—one that doesn't feel like a "diet" but rather like a lifestyle. The Alpha Fuel Solution isn't a diet. It's a healthful and natural pattern of eating based on our simple Fuel Rules. It's convenient, practical, and delicious. It's the way men were meant to eat.

Prehistory 101

The rise and spread of civilization has brought us lots of sweet stuff, such as comfortable couches, cable TV, cornflakes, and cupcakes (this is not *our* idea of the four Cs). Chasing down and spearing your dinner on a grassy plain was a lot tougher than pulling open the refrigerator door. As the intense physical demands on our species disappeared, so ultimately did the abdominals of the average Joe Six-Pack.

How did the dietary habits of early humans compare to our diet today? Anthropological nutritionists believe ancient eating styles tell us plenty about living a healthy and intuitive lifestyle. There were no fast-food joints back then, no pastry aisles, and no microwaves. For most of the millennia of human existence, we survived without the assistance of fire. Prehistoric humans wandered in tribal groups after herds of game mammals—nomadic hunters in pursuit of prey. Walter L. Voegtlin, MD, FACP, author of *The Stone Age Diet* in 1975, was one of the first to conclude that our primitive diet was mostly protein and fats from wild game.

Loren Cordain, PhD, a professor at Colorado State University and an expert in Paleolithic nutrition, avers that while it's difficult to be certain from fossil records exactly what proportion of animal to plant foods comprised the prehistoric diet, meat was likely a major human food source from when the Paleolithic Age began more than 2.5 million years ago until it ended around 10,000 years ago. In books such as *The Paleo Diet: Lose Weight* and *Get Healthy by Eating the Food You Were Designed to Eat,* Dr. Cordain concludes that vegetarianism is a far cry from our ancient culinary heritage.

Of course, this probably doesn't sit well with our plant-munching amigos. We like vegetarians. Their concerns about cruelty and barbarism concerning the upkeep and slaughter of livestock are respectable. If the choice to avoid meat is based on religious, moral, or ethical reasons, we won't argue the point. On the other hand, if vegetarians believe that they're eating in a more "natural" manner, they miss the mark. Their bodies, like yours and ours, are the result of more than 2.5 million years of adaptation. Human digestive systems can't break down the tough cellulose material or "dietary fiber" found in plants. In contrast to grazing herbivores, like cattle and sheep, we don't regurgitate and chew our cud. We have canine teeth, ridged molars, and incisors in both jaws, which move vertically up and down to crush and tear. Like it or not, we are carnivorous.

Of course, early man didn't live by meat alone. He supplemented his diet with fish, nuts, fruits, wild berries, and vegetables, especially when meat was in short supply.

In light of our evolutionary history, how have so many Americans come to rely on corn chips and cupcakes for subsistence? According to scientists, the problem started between 10,000 and 20,000 years ago. They speculate that prehistoric man sought alternative nutrition after the worldwide extinction of large mammals. Simultaneously, the human population grew, and meat was too scarce to feed everyone. Nomadic people the world over were forced to develop a novel and reliable method to feed everyone and replace meat as a primary food source. About 10,000 years ago, our ancestors started to domesticate wild grasses. Agriculture was born.

GRAINS AND GEARS

The agricultural revolution radically changed the human lifestyle. Instead of pursuing wild game, our ancestors settled and began to plant, raise, and store cereal grains and keep dairy livestock. Agriculture made civilization possible. Without it, we'd still be on the grasslands, if our species had survived at all. Globally, the majority of food is provided through contemporary agriculture—cereal grains are our species' primary source of energy worldwide. Without cereal grains, mass starvation would plague the earth.

But before we give agriculture a standing ovation, let's think this through. Our species ate a lot of meat and fish for more than 2.5 million years, and human physiology adapted to that diet. According to anthropological nutritionists like Dr. Cordain, our genetic makeup, or genome, hasn't changed much in 40,000 years. Our genes today are pretty much the same as those of our ancestors. Yet we consume a vastly different diet. Grains and dairy were not part of the human diet until about a mere blink of an eye in the grand adaptive scheme of things. The dietary shift from meat to crops radically altered the composition of our nutrition. Instead of relying on protein and fat for the majority of energy needs, our ancestors' new agriculturally driven diet provided carbohydrates in force. Although our species is resilient enough to adapt to new proportions of protein, fat, and carbohydrate, adaptation takes time. Our bodies aren't well adapted to the low-fat, high-carbohydrate, grain-centered diet recommended by most modern-day nutritionists.

The agricultural revolution had a profound effect on human nutrition. But a more recent revolution struck a fresh blow to human health: industrialization. Technology and industrialization obliterated physical activity and also radically changed our diet. Over the past 200 years, we've invented complex machinery and erected mass-production facilities to refine sugar and flour, which we add to a limitless array of canned, boxed, and bagged edibles. We've also invented novel, lab-created food materials, including trans fatty acids and high-fructose corn syrup. And our bodies are rebelling.

A nutritional foundation based on the way our ancestors ate is the way to get lean, strong, and healthy. More protein means more muscle. More healthy fats mean more testosterone and manliness. More fruits and vegetables means a reduced risk of cancer. Fewer processed foods, including HFCS, trans fats, and refined grains, means less of the symptoms of the Great American Diet Disaster. It's perfectly simple. There's no counting calories or complicated food plans. The nutrition plan to follow isn't a dieting gimmick or get-slim-quick scheme conjured up to profit from the diet craze. Look at it this way . . . if it's a fad diet, it's based on a 2.5-million-year-old fad.

SO EASY A CAVEMAN COULD DO IT

If you're concerned that the Alpha Fuel Solution will have you stark naked eating raw bone marrow in a grassy savannah, don't worry. Unless the woolly mammoth is magically resurrected, it would be impractical, if not impossible, to follow the exact diet of our nomadic ancestors. Nor would you necessarily want to. Some contemporary nutrition choices that were't available on the ancestral menu (e.g., whey protein, nonfat Greek yogurt, and olive oil) can be beneficial additions to your diet. Our solution to the Great American Diet Disaster goes beyond Paleolithic principles and adheres to the philosophy underlying the entire Alpha Male Challenge: that each of us is capable of adapting.

The Alpha Fuel Solution isn't about falling back into the past—it's about bravely moving into the future. To the relief of every woman in America, guys can't go back and act like cavemen . . . and we can't eat like them. However, we can learn from their habits, and apply it all to contemporary life.

Our approach will change the way you eat.

THE RULE OF THIRDS

"Although the proportion of macronutrients when following the Alpha Fuel Solution dietary guidelines falls roughly in the range of 33/33/33, the metabolic advantage and real power behind the plan lies in the seamless fabric created by functional, nutrient-dense food choices, controlled portions, and micro- and macronutrient intake—all enhanced with nutrient timing and performance nutrition. There is already a substantial body of scientific evidence indicating the health benefits of the model on which Alpha Fuel principles are founded, and it will continue to emerge for decades to come. For people without specific medical problems, the Alpha Fuel Solution is a phenomenal nutritional prescription for optimizing health, longevity, body composition, and human performance in day-to-day life for men around the world."

—Hector Lopez, MD, MS, CSCS

We've designed the Alpha Fuel Solution not as a "diet" but simply as an improved method of choosing what to eat, and how much of it to eat. It combines the best of our ancient eating patterns with the latest nutritional science to help you reach your true Alpha Male potential. Combined with the other components of the Challenge, it will help you naturally raise testosterone levels, build muscle, and burn fat.

Let's talk about the specific "how" of eating, and, just as important, the "how much." Your body requires the right nutrients in the correct quantities to operate at peak performance. Our model is founded on the nutrition your body was designed to eat, updated for top performance in the world of today and tomorrow. Basically, we're talking about roughly one-third of your daily calories, averaged out over a few days, from each of the three macronutrients: protein, fat, and carbohydrates. It's as easy as that. You'll notice that the protein is a bit higher than in the "average" popular diet, but it's perfect for an active guy who exercises. A 1:1 ratio of protein and carbs is a terrific way to improve your body composition over a higher carb diet with the same number of calories. Note, too, that the proportion of healthy fats is a tiny bit higher than in other popular diets, but it's exactly right to support optimal testosterone levels.

BEYOND CALORIES

Maintaining body weight means taking in neither more nor less energy than you burn throughout the day. If you want to build manly muscle, you need to take in more calories than you burn. If you want to shed excess pounds of fat, you need to burn more calories than you take in. Even if your goal is to shed body fat or maintain your current body weight, you should strive to maintain or build lean muscle. Muscle constantly burns calories and looks good, so never work to

lose muscle weight. Though it may seem like progress to see the number on the scale go down, rapid weight loss will result in the loss of a lot of manly muscle. As a result, your total energy needs go down too, and it's much easier to regain weight. Weight regain after quick loss is mostly fat. In the end, you're just fatter at your original weight.

Many diet plans used to tout calorie counting as the be-all and end-all of winning the battle of the bulge. Not true; instead of obsessing over calories, the Alpha Fuel Solution targets taking in the right types and appropriate portions of macronutrients to build a stronger body. All calories are not created equal. Calories from carbohydrates are handled differently by the body than protein calories; protein calories are treated differently than fat calories, and so on. Your daily meals and overall dietary intake should be the right number of calories, but also an optimal combination of protein, fats, and carbs.

What quantity of food you should be eating depends on your current size, condition, and goals. Are you trying to build some muscle bulk? Or are you trying to drop the excess baggage you've accumulated? The long look in the mirror you took at the start of this book should provide your answer, but if you're still not sure, check out your MaleScale baselines. Depending on your chest-to-waist differential, you may need to focus primarily on gaining muscle or on losing body fat. If your chest-to-waist differential is fewer than 6 inches, or if your waist is more than 38 inches, there's no doubt you should be targeting fat loss.

Our prehistoric ancestors didn't methodically weigh ounces of bison. They didn't measure grams of almonds. They didn't count calories. Yet they were by far leaner and more conditioned than modern man. So don't "count" yourself out by calorie counting! Leave the weigh-ins for just before a fight. The Alpha Fuel Solution is composed of basic principles to automatically keep your energy intake in the range of 1,900 to 2,500 calories, which will work for most guys. And it will do it without you weighing anything and without you ever needing to think about it.

FUEL TOOL: MAN-HAND YOUR MEALS!

We offer a simple, effective, and manly means of assessing how much food you need. You may have heard the advice to eat small meals throughout the day. But that's hardly specific enough for most guys. What exactly does that mean? To keep things as simple as possible, the Alpha Fuel Solution offers you a convenient tool called the Man-Hand method of measuring food intake. It's an easy technique that's been used by nutritionists to teach appropriate portions for years. It's perfectly primitive, and it works. Our ultimate goal is to make you good at simply eyeballing the right portions, without stocking your dishwasher full of cup measures. In the beginning, you'll use your hand as a measurement tool because the size of your hand is often related to your body size. Basing the portion size of solid food on the size of a man's hand—your own hand—will help you meet your specific nutrient needs while satisfying your hunger.

NO COUNTING CALORIES, FAT GRAMS, CARBOHYDRATE GRAMS, OR PROTEIN GRAMS

Here's how it works. Let's say you're getting ready to eat a meal. Start by choosing a **protein** that is about the size and thickness of the palm of your hand, or just a little bigger. That's roughly 5 or 6 ounces of protein. Now let's determine what portion size of **carbohydrates** you'll need. Loosely clinch both of your fists and hold them side by side; a portion of a low-glycemic carbohydrate (such as broccoli or cauliflower) equal to the combined size of your fists belongs on your plate. That's about 1 to 1¼ cups of carbohydrates. Salad greens take up a lot more space than other low-glycemic carbohydrates, so filling a medium-size or large bowl with lettuce or spinach will give you an appropriate portion size. If you choose to add a higher glycemic carbohydrate to your meal, have only one, and make it the size of just one closed fist.

Next, we'll move on to a good portion size for healthy **fats.** We've developed a simple method to eyeball fat portions with good accuracy. For solid types of good fats, and for liquid fats like olive oil or macadamia nut oil, use the tip of your index finger and tip of your thumb to form an "okay" sign. The size of the circle formed (the O) is the guide for fat portion size. For liquid fats, that's about a tablespoon. Now, for foods like nuts and seeds, which may be a combination of both fat and

---

WHAT ABOUT ALCOHOL?

Alcohol in the diet can contribute energy in the amount of 7 calories per gram.

Though excessive and inappropriate types of alcohol promote the dreaded "beer belly" look, some forms of alcohol, in moderation, provide antioxidant compounds and support a healthy body.

From a historical perspective, even primitive man had access to fermented fruit, or, in other words, wine. An occasional glass of wine is perfectly fine. On the other hand, alcohol that provides excess calories and little nutritional value, such as high-sugar mixed drinks and high-carbohydrate beers, should be avoided.

protein, a small to medium-size handful is an adequate portion size. Although the Alpha Fuel Solution incorporates healthy amounts of the right fats, fat portion distortion happens easily. If you think the portion size is too much, it usually is. And it goes without saying that while you can devour every bit of food on your plate, *going back for seconds is not permitted*. If you Man-Hand your meals, second helpings are overeating and an almost certain way to lose control and ruin any diet plan.

It's not necessary to be obsessed with your foods' nutritional values once you become adept at eyeballing a good meal based on Man-Hand portions. Eventually, you will be able to automatically combine healthy foods in the right ratios and make smart decisions with minimal effort—pretty much like your unconscious handles a lot of your moment-to-moment living by running in the background like an autopilot program.

MACRONUTRIENTS 101

Primitive man's diet consisted of the same three basic macronutrients as ours: protein, carbohydrates, and fat. Add up the macronutrients, add water, and you've pretty much got the basic stuff we all eat, and have eaten, for 2.5 million years.

We get all the energy we need from the macronutrients. Calories (or more scientifically, "kilocalories") are the units of energy contained in all foods. When you eat protein, carbohydrates, and fats (or when you drink alcohol), you take in calories, which you can store as energy for later use. Throughout the day, your body burns calories for energy. The simple equation we've all heard is: calories in, calories out.

There are calorie differences between the macronutrients. Protein and carbohydrates have the same calorie energy per gram. Fat has more than double the energy of the other macronutrients.

MACRONUTRIENT	CALORIES PER GRAM
Protein	4
Carbohydrates	4
Fat	9

The higher number of calories per gram of fat was a factor that led to the "low-fat" and "fat-free" revolution in dieting that is partially responsible for the Great American Diet Disaster. But there's more to packing on muscle and stripping away body fat than just calories. Let's take a closer look at each of the macronutrients. Be aware that in the real world, many foods don't fit neatly into one of the three macronutrient categories. For example, meat, fish, and nuts all provide combinations of protein and fats, and fat-free dairy and legumes have protein and carbs. Nevertheless, an overview of each macronutrient category is essential for the practical knowledge you'll need to send your Alpha Factor soaring.

Protein

Proteins are compounds made up of amino acids, and we humans, in turn, are creatures made up of proteins. Your muscles are made up mostly of protein and water; the matrix of amino acids in the human body is unique to our species. Proteins play a huge role in the development of our bodies. They help build our muscles, bones, blood, skin, and hair. They help us resist diseases. Lean red meats, poultry, fish, egg whites, and a small amount of nonfat dairy are good sources of muscle-building protein.

Your body can convert the protein you eat into carbohydrates and fats. But your body only has the ability to make 11 out of the 20 standard amino acids, leaving 9 "essential amino acids" that your body can't make. "Complete" protein foods contain *all* of the essential amino acids. In general, animal proteins (meat, eggs, poultry, fish, and nonfat or low-fat dairy) are considered good complete protein sources. Protein sources that lack any of the nine essential amino acids—many vegetable sources—are "incomplete." For your body to use incomplete proteins, they must be combined with foods that have the missing essential amino acids to collectively be a complete protein.

How does the protein in your diet boost your score on the MaleScale? Without a minimal amount of protein, you would become malnourished and die. Without *enough* protein, your body can't conduct its business of repairing damage and packing on bigger, stronger muscles. According to Jeff Stout, PhD, FACSM, FISSN, FNSCA, CSCS*D, a nationally recognized nutrition expert, author of six sports nutrition textbooks, and director of the Human Metabolic and Body Composition Laboratory, increasing the ratio of protein to carbohydrates in your diet will work together with your resistance training to pack on more muscle. It'll also improve thyroid hormone levels and insulin response. He concludes from his research at the University of Oklahoma and his review of the literature that adjusting the daily ratio of grams of protein to carbohydrates closer to 1:1 may be the optimal mix for accelerating muscle growth without a gain in fat.

The importance of damage repair takes on particular significance within the Alpha Male Challenge. Resistance training breaks down muscle tissue, provoking the body to send biochemical reinforcements to shore it back up. With proper nutrition, your body will rebuild your muscles even thicker and stronger. It's the nutritional version of Selye's general adaptation syndrome and validation of Nietzsche's famous quotation, both mentioned in our Alpha Attitude chapter. Protein not only makes you larger, but it also makes you leaner. How? Even the process of digesting food takes energy—in other words, burns calories. That's called the "thermic effect of food." Roughly 10 percent of the calories you burn in a day are used up digesting and using food. Protein uses up more energy than the other macronutrients due to extra steps needed to break it down, so eating protein burns more calories than eating carbohydrates, and burns a lot more than eating fats. That's how eating protein boosts metabolism (by 20 percent compared to carbs). Hector Lopez, MD, MS, CSCS, founding partner and medical director of Performance Spine and Sports Medicine, LLC, and Northeast Spine and Sports Medicine, PC, in New Jersey, which integrate medicine, chiropractic, physical therapy, and nutrition, reports: "Interestingly, there is recent evidence showing that increased protein consumption after a period of aggressive weight loss may help prevent or limit weight regain. More importantly, these studies indicate that weight regained in most cases is in the form of fat-free mass—i.e., mostly lean muscle! How's that for a true 'Alpha Advantage'?"

Proteins are complex molecules that require plenty of effort to digest. When you eat protein and carbohydrates together in the same meal, the digestion of the carbs is slowed down because the body is busy working on the protein. Think of it as a time-release effect on the carbs. According to research published in the *American Journal of Clinical Nutrition*, protein brings down the glycemic index of the carbs. Mixing protein with carbs means less of an insulin spike and less fat storage—good news for your abs. Also, according to Dr. Lopez, "Protein is more satiating than carbohydrate or fat in both the short-term and long-term, which is also great news for your weight and waistline."

Carbohydrates

Carbohydrates are the primary source of energy for the brain and body. You'll find them in fruits, vegetables, bread, pasta, and dairy products. You'll also find them in candy and cookies and crackers and cupcakes and corn chips . . . and simple table sugar. A hefty load of processed carbs is the staple of the typical couch potato's diet and a reason for his ever-expanding waistline. Understand that it's not that all carbohydrates are bad for you; they're not.

MISSION MINE SWEEPER

The diet industry doesn't make it easy to make good decisions about proper eating. The hard truth: Most of these "fat-free" foods are just as bad if not worse than their "fat-full" counterparts. They are often filled with sugar or high-fructose corn syrup, along with endless ingredients seemingly named in a foreign language.

Our solution is an exercise that will do away with these imposter health foods and assorted other dietary detriments. We call it "Mission Mine Sweeper," and you'll perform it during your very first week of the Challenge.

It's time to sweep out the land mines that can blow up your plans and derail your goals. Here's how:

◎ Sift through your kitchen pantry, cupboards, cabinets, and refrigerator, and scour your tabletop and countertops for any "enemy" foodstuffs—the highly refined and processed, heavily sweetened stuff that'll sabotage your strength, health, and appearance.

◎ Seek out foods that come in sealed, shelf-stable bags and boxes and have long lists of ingredients. Beware of lots of sugar, high-fructose corn syrup, salt (sodium), or partially hydrogenated oils. Also, if you can't pronounce half of the ingredients, that's a hint that it might not be a good choice. Remember, there's no list of ingredients on an apple. Get the point? Here's a more specific but nonexhaustive list of examples of what to get rid of:

◎ White bread (and all non–whole grain breads)

◎ White rice

◎ Pasta (other than whole wheat)

◎ Cookies, pastries, cakes, pies, bagels, muffins, Pop-Tarts

◎ Ice cream, frozen yogurt

◎ Sweetened cereals, including supposedly "healthy" ones (look for sugar on the label)

◎ All regular (non-diet) soda and high-carb juices and juice cocktails

◎ Candy (other than a little dark chocolate)

◎ Potato chips, crackers, corn chips, and other salty snacks

◎ Foods labeled "fat-free" (other than dairy), "diet foods," or "light" foods

◎ Frozen "crap," such as frozen pizzas, frozen premade meals, frozen breaded chicken/fish sticks, frozen hot/"lean" pockets, and frozen burritos

◎ If you share your home with others, discuss your mission with them in advance. Get their participation! The truth is, this stuff is no healthier for them than it is for you. If you can identify and exterminate the enemy foods, you can enhance not only your own health, but the health of your loved ones, as well.

◎ If you keep any food at work, be sure to do the same purge there.

Carbs are so easily metabolized that they are often called the body's "preferred fuel source." In other words, your body loves to use them—and store them—for its energy needs. Carbs were formerly classified as "simple" or "complex" based on their chemical structure, but the distinction mostly confused people. (The USDA abandoned the distinction in its 2005 *Dietary Guidelines for Americans*.) For practical purposes, the chemical structure of a food matters a lot less than what your body does with it. All carbs are ultimately absorbed as sugar.

So a new way to think about carbs emerged: glycemic index (GI) and glycemic load (GL). Remember, the GI is a scale that ranks carb-containing foods based on the speed at which foods are broken down, absorbed, and turned into blood sugar. A food's value on the GI scale is based on a comparison to a reference standard (from glucose or white bread). When a food with a high GI is eaten, it is quickly digested and absorbed, which causes your blood sugar content to spike. A high concentration of glucose in your blood can damage your organs, so your body's ever-vigilant pancreas responds by sending a flood of insulin into the bloodstream. Insulin clears the blood of glucose; some of the sugar is used as energy, but the rest is stored . . . as *fat*.

The GI uses a uniform unit of 50 grams of carbs as its basis. The amount of a specific type of food needed to get 50 grams of carbs will vary widely, depending on the amount of carbs in the food. The glycemic load (GL) of a carb takes into account the typical *serving size* of carbohydrate foods that we eat. Take carrots, for example. They have a sky-high GI of 131, but the GI of carrots is based on the effect of eating 1½ pounds of them. Unless you're Bugs Bunny, the GI of carrots is misleading at best. By taking into account typical portion sizes, GL is the better guide for which carbs to eat.

Carbohydrate foods that fall within a GL range of 1 to 10 (strawberries, oranges, and carrots, for example) are considered low GL; foods within a range of 11 to 19 are medium GL (bananas, sweet potatoes, and wild rice); foods with a rating of 20 or more are high GL (macaroni, white rice, and cornflakes).

Some foods are both high GI *and* high GL, and these are the culprits to avoid the most (baked potatoes and cornflakes, for example). Have these only in limited amounts at very specific times (see page 118). The Alpha Fuel Solution is designed to minimize these foods in your diet without overthinking it.

Carbohydrates are also an important source of fiber. When most American guys think of fiber, they think of cereal grains and whole wheat bread. But eating a diet based on grains is not the only way to meet fiber requirements. Including more fruits and vegetables, along with some legumes and a small amount of healthy grains, will easily provide the recommended 30 grams or more of fiber and provide a lot more overall nutrition. Yup, that's how we roll.

Fats

Like we said before, eating fat in your diet doesn't necessarily make you fat. Many overweight people pile "fat-free" baked goods and other "low-fat" stuff into their supermarket carts, brainwashed to believe that any and all dietary fats are to be avoided. Big mistake, because most fat-free processed foods replace the fat with loads of insulin-spiking sugar and corn syrup.

We've already discussed staying far away from the partially hydrogenated oils known as trans fats, and limiting (but not eliminating!) your intake of saturated fat, which you need for optimal testosterone levels. The good fats you want to eat most of generally fall into the categories of polyunsaturated and monounsaturated fats.

Polyunsaturated fats don't adversely affect cholesterol levels. In the same way that there are certain amino acids that are essential, there are also some fats that our body can't make. We need to get these from our food. These "essential fatty acids," or EFAs, are the omega-3 and omega-6 fatty acids we talked about earlier in the context of their imbalance in the Great American Diet Disaster. A goal of the Alpha Fuel Solution is to get both types of EFAs, but to increase the omega-3 essential fatty acids (including the healthful alpha-linolenic acid [ALA], eicosapentaenoic acid [EPA], and docosahexaenoic acid [DHA]) from sources like flaxseed and fish oil. Fish oil EFAs have anti-inflammatory properties, as well as fat-burning, muscle-building, antioxidant, and energy-production properties. They can:

- Lessen inflammation throughout your body
- Reduce excessive blood clotting
- Lower your cholesterol and triglycerides
- Protect against thickening of the arteries

Monounsaturated fats in the diet actually *lower* the so-called bad cholesterol, improve insulin sensitivity, and reduce the risk of heart disease. They also offer antioxidant properties and provide fatty acids for healthy skin and the development of body cells. Olive oil is probably the most popular monounsaturated fat today, but many nuts, such as pecans and almonds, are also good sources. They maintain healthy and manly testosterone levels. There is mounting evidence of the power of displacing dietary carbohydrates and saturated and trans fats with monounsaturated fats to maintain healthy waistlines and decrease mortality.

Fat is of utmost importance to your Alpha Factor. If all fats are eliminated from your diet, your brain won't be able to operate efficiently and the production of some hormones, like testosterone,

will suffer, too. Without enough of the *right* fats, testosterone levels will melt faster than the polar ice caps, simultaneously sinking your sexual function and performance.

In sum: Low-fat diets lower testosterone and contribute to the de-masculinization of the modern man! Replacing unhealthy saturated and trans fats with EFAs and monounsaturated fats is one of the most important things you can do to improve your diet, health, testosterone, and Alpha Factor. Roughly one-third of your calories should come from good fats. Much less than that, and your testosterone production just won't be optimal, which could adversely affect your ability to pack on lean muscle. But exceed 40 percent of your calories from fat, and guess what your body will start accumulating? Plenty of body fat!

FUEL FOODS: WHAT TRUE ALPHA MALES EAT

Choosing the right foods is going to be a lot easier now that you've purged your pantry of all the garbage. Now you have room for all the delicious and nutritious foods you'll go out to hunt, gather, and bring home to replace the junk. Many if not all of these items are most economically purchased at a discount bulk warehouse, such as BJ's, Sam's Club, or Costco.

Here's your shopping list of the Fuel Foods that will be your staples in the Alpha Fuel Solution.

Your Shopping List

Fill your basket with lean proteins, fruits, and vegetables:

- Whole roasted chicken (cooked/uncooked)
- Frozen chicken cutlets (uncooked, boneless, and skinless)
- Fresh turkey (whole or breast)

- Turkey (chopped meat)
- Lean fresh beef/steak, favoring grass-fed (see "Eat Meat!" on page 106)
- Lean chopped beef
- Lean pork (see "Eat Meat!" on page 106)
- Lean chopped bison/buffalo
- Veal sirloin
- Deli-sliced roast beef
- Deli-sliced turkey breast
- Deli-sliced low-sodium ham
- Canadian bacon
- Low-sodium turkey bacon or turkey sausage
- Green and black olives
- Fresh fish (any kind, favoring wild over farm raised)
- Canned tuna in water
- Smoked salmon (preferably Alaskan wild salmon)
- Frozen tail-on shrimp
- Scallops
- Omega-3-enriched eggs
- Egg whites (large carton)
- Lots of fresh veggies (all kinds, including cabbage, cauliflower, broccoli, zucchini, spinach, and kale, preferably organic)
- Salad fixings (romaine lettuce, grape tomatoes, baby carrots, radishes, cucumbers)
- Lots of fresh fruits (a wide variety, preferably organic)
- Frozen berries in bulk
- Nuts and seeds (a variety)
- Fat-free cottage cheese
- Plain Greek nonfat yogurt
- Nonfat/low-fat string cheese
- Nonfat/low-fat cheeses
- Oil (olive, flaxseed, macadamia nut)
- Low-sodium canned beans
- Fresh beans, string beans
- Whey protein
- Sweet potatoes
- Salsa
- Frozen fruit for smoothies

- Natural peanut butter
- Almond butter
- Frozen fruit bars—100% juice
- Low-sodium beef jerky
- Lentils
- Hummus
- Nonfat cream cheese
- Pam organic canola spray

Now add some beverages to keep you hydrated:

- Bottled water (your main drink of choice!)
- Carbonated unsweetened water (lemon or lime flavored)
- Skim milk (optional: fat-free half-and-half for your coffee)
- Diet soda, Crystal Light, and other artificially sweetened 0-calorie drinks (limited)

To give all these delicious foods some extra flavor, you can throw some of the following items into your shopping basket:

- Powdered spices (nutmeg, cinnamon, paprika, chili powder, ginger, hot red pepper flakes, and any others you like)
- Fresh scallions, onions, cilantro, parsley, dill, and other herbs
- Light soy sauce (low-sodium)
- Dijon or horseradish mustard
- Bottled or fresh salsa
- Marinara sauce
- Tikka Masala sauce (limited)
- Flavored vinegar (balsamic, red wine, ginger rice, red raspberry)
- Garlic cloves (fresh or prechopped in jars)
- Shredded coconut
- Sun-dried tomatoes
- 100% fruit preserves
- Sugar substitute(s) (optional)
- Cocktail sauce
- Wasabi mustard
- Nonfat/low-fat mayonnaise

You can also add the following optional foods to your basket, if you wish, but in much more limited amounts:

- Raisins, prunes, and other dried fruits (unsweetened only)
- Oatmeal (steel-cut)
- Ezekiel 4:9 Bread
- Whole grain wraps
- Bran crisp bread
- Dark chocolate

Bought in bulk, some of these items will last for several weeks or even for the entire Challenge. Others, like meats, fish, and fresh fruits and vegetables, will perish more quickly and will require weekly shopping—or some extra space in your freezer.

Finally, you'll want to pick up two or three 5-pound containers of whey protein powder (see "The Handshake Diet" on page 117). Whey protein will become an important part of the Alpha Fuel Solution during your Challenge. Also, pick up a convenient plastic shaker online or at a local health food store—it'll allow you to fully mix a tasty and nutritious shake in less than a minute. Visit www.alphamalechallenge.com for the skinny on whey protein.

FUEL RULES: EATING AS NATURE INTENDED

By sticking to the shopping list provided, you'll be eating more healthfully than ever before. We'll delve deeply into the details to support the guidelines for the Alpha Fuel Solution in the pages that follow, but our most simple recommendations for a lifestyle of healthy eating for everyone who wants to be their best boil down to 12 simple edicts:

Fuel Rules

1) Eat three or four meals and one or two snacks daily, spaced 3 to 4 hours apart.

2) Include a lean protein, fibrous carbs, and healthy fats in every meal.

3) Measure portions using the Man-Hand method.

4) Eat more fish ($\geq$ twice weekly).

5) Eat less dairy (other than nonfat or low-fat).

6) Avoid white: sugar, rice, bread, and pasta.

7) Eat lots of veggies daily (organic, if possible).

8) Do not eat greasy, salty, or sugary junk foods or sweetened cereals.

9) Snack on raw veggies, fruits, and nuts.

10) Do not drink regular soda, processed juices, or juice cocktails.

11) Do not eat fast food/fast frozen products (pizza, tacos, burgers, etc.).

12) Drink plenty of water!

So now let's get specific on the foods you ought to buy and eat to be your best.

Fish

Fish is one of the healthiest Fuel Foods you can eat. It's a great source of both protein and heart-healthy omega-3s, and it's lower in saturated fat than meat and poultry. Of course, we're *not* referring to fat-soaked fried and breaded fish sticks. If you like fresh fish, you're way ahead of the game.

Oily fish, such as wild salmon, herring, mackerel, sardines, anchovies, and eel, are packed with lots of heart-healthy EFAs. White, nonoily fish, including cod, haddock, sole, snapper, and monkfish, are lower in omega-3s. Most *any* grilled, poached, steamed, or broiled fish is a good source of complete protein and vastly better than what most couch potatoes put in their mouths. For a tasty treat, try the Wild Dijon Salmon recipe on page 305.

And don't forget shellfish like shrimp and lobster, which are good sources of protein, too. We've heard some guys worry about eating shrimp because of the high cholesterol content. Shrimp has 166 grams of cholesterol in a 3-ounce serving. But unlike saturated fat or trans fatty acids, the dietary cholesterol in shrimp may have little or no impact on cholesterol levels in your blood. Shrimp contains *no* saturated fat (and, of course, no trans fats). So munching away on shrimp is a healthier choice than eating fatty red meat for those worried about the heart. Oysters, either raw or cooked, provide a combination of protein, magnesium, and zinc, and may help boost your libido. Muscles, clams, scallops, and calamari (steamed, not fried!) are also a healthy part of the Alpha Fuel Solution.

What about sushi? Eating uncooked fish does present health risks, including the risk of parasitic organisms embedded in the flesh. But we enjoy sushi and especially sashimi occasionally, and we attempt to limit the risks by dining regularly only at trusted local restaurants where the fish is stored at proper temperatures.

If you check out the labels at the supermarket, you may see catfish and salmon that are "farm raised." Fish farmers breed and raise fish just like ranchers raise cattle. Fish farms are small pondlike quarters containing antibiotics, pesticides, chemicals, and wastes. The greatest profits are achieved when the stock grows as big as possible, at the fastest possible rate. Farmed fish are plumped up fast by both fish meal and fish oils, which contain PCBs (polychlorinated biphenyls), a toxic chemical common in fish from highly polluted waters. Although farmed fish still offer heart-healthy omega-3s, it's better to choose wild-caught fish over farm raised if you eat a lot of fish. We recommend you eat packaged wild Alaskan smoked salmon regularly, but we also suggest you throw in a meal of farm-raised catfish or salmon once a week (or even twice, in these cost-conscious times).

When it comes to eating wild-caught fish, size matters. The toxic chemicals, including methyl-

mercury, that small fish accumulate from household wastes and industrial runoff are passed up the food chain in greater concentrations. Generally, the higher a fish is on the food chain, the longer it lives and the more toxic chemicals it accumulates. Still, methylmercury poisoning from fish may take a backseat to the greater health risk of too few heart-healthy omega-3s in the diet. A study conducted by researchers at the University of Rochester School of Medicine and Dentistry in New York, published in the *Journal of the American Medical Association,* found that island people with 10 times the mercury levels of most Americans did not present with harmful side effects. We think there's enough concern to avoid eating too much freshwater lake fish and limiting your cumsumption of big predatory fish like shark, tilefish, king mackerel, and swordfish. Jean Jitomer, MS, RD, suggests no more than one 3-ounce serving weekly of these high-mercury fish. Otherwise, eat fresh fish regularly without fretting too much about toxins.

It's very easy to prepare fresh fish and it will take you less time than you think. In a hurry? Check out the simple preparation suggestions in Appendix B.

Chicken and Turkey

Poultry is a staple Fuel Food. Chicken and turkey are both terrific low-fat sources of great taste and enough protein to kick-start your Alpha Factor. We're not talking about chicken "fingers," "nuggets," or deep-fried wings here. We're talking about roasted, grilled, or broiled poultry, and with the skin removed. The majority of fat is found in the bird's skin. A chicken thigh with the skin on has triple the fat of an equal portion without skin. Still, even chicken with the skin on has less fat than most red meats.

White meat chicken is extremely healthy. A classic choice is the chicken breast, which is easy to prepare in a variety of ways. (For example, check out the Turbulent Thai Chicken recipe located on page 304.) The average boneless, skinless chicken breast weighs about 4 ounces and contains 35 grams of protein and 4 grams of fat. Most of that fat is monounsaturated fat—only 1.1 grams is saturated.

Dark meat has even more protein and B vitamins than white meat, with only a few extra grams of fat. The difference in color between white and dark meat is due to the predominance of the types of muscle fibers within the meat.

If you have the option of purchasing "free-range" chicken from your local market, consider going for it. Chickens that forage naturally are lower in fat than those that are pumped full of feed. "Organic" chickens that are free of antibiotics and chemicals are an even better bet, especially if you eat a lot of chicken and if you can splurge for the extra cost. Check out the simple chicken preparation suggestion on page 303.

Turkey is also a terrific choice, because it is high in protein and low in saturated fat. White meat turkey has even less fat than chicken breast. Turkey breast is 94 percent protein and only 6 percent fat. There's not much difference between dark and white turkey meat. Joy Bauer, MS, RD, CDN, compares 3 ounces of each choice:

- 3 ounces skinless breast meat = 115 calories, 1 gram fat
- 3 ounces skinless dark meat = 135 calories, 3 grams fat

Lean Meat

Lean red meats are a great Fuel Food to naturally raise your testosterone level. Lean beef provides a combination of protein, zinc, magnesium, iron, and B vitamins (especially B_{12})—all good stuff for your Alpha Factor. Other meats, including lean pork loin, are also amazing sources of protein and help build muscle. It is easy to find lean meat choices at most restaurants and eating establish-

ments. Just be sure to tell the waiter/staff to put the gravy/sauce on the side.

Now, before you start bingeing nightly at the local steakhouse, note that we said *lean* meats. Research conducted by the Center for Science in the Public Interest found that a "decent meal" can be built around a sirloin steak or a filet mignon, but that wasn't the case with any other steak tested. Their nutritional analysis concluded that a rib-eye has the fat of two sirloins and that a T-bone has the fat of three sirloins, while a porterhouse steak or prime rib has the fat of four. What about the ever-popular New York strip? Be aware that you're eating 18 grams of saturated fat, which is more than double the sirloin.

You need saturated fat, but too much saturated fat in our diets is why the USDA advises limiting red meat. A 22-ounce T-bone steak at a Ruth's Chris Steak House has a whopping 48 grams of saturated fat—more than double the recommended daily amount. (Some of that fat, points out PhD student and nationally ranked bodybuilder Jean Jitomir, MS, RD, is due to added butter rubs, a common if not standard practice in steakhouses.)

Aside from the butter rubs, you can blame some of the problem of red meat's excess saturated fat content, ironically enough, on the agricultural revolution. The red meat we eat today isn't the same as the kind our ancestors ate. Today's fattened-up domesticated animals are fed grains and corn feed, which can infuse a 16-ounce porterhouse steak with 88 grams of fat, 40 percent of which is saturated fat. That makes it 19 percent fat by weight and 65 percent of its calories from fat. Wild game, like the meat sources eaten in Paleolithic times, primarily feed on grass and plant foods and have 2 to 4 percent fat by weight (15 to 20 percent of calories), much of which is healthy monounsaturated fats. To highlight the rapidly changing nature of our food sources, think of this: Before World War II, all beef cattle in the United States were grass-fed; now 75 percent are *not*.

However, none of this means you should eliminate saturated fat! A sufficient amount of saturated fat is a friend to your Alpha Factor. Precisely how much remains open to debate. "Red meat has been maligned now for the past few decades," says powerlifting champ and diet expert Mauro DiPasquale, MD, author of *The Metabolic Diet*.

But the tide is turning and research is showing that red meat has been undeservedly maligned. After all, red meat has been a staple in our diets since the beginning of our time. So why all of a sudden is it poisonous to us? Red meat contains as much oleic acid, the same monounsaturated fat as in olive oil, as it does saturated fat. Oleic acid is considered to have significant health effects and is also felt to act as a sensing nutrient to decrease appetite. As well, red meat, with its saturated fat, increases serum testosterone levels. I've seen this in clinical studies that I've done on patients and athletes who I've put on my diets, with the emphasis on red meat.

So eating meat isn't a health concern, per se. The problems arise when fatty meat is a dietary mainstay, especially when the meat comes from

EAT MEAT!

Most types of meat, poultry, and fish can be healthy, protein-packed additions to your menu. The trick is selecting the cuts that are lowest in saturated fat. Generally speaking, all flesh foods will be healthier and lower in fat when 1) the skin is removed; 2) all visible fat is trimmed off; 3) you buy the meat from a store and cook it yourself; and 4) you cook the meat without a lot of added fat, particularly butter.

It's important to cook meats yourself most of the time because restaurants typically add extra fat, usually in the form of butter, cheese, and cream sauce. So even though the cut of meat you order may be lean, and the menu states that it's "grilled," the meal you're served may not be lean!

At home, try preparing your meat on an indoor or outdoor grill. Also, a top round beef roast or center-cut pork tenderloin makes a tasty roast, providing you with enough meat for 2 or 3 days.

All cuts listed below contain 5 grams of fat or less per 4-ounce serving. When purchasing a lean meat, make sure that the name is exactly the same as those listed below. For instance, "sirloin tip" is not the same as "top sirloin."

PROTEIN SOURCE	ACCEPTABLE CUTS
Beef	Bottom round, brisket flat half, eye round, lean ground beef, sirloin tip side, top round, top sirloin,
Lamb	Leg shank half, loin
Pork	Sirloin roast, tenderloin, top loin
Veal	Leg top round, sirloin
Wild Game*	Antelope, bison (buffalo), boar, caribou, duck, elk, goat, grouse, moose, ostrich, pheasant, squirrel, turkey, venison, water buffalo

* Most wild game trimmed of fat is acceptable.

—Jean Jitomir, MS, RD

livestock subsisting on the same grains and corn we're trying to limit in our own food plan. How do you solve the problem? Some advocates of Stone Age eating recommend exotic wild game in lieu of more traditional meats, and if you have the taste for them and can bear the higher cost, we think it's a great idea. Elk, antelope, buffalo, and kangaroo are high in protein and low in fat. But try finding wild boar at the local supermarket. For most guys, if it's not readily available among your local shopping options, it's an impractical choice, other than every rare once in a while.

Organic meats are another option, but their sky-high cost and restricted availability make them an impractical everyday option. (Certified Organic animals must be fed certified organic feed, which is very expensive.) If you can find and afford Certified Organic meat, you can try it—but be aware that if the animal was fed grains rather than grass, you're probably not getting the benefits you want. A 16-ounce organic strip steak still has 1,100 calories and 68 grams of fat, 40 percent of which is saturated fat, and 55 percent of calories from fat. A better approach is to check out the growing number of ranches that offer an improved, although still more pricey, option: meat from cattle that graze on grass. "Grass-fed" beef is a much healthier choice—less fat, fewer calories, 60 percent more omega-3 EFAs, and lots of beneficial conjugated linoleic acid (CLA)—than typical supermarket steaks. Fortunately, more and more specialty stores are stocking this nutritional powerhouse. Many ranchers of grass-fed "natural" cattle also use no antibiotics, hormones, or animal by-products in the feed. Be aware, however, that the term *grass-fed* isn't regulated; cattle that graze in the fields for a brief term prior to slaughter can be called grass-fed even though they were fed corn and grains for most of their lives. Look

for grass-fed beef that grazed for long periods, rather than just before slaughter. Several ranches offer this kind of beef and are worth trying out if your wallet permits!

For the rest of us, limiting supermarket red meat to a few times a week, choosing the leanest cuts, and trimming the visible fat is the most practical option. You won't get rid of all of the fat (nor would you want to!) because it's marbled all through the meat, but you'll get the excess off.

How you cook meat is crucial. Under high heat, the fat in the meat will liquefy. Cooking methods that let the fat drip away and be discarded can reduce the saturated fat content. Grilling and broiling are two such methods. However, grilling steaks or other types of animal meat on open-flame grills leads to the production of chemicals called heterocyclic amines (HCAs) and polycyclic aromatic hydrocarbons (PAHs). HCAs are formed when amino acids react with creatine at high cooking temperatures; PAHs are formed when fat drips onto hot charcoal and is then carried back to the meat via smoke. Both are cancer-causing agents that in recent years have led to a public backlash to barbecuing. Although the concerns may well be overstated, you can take simple but important steps to dramatically reduce the number of carcinogens that are formed when grilling. Studies have shown that even briefly marinating meat can dramatically reduce the formation of HCAs by upwards of 92 to 99 percent. Although scientists are not completely positive as to why there is such a dramatic difference, it may be because the marinade acts as a barrier to the open flames. Also, several natural ingredients in marinades, including vinegar, citrus juice, herbs, spices, and olive oil, all seem to contribute to lower HCAs. To combat PAHs, scientists and the American Cancer Society suggest using leaner cuts of meat, flipping regularly, and putting down aluminum foil with holes in it to prevent flare-ups when fat drips. An alternative to grilling is to cook the meat very slowly over an extended time, avoiding exposure to open flames. Check out page 299 for simple advice on meat preparation.

Eggs

The egg is a winner when it comes to the Alpha Fuel Solution. Eggs are a relatively inexpensive source of the very highest quality protein that money can buy. An omelet with turkey and some spinach or broccoli is a great way to start the day; boiling up a dozen eggs on Sunday night takes virtually no effort and will provide meal and snack versatility for most of the week.

There was a period during which eggs were on the "do not eat" list in many households because of the egg's high proportion of calories from fat—over 60 percent of daily calorie intake. Moreover, a large egg contains about 215 milligrams of cholesterol—more than a comparable portion of any other food. But guess what: Testosterone is derived from cholesterol. Without cholesterol, you'd be fresh out of the manly hormone—not our idea of a good time. Plus, egg yolks are a top source of choline. As pointed out by Jonny Bowden, PhD, CNS, in *The 150 Healthiest Foods on Earth,* "The choline in the egg yolk actually helps *prevent* the accumulation of cholesterol and fat in the liver!" And the newest generation of eggs has been tweaked to improve the ratio of omega-3s. Now available in supermarkets everywhere, these new "super eggs" are a terrific diet mainstay—as long as you don't overdo them. If you want to err on the side of caution, try breakfast omelets with one or two whole eggs and the balance in egg whites, which have no fat and no cholesterol. If you're willing to spring for the extra cost of organic eggs, go for it. These eggs are obtained from chickens that aren't pumped full of antibiotics and chemical feed.

If you have a seasoned cast-iron pan, you can make an omelet without excessive oil and without eating the tiny amounts of carcinogenic material that can flake off cheap Teflon pans. Or you can boil up some eggs and try our egg salad recommendation in Appendix B.

Dairy

Primitive man didn't drink milk. If he managed to catch a wild animal, he ate it. The process of holding the beast still and trying to pull its udders would have never crossed his mind. It wasn't until the agricultural revolution and the domestication of livestock that whole dairy products became a staple in many folks' diets. The older guys among us were urged as kids to drink milk for strong bones and teeth, without much talk about the negatives associated with whole milk products. Of course, whole milk is high in saturated fat. Drinking lots of whole milk and eating ample cheese can increase your cholesterol and lead to heart disease.

Do you need milk for the calcium required to maintain strong teeth and bones? There are many other sources of dietary calcium to ensure an adequate daily intake. Calcium/magnesium dietary supplements provide one way to augment your nutrition, and there are plenty of nondairy calcium-rich foods, such as canned red salmon, rhubarb, sardines, collard greens, spinach, turnip greens, okra, white beans, and broccoli. Further, in many parts of the world where dairy isn't a staple food, the people often have fewer cases of osteoporosis and fewer bone fractures than Americans. What's interesting is that these populations also maintain healthy bodies at less than half the levels of calcium recommended for Americans. Neither the World Health Organization nor the Canadian government recommend as much calcium as the American government does.

Dairy products can provide a high-protein content at a very reasonable cost, along with calcium and vitamin D. Given the crucial role that protein plays in the Alpha Fuel Solution, we recommend that you keep dairy on your menu, but in modest amounts, and mostly in low-fat or fat-free forms. (You'll be getting enough healthy fats from the rest of your menu.) Low-fat or fat-free dairy is generally an exception to the rule of avoiding "fat-free" foods. But beware that commercial yogurt with fruit, or packaged cottage cheese with pineapple, are far from great diet foods, even if they're low-fat or fat-free. The "fruit" is mostly fruit-flavored sugar or fruit concentrate with added HFCS, colors, and thickeners. If you love some yogurt occasionally, you're much better off buying plain and adding your own delicious mix of fruit and nuts.

However, that's not the case with low-fat and fat-free milk. Manufacturers strip the dairy of fat and leave the protein. In fact, some "skim plus" milk products add extra protein in place of fat to thicken the product, which gives it a mouthfeel comparable to that of whole milk. Ask your favorite local coffee shop to stock it!

Fruits and Vegetables

By now you understand the reasons why bread, cereal, and pasta should *not* be the main part of your daily diet. Fruits and vegetables provide the bulk of the carbs needed to fuel Alpha performance. They have a variety of vitamins, minerals, and antioxidants, as well as fiber. A diet that eliminates them also eliminates most sources of fiber, and most guys should get at least 30 grams of daily dietary fiber (15 grams for every 1,000

CARB RULES: GLYCEMIC LOAD

The Fuel Rules of carbohydrate consumption are pretty simple. Packaged, processed carbohydrates and junk foods are to be avoided. Most cereal grains, pasta, bread, mashed potatoes, and rice cakes are high-glycemic carbohydrates that quickly elevate blood sugar, causing a spike in insulin that promotes fat storage and may promote the development of type 2 diabetes. They should be consumed sparingly, and the refined kinds avoided completely. What are the worst in glycemic load? The glycemic load of white bread has provided a good place to draw a line because virtually all the junk is over that and almost all the good stuff is below that. Compared to a reference standard of a slice of white bread (100), a few of the highest GL examples include a cup of spaghetti (213), a cup of gnocchi (260), a cup of white rice (283), a corn muffin (299), and a medium-size bagel (340). Think about that the next time a bagel seems like a health food to you.

According to Dr. Rob Thompson, author of *The Glycemic Load Diet,* "The total glycemic load of the starches in the average American's diet is more than 20 times that of any other food including sugar and candy. That means if you eliminate flour products, potatoes and rice—even if you compensate by eating more of other foods—your glycemic load and the amount of insulin your body has to make will be a fraction of what it was before."

Frankly, we think that virtually all fruits and vegetables are nutritious, regardless of their glycemic load, although you'll need to limit the dried fruit a bit.

For getting and staying lean, we want to stick with the lower glycemic fruits and vegetables throughout the day—those that are released more slowly. You should eat higher glycemic carbs—those that are released more quickly—immediately before or after a workout. That's when your body needs fast-acting carbohydrates to replenish those burned and to prime the muscle-building process. For a list of low glycemic carbohydrates, see alphamalechallenge.com.

calories you eat, as recommended by the United States National Academy of Sciences, Institute of Medicine).

People who eat five or more servings of fruits and vegetables daily have half the cancer risk compared to those who eat only two servings. Raw cruciferous vegetables such as broccoli and cabbage are rich in cancer-fighting compounds, and so are delicious fruits like blackberries.

Start each day by washing some fruit and leaving it in a bowl on the table or counter for snacking. *Always* keep some fruit in plain sight!

Seedless grapes make a great snack—leave them where you (and others in the household) can readily see them, rather than hiding them in a refrigerator drawer. You'll find that they become your *first* snacking choice.

Your local supermarket provides a dizzying array of fruits and vegetables; here's how to make smart selections. Some fruit and vegetable selections are labeled as "genetically modified" (GM). This means that the growers have manipulated the product's genes to help improve some of its traits. A common reason for genetic modifications is to create resistance to insects and viruses;

"ONCE FORBIDDEN . . . NOW FORGIVEN"

4 Previously Condemned Dietary Delights to Enjoy in Moderation

1) **Red Wine:** Remember the time when this delightful beverage was vilified for being nothing more than a source of "empty calories" that would prevent you from getting lean? Well, we've come a long way since then. When consumed in moderation, the alcohol in wine is known to decrease heart attack risk, as well as increase HDL cholesterol (the good cholesterol). To top that off, a glass of red wine (pinot noir, for example) is chock-full of many antioxidants called polyphenols, including resveratrol, which have potent health-promoting effects. From acting as antioxidants, improving blood circulation, and reducing inflammation to controlling the expression of survival genes, red wine polyphenols are key biochemicals that pack a powerful punch!

   Bottom Line: You can indulge in the occasional glass or two of red wine and still maintain or even boost your Alpha Factor. During your 10-week Challenge, however, you are limited to two glasses per week while on the Handshake Diet and none while on the Spartan Diet.

2) **Dark Chocolate:** Here is a tasty treat that was disparaged in the past for being the prototypical "junk food." Now there is strong scientific evidence showing that the flavanoids found in cocoa possess antioxidant benefits, improve blood vessel health and bloodflow to the heart and other organs, reduce blood pressure, decrease inflammation, and improve blood sugar metabolism by improving insulin function. That is quite the list, and it doesn't even include additional benefits from the fiber and rich mineral content. You may be asking, "What about the fat?" More than one-half of the saturated fat is stearic acid, which is known to have a neutral effect on total cholesterol; one-third of all the fat is oleic acid, the monounsaturated fatty acid found in olive oil that is also known for its heart-healthy benefits. Just be sure to look for dark chocolate that is greater than 85 percent cacao, and ideally 100 percent, to maximize the health benefits, and keep it under 20 grams (under the size of two small cookies).

   Bottom Line: Unless you are on the Spartan Diet, consider treating yourself to some decadent dark chocolate on occasion . . . but keep the portion under control or the calories start to mount quickly with this energy-dense food.

you may already eat GM foods! There are no regulations that make growers label their produce with "GM."

One way to avoid GM foods is to go organic. Are organic fruits and vegetables worth the extra cost? We think so, assuming you can spare the extra dough, but only for some products. Sticking to organic apples, peaches, and pears is a terrific way to limit your intake of pesticides and exposure to GM foods. On the other hand, for foods with thick outer skins that you don't eat, such as bananas, going organic is probably not worth the extra cost.

Looking for a wonder Fuel Food? Broccoli easily makes it to the top of the carbohydrate list for peak male health and performance. Why? There's a component of broccoli, called indole-3-carbinol, that has been found in clinical studies to regulate estrogen. Wow! Broccoli acts as an antiestrogen, keeping those female hormones in check and your Alpha Factor high. The green wonder may also be an important tool in fighting certain cancers due to its ability to either block or change bad estrogen into safer forms.

Cabbage is another cruciferous vegetable that has proven to help fight estrogen buildup and is a

---

3) Coconut: This food was often maligned for containing so much saturated fat that your heart would be pumping sludge through your arteries. However, not all fat—or saturated fat, for that matter—is created equal! More than half of its saturated fat is lauric acid (a 12-carbon fatty acid), which has displayed antimicrobial activity in addition to increasing HDL cholesterol, with some studies showing decreased heart disease risk. Much of the remainder of coconut's fat content is in the form of medium-chain triglycerides (MCTs), which have no real effect on blood cholesterol levels. Due to its high fat saturation, coconut makes for a very stable fat or oil during high-temperature cooking. Again, be mindful of your portion size here—the calories add up in a hurry.

Bottom Line: Unsweetened coconut in moderation will provide some welcome variety to your diet, whether you use it as a stand-alone snack in its shredded form or as part of one of your Alpha Fuel meals.

4) Jerky: (beef, venison, buffalo, and even wild salmon) The first thing that comes to mind for most people with any type of jerky is that it's high in sodium and fat. How can a food so evil possibly contribute to improving your waistline and health? Once again, not all fats and, in this case, "jerky" is created equal. The key is to look for the variety that is not loaded with MSG, nitrates, or sodium. Also, be sure to find brands that specialize in providing grass-fed as opposed to grain-fed beef, buffalo, or venison. This will help optimize the omega-6 to omega-3 ratio within the meat and minimize the most "heart-unhealthy" of the saturated fats (palmitic acid). Alaskan sockeye salmon jerky may just be the absolute champion of jerky products, with its power-packed combo of EPA/DHA omega-3 fats plus plentiful protein, to boot.

Bottom Line: The right beef or salmon jerky product gets a "pass" as a safe Alpha Fuel food to snack on when you are on the run and pressed for time; it provides healthy fats and muscle-building protein, while keeping your hormonal environment primed for fat loss.

There you have it. Four snacks that were previously classified as taboo for the man looking to get lean have risen from bottom-of-the-barrel "junk food" to actually being labeled as "functional foods" *in moderation* (strongly emphasized), with numerous health benefits.

—Hector Lopez, MD, MS, CSCS

great source of fiber. The unpopular scents of all vegetables in this family (cauliflower, Brussels sprouts, kale) are due to the indole-3-carbinol compound—but they're outright terrific for you!

Spinach is loaded with vitamins and is a great source of vitamin K, which is important for building strong bones, all in the lowest-calorie package you can imagine.

If we chose to include only one grain in the Alpha Fuel Solution, it would be oatmeal. Oatmeal is one of the few grains we like a lot; it's a great source of vitamins, protein, and both soluble and insoluble fiber. It has a very low glycemic load, so it won't send your blood sugar soaring. But make sure you get steel-cut oats or old-fashioned rolled oats; the instant oatmeal in most supermarkets isn't worth eating.

We also think beans and legumes are great, in moderation. There's no denying that they are a great source of protein, zinc, and fiber, and they have powerful testosterone-raising attributes. Examples of healthy bean choices are lima beans, navy beans, black beans, pinto beans, and kidney beans.

Oils, Seeds, and Nuts

We've grouped these items together because they all contain healthy fats that can have a place in your Fuel Food arsenal.

When it comes to oils, we think of fish first. The benefits of fish oils are now well documented, and we recommend that you get them by eating plenty of fish and taking supplements, as well. For cooking over medium to high heat, opt for oils rich in monounsaturated fats. Extra virgin olive oil (from the first pressing of the olives) is rich in monounsaturated fats, mostly oleic acid, which has been shown to be great for your heart. So is macadamia nut oil—in fact, it's even richer in monounsaturated fat than olive oil.

Keep in mind that portion control is important when adding fats to food. "I see some guys pouring ½ cup or more of olive oil into salad or to baste meats because they think it's healthy. More seems better," notes dietitian Jean Jitomir. The key is to remember that a little goes a long way!

Consuming seeds and nuts is a great way to get healthy antioxidants like vitamin E, in addition to

---

MONOSATS: EXTRA VIRGIN OLIVE OIL AND MACADAMIA NUT OIL

EXTRA VIRGIN OLIVE OIL, the staple of the Mediterranean diet, has recently gained tremendous prominence in the health and dieting field. The reason is that olive oil contains an extremely high concentration of monounsaturated fats. These omega-9 fats—specifically oleic acid—reduce LDL cholesterol, decrease C-reactive protein (a marker for inflammation), and provide the body with a bevy of antioxidant-rich phenolic compounds that help combat cancer, heart disease, and chronic inflammatory diseases. If you're not consuming extra virgin olive oil (cold pressed and immediately bottled), you won't get all the previously mentioned health benefits. The reason is simple: Olive oil is an extremely reactive oil that's sensitive to light, heat, and environmental chemicals. Authentic Italian chefs never cook with olive oil; they add it for extra flavor once the dish is prepared.

MACADAMIA NUT OIL has the highest concentration of monounsaturated fats currently available. In fact, macadamia nut oil is so high in monounsaturated fats (84 to 85 percent) that it even surpasses olive oil (65 to 74 percent). Macadamia nut oil's extremely high smoke point makes it excellent for stir-frying and baking; olive oil has a much lower smoke point and degrades when used in cooking. Macadamia nut oil has a sweet buttery taste, and it contains an extremely high amount of vitamin E (four times higher than olive oil). Perhaps the only drawback to using macadamia nut oil is the fact that the world's supply of the stuff is limited and when the growing season comes to an end, there's no more left until the following year.

—Dave Palumbo, BS, CPT, owner of Species Nutrition

MAJOR BENEFITS TO DRINKING THE RIGHT AMOUNT OF WATER:

⊙ Decreases dehydration to help keep you clear and focused

⊙ Eliminates toxins

⊙ Is a medium for digestive enzymes

⊙ Helps maintain healthy skin and hair

⊙ Is essential for absorbing vitamins and minerals

omega-3 EFAs. Although nuts and seeds tend to be skewed high toward omega-6s, walnuts and macadamia nuts do have plenty of omega-3s. Cashews, hazelnuts, pecans, and pistachio nuts are all healthy snacks and better alternatives to any junk food option. As with all fat sources, don't overdo it—keep the portion to a handful or two, and go for the unsalted varieties. Of course, avoid nuts completely if you have nut allergies.

HYDRATING THE TRUE ALPHA MALE

We've talked about eating, but what about drinking? No, we're not talking about boozing it up at the local watering hole, but about providing your body with the fluids required to keep it healthy and strong. During the heightened demands of the Challenge, you need hydration more than ever!

Water

Water is essential to human existence. Water functions as a solvent for all the biochemical reactions taking place in the body; it also acts as a coolant, a means for release of toxins, and a lubricant. Water accounts for about 60 percent of the average guy's body weight. For the lean and sinewy True Alpha Male, it's closer to 70 percent. Research shows that more water increases fat burning, while dehydration increases protein breakdown and insulin resistance.

Water is an essential part of body temperature regulation. Even while working out in the cold, a good amount of water is lost through sweating. The World Health Organization recommends nearly double the amount of water for men who are active in a hot environment, so go ahead and feel free to drink more in hot conditions or when you're exercising.

DRINKING ADVICE (WATER OR OTHER FLUID) THAT'S EASY TO SWALLOW

⊙ Drink about 10 ounces of water approximately 2 hours before a workout.

⊙ Drink another 5 ounces immediately before the workout.

⊙ Be sure to drink about 5 ounces every 20 minutes during your workout.

⊙ After your workout, weigh yourself and replace your lost water (sweat) with a full bottle of water for each pound lost.

⊙ Don't wait until you're thirsty to have a drink—you may already be dehydrated. If you're thinking about it, take a sip!

⊙ Hate the (lack of) taste of water? Try squeezing some lemon in it to give it a little flavor!

Although it's difficult to confirm whether drinking a glass of water before a meal really helps satiate hunger, what is supported is the fact that high-water-content foods such as fruits, vegetables, and even lean meats will help reduce total calorie intake and diminish hunger pangs. Because we tend to eat the same amount of food every day, a diet composed of food with a high water content reduces overall energy intake automatically.

HOW MUCH WATER SHOULD I DRINK?

According to *ScienceDaily* and the Mayo Clinic, your water requirements depend heavily on lifestyle factors, including your personal activity level, age, living climate, and altitude—a warmer climate, high altitude, and older age all increase water demands. For a larger guy engaged in an intense training program like the Challenge, adequate daily intake could easily exceed 8 cups per day.

Too much alcohol or coffee, both natural diuretics, will instigate dehydration. If you do frequently consume these in excess, it's important to replace the water that's lost from them.

If the taste—or lack of taste—of water doesn't suit you, try adding in some lemon juice for flavor. If you need even more flavor and sweetness, add some Crystal Light. (But be aware that controversy over the safety of artificial sweeteners continues, so don't consume them to excess.) Bottled non-calorie fruit drinks are fine occasionally, but be aware that excessive drinking of carbonated diet soft drinks may damage tooth enamel. You can also try your own brewing concoctions, such as iced green or herbal teas.

Is Fruit Juice Okay?

Fruit juice beverages are hawked to the public as healthful alternatives to sugary soda pop and soft drinks. But most are filled with HFCS, so other than some vitamin content, they're really not much better at all. Even if the juice has no added HFCS and is 100 percent fruit juice, it's been stripped of a primary benefit of fruit: the fiber. Without the fiber, the product hits your body with a high glycemic load. Keep your consumption of fruit juices to a minimum. Eat the fruit itself.

THE PERFECT MEAL PLAN SCHEDULE

Spacing out your Fuel Food intake throughout the day assures that you're never too full and never too hungry. It allows your body to properly digest and utilize the nutrients you consume. Ideally, you'll want to consume about five or six small meals per day, every 3 hours, starting with breakfast. For some guys, eating five or six meals a day will be an effort. However, once you experience a faster metabolism and more even blood sugar, you'll be motivated to continue frequent eating based simply on the benefits.

In order to be successful, it's important to plan ahead and form a routine that fits into your everyday lifestyle. For example, a balanced breakfast can improve metal clarity, energy level, and mood. If you skip the morning meal, stamina and endurance suffer and you are more susceptible to overeating processed foods later in the day. Eating breakfast also boosts metabolism; therefore, you will burn calories more efficiently throughout the day.

Basically, plan to have three full meals at breakfast, lunch, and dinnertime. Snacks, which may be another Man-Hand meal or a convenient protein shake (see "The Handshake Diet" on page 117), fill the voids between breakfast, lunch, and dinner, for a total of five or six eating times.

A Sample Alpha Fuel Day

The brilliance of the Alpha Fuel Solution is that you don't have to follow a rigid diet, only the general Fuel Rules we've discussed. But as a guide, we offer two examples of what a menu

MEAL PLAN FOR A 170-POUND MALE
2,000 CALORIES

MEAL 1 (BREAKFAST)	CALORIES	CARBS (G)	PROTEIN (G)	FAT (G)
3 egg whites	51	2	11	0
1 whole egg	70	1	6	5
1 cup skim milk	90	12	8	0
½ cup oatmeal	150	27	5	3
walnuts (small handful)	50	1	2	5
raisins (small handful)	33	8	0.5	0
20 ounces water	0	0	0	0
2 tablespoons flaxseed	90	4	0	7
Meal Total	534	55	32.5	20
MEAL 2 (MIDMORNING SNACK)				
½ cup dried cranberries	30	8	0	0
1 ounce (28 almonds)	170	5	6	16
1 cup grapes	62	16	0	0
20 ounces water	0	0	0	0
Snack Total	262	29	6	16
MEAL 3 (LUNCH)				
6 ounces salmon, chinook, raw	304	0	34	18
2 cups steamed broccoli	70	10	2	0
Meal Total	374	10	36	18
MEAL 4 (MIDAFTERNOON SNACK)				
apple	95	25	0	0
1 tablespoon almond butter	94	3	4	8
20 ounces water	0	0	0	0
Snack Total	189	28	4	8
MEAL 5 (DINNER)				
6 ounces chicken breast	282	0	58	4
2 cups asparagus	54	10	6	
20 ounces water	0	0	0	0
Meal Total	336	10	64	4
MEAL 6 (POSTWORKOUT SNACK)				
1 banana	92	27	0	0
2 scoops protein powder	300	8	40	10
16 ounces water	0	0	0	0
Snack Total	392	35	40	10
DAY'S TOTAL MACRONUTRIENTS		167(g)	182.5(g)	76(g)
Total Calories	2087	695	725.2	675
Percentage Breakdown		33%	35%	32%

would look like for a sample day. First, we're using a guy who weighs about 170 pounds here and is following the Alpha Wave Basic Training program. Here's a sample of the food content (about 2,000 calories) he'd need to maintain his current body weight. The point is to simply give you an idea of what a typical day might look like in terms of food. To help you better understand the macronutrient content of the foods you eat, we've broken that down for you, too. To add

MEAL PLAN FOR A 220-POUND MALE
2,750 CALORIES

MEAL 1 (BREAKFAST)	CALORIES	CARBS (G)	PROTEIN (G)	FAT (G)
5 egg whites	85	3	18	0
1 whole egg	70	1	6	5
2 cups skim milk	180	24	16	0
1 cup oatmeal	300	54	10	6
1/8 cup walnuts	100	3	4	10
1/8 cup raisins	65	16	0.5	0
20 ounces water	0	0	0	0
2 tablespoons flaxseed	90	4	0	7
Meal Total	890	105	54.5	28
MEAL 2 (MIDMORNING SNACK)				
1/12 cup dried cranberries	30	8	0	0
1 ounce (28 almonds)	170	5	6	16
2 cups grapes	124	32	0	0
20 ounces water	0	0	0	0
Snack Total	324	45	6	16
MEAL 3 (LUNCH)				
8 ounces salmon, chinook, raw	405	0	43	24
2 cups steamed broccoli	70	10	2	0
Meal Total	475	10	45	24
MEAL 4 (MIDAFTERNOON SNACK)				
apple	95	25	0	0
1½ tablespoons almond butter	140	5	5	12
20 ounces water	0	0	0	0
Snack Total	235	30	5	12
MEAL 5 (DINNER)				
8 ounces chicken breast	376	0	77	5
2 cups asparagus	54	10	6	0
20 ounces water	0	0	0	0
Meal Total	430	10	83	5
MEAL 6 (POSTWORKOUT SNACK)				
1 banana	92	27	0	0
2 scoops protein powder	300	8	40	10
16 ounces water	0	0	0	0
Snack Total	392	35	40	10
DAY'S TOTAL MACRONUTRIENTS		235(g)	233.5(g)	95(g)
Total Calories	2746.61	933	933	853.75
Percentage Breakdown		34%	34%	31

some muscular body weight, he'd add another meal to the equation or just eat 20 to 25 percent larger portions.

Note that we have three full meals, two convenient snacks, and a protein drink that can be consumed right after training (or split up by taking half before the workout and half after).

In case you're wondering, the fiber total in this sample meal is 38.92 grams—an amount that equals or exceeds the current government recommendations for fiber intake. The saturated fat content is 14.55 grams.

Now, let's say that you're a guy who weighs 220 pounds. You'll need 2,750 calories to maintain your weight during the Challenge. The sample below shows how much larger the portions would need to be to sustain you. If you wanted to lose excess fat, you'd reduce the portions a bit; it's as simple as that.

The total fiber is 45 grams. The total saturated fat is 19 grams. The appendix gives you specific ideas for cooking methods and delicious Alpha Fuel recipes. These are generally high-protein, low-carb, and low-fat choices balanced with snacks that are more weighted toward unprocessed carbs, such as fruits, and healthy fats, such as nuts.

THE HANDSHAKE DIET

The Alpha Fuel Solution is a simple, healthful way of eating that you can use for life. Follow our Fuel Rules and stick with Fuel Foods in Man-Hand portions, and you'll improve the way you look and feel. But for the radical and dramatic transformation you're seeking over the next 10 weeks, we have a slightly modified version for you to follow.

The Handshake Diet is a convenient variation on the Alpha Fuel Solution designed to meet the intense demands of the Challenge. You'll still be eating three or four Man-Hand-sized meals and one or two snacks each day, each consisting of the healthy food choices that we've discussed. But you be substitute a high-protein/low- or no-carbohydrate "shake" for either one meal (typically breakfast for most guys, because it's quick and convenient) and one snack, or for two snacks, each day. You have the choice of either purchasing a protein powder or a ready-to-drink (RTD) packaged protein product. Both are available online, in health food stores, and in many fitness clubs. A selection of RTD brands is now also available at your local convenience store.

The most economical approach is to buy a 2- to 5-pound canister of chocolate or vanilla powder and make the shakes yourself in a plastic shaker (with 8 to 10 ounces of water) or an electric blender (adding ice and other healthy ingredients, as suggested in the 10-week plan). One scoop of powder contains approximately 20 grams of protein.

Why shakes? A higher protein intake is *crucial* during the rigors of Alpha Wave Basic Training. Supplementing your solid food meals with liquid protein shakes is a great way to ensure that you get the protein your muscles need to repair themselves and grow stronger. The Handshake Diet will supply you with the protein you need.

Protein powders come from a variety of sources. There are soy protein powders, but because of the phytoestrogens (dietary estrogens—remember the problems with estrogens discussed in Chapter 1?) contained in soy, we'd rather you didn't *overuse* soy in your diet. If you use soy proteins due to an allergy to dairy, experts such as Dr. Lopez suggest keeping the concentrated soy protein intake to fewer than 40 grams per day.

The choices for dairy-based protein products are generally made from whey, casein, or a combination of both. High-quality whey is quickly and easily digested, so it's a great way to get protein to your muscles fast. But combining whey with casein gets high marks, too, especially right after a workout, because the longer-digesting casein keeps feeding protein to your body even after the whey is digested. What's best for you? Scout out the options at www.alphamalechallenge.com and decide for yourself.

A study at Baylor University examined the effects of supplemental protein and amino acids on muscle performance and markers of muscle anabolism over 10 weeks of resistance training. Guys were randomly assigned to receive either 20 grams of protein (14 grams whey and casein protein, 6 grams free amino acids) or 20 grams of dextrose placebo (sugar!) an hour before and after exercise. The guys lifted intensely four times a week. The results? The protein supplement resulted in greater increases in total body mass, fat-free mass, thigh mass, muscle strength, and other anabolic markers.

Many of the whey products or combination whey and casein products on the market have added benefits: rich concentrations of branch chain amino acids (BCAAs) and glutamine. Glutamine is a conditionally essential (i.e., you need more of it during times of heavy stress) amino acid that has been shown to support the immune system.

Ready for one of the most powerful body composition improvement strategies we know? It's not just what you eat, it's when you eat. We're talking about the most important time of the day: before and after your Alpha Wave Basic Training. Knowing what to eat—not only before a workout, but also after—can be just as important as the workout itself. For both pre- and postworkout meals, you want a mix of protein and carbs. Immediately before and after your workout are the only times you'll benefit from consuming a high-glycemic carbohydrate. A protein shake *before* a workout has also been shown to stimulate the metabolic processes that dramatically increase muscular size and strength. A protein drink with a high-glycemic carbohydrate consumed within 15 to 30 minutes postworkout is critical to rebuilding muscles and preventing a flood of stress hormones that break down the body. At that critical time, the dextrose stimulates an insulin spike that helps shuttle protein and other supplements (e. g., creatine and BCAAs) to the muscle. The carbohydrates replenish energy stores while the protein is left for muscle building. Avoid fats immediately postworkout, because they will slow the movement of nutrients into the body. Also, drink plenty of water to help rehydrate your body.

So on your Alpha Wave Basic Training days, time your shakes to provide your body with protein when it needs it most.

Here are the Fuel Rules for pre- and postworkout protein intake, courtesy of Dr. Lopez:

- If you're replacing a meal with a shake or if you're drinking one 15 to 30 minutes after a workout, use two scoops of protein (or about 40 grams of protein) with a high-glycemic carbohydrate.
- If you're replacing a snack with a shake or drinking a shake 15 to 30 minutes before a workout, use one scoop (or about 20 grams of protein) with a low-glycemic carbohydrate.
- A glass or two of skim milk has the potential of stepping in to fill the role of a postworkout recovery drink when you don't have access to supplements. Also, dried, nonsugared fruits offer a convenient and practical whole food carbohydrate alternative immediately following exercise.

Note: Eat a whole food Alpha Fuel meal 60 to 90 minutes postworkout, with functional fats and fibrous vegetable or fruit carbohydrates to encourage a slower assimilation, or "trickling," of amino acids and carbohydrates for continued muscular recovery.

The Feast Meal

Following the basic Alpha Fuel Rules is how our species should be eating, pure and simple. We do believe, however, that in following the Handshake Diet the occasional deviation from the model is not only permissible, but also beneficial. Besides, if you've stayed on the program all week long, you're among a tiny percentage of American guys eating smartly, and you should be rewarded. Here's the deal. For one meal each week (Sunday dinner, for instance), go ahead and have whatever you want to eat. Whether it's pasta or bread along with a delicious sweet dessert, go ahead. It's not "cheating" on your diet because you're not *on* a diet. So don't sweat it. Go to your favorite restaurant and eat what your heart desires, if you like. Just remember, it's just one meal—one appetizer, one entrée, and one dessert.

If you deviate from the Handshake Diet more than once a week, you will step backward. On the other hand, a single Feast Meal may help you adhere to the plan by reducing your sense of self-deprivation.

Now, the weekly Feast Meal isn't for everyone, especially if you want to maximize your progress. Here's the crucial caveat: *If your chest-to-waist differential is less than 6 inches or your waist circumference is more than 38 inches, you should limit yourself to one Feast Meal every other week for now. Think of the reward that lies ahead if you can burn that stubborn fat!*

Some individuals may find it difficult to reestablish wholesome eating after indulging in even one Feast Meal. Despite good intentions, a small number of guys may fall into a pattern of eating unhealthy, processed foods for days or weeks. Don't beat yourself up if you fall into this category. If you think you could be unduly tempted, here are a few suggestions:

- Try having the Feast Meal out at a restaurant instead of bringing junk foods into your home.
- Buy the food as take-out and bring it to a park or someplace where it's hard to get more of it.
- Eat your Feast Meal with a friend who knows your intention to stop after one food or meal; they can provide social support to help you be strong.

- Stay away from Feast Meals for now and work harder on your commitment exercises. In time, you'll boost both your muscle and your willpower.

You'll be following the Handshake Diet throughout the 10-week Challenge if you are seeking more muscular size, endurance, strength, and power but do not seek to lose body fat. However, if, like the vast majority of American guys, you're looking to build muscle *and* torch body fat, you'll deviate from the Handshake Diet only in Weeks 5, 8, and 9. In Week 5, and Week 5 only, you will simply avoid all bread, cereal, rice, and pasta, even including whole grain products. And in Weeks 8 and 9, you will be following a more rigorous version of the Alpha Fuel Solution we call the Spartan Diet.

THE SPARTAN DIET

The Spartan Diet is a ketogenic-style or very low-carb variation on the Alpha Fuel Solution. As part of the 10-week Challenge, it is a much more restrictive menu than the Handshake Diet and it kicks in only during Weeks 8 and 9. We added it to the Challenge to take a blowtorch to any stubborn body fat

---

OMEGA-3 ACIDS: INTERACTIONS WITH HERBS AND DIETARY SUPPLEMENTS

According to the National Institutes of Health, omega-3 fatty acids can have adverse interactions with herbs and other supplements or drugs because they may:

- ☉ theoretically increase the risk of bleeding when taken with herbs and supplements that are believed to increase the risk of bleeding
- ☉ lower blood pressure, and theoretically may add to the effects of agents that may also affect blood pressure
- ☉ slightly lower blood sugar levels
- ☉ lower triglyceride levels, but may slightly increase LDL ("bad cholesterol") levels by a small amount
- ☉ over extended periods cause a deficiency of vitamin E

Men taking multivitamins regularly or in high doses should discuss risks with their health care practitioners.

you're hoarding as you near the Destination of your Challenge. The Spartan Diet isn't applicable to you if you are solely looking to build muscle; you should just stick to the standard Handshake Diet. But if you seek a leaner body with abdominals you can be proud of, the Spartan Diet is for you!

If you're familiar with diets like Atkins or South Beach, then you have an idea of what a ketogenic-style diet entails. Unlike those diets, however, the Spartan Diet we offer in the Challenge isn't open-ended—it lasts for only 2 weeks. While long-term ketogenic-style diets remain a subject of some controversy, the very brief term of the Spartan Diet makes it both healthy and mentally manageable for most any guy.

The Spartan Diet is perfectly timed in the Challenge, both physically and psychologically. From the physical perspective, many guys will lose the greatest number of pounds in the very first week of the Challenge. The sudden and intense demands of the program will shock the body into shedding excess fat and water right away. In the weeks that follow, fat losses will vary. Although some guys will see steady fat losses throughout the Challenge, others may reach a plateau by Week 8. The Spartan Diet kicks in to present a whole new shock to the body, jump-starting the fat loss process all over again. Also, because ketogenic diets may reduce exercise intensity capacity for some guys, the Spartan Diet coincides with the 3rd Wave of training, when overall training volume is lowest.

From the psychological perspective, introducing the Spartan Diet in Week 8 makes perfect sense, too. Rather than foisting a strict "induction" phase at the very start of a new diet plan, when old habits are freshest in your mind, the Spartan Diet takes hold when guys have already invested 7 full weeks into the Challenge. Old habits have already been broken and a healthier lifestyle and Alpha Attitude is already becoming part of everyday life. Given all the time and effort already invested, why quit now?

To understand what happens inside your body on the Spartan Diet, let's talk about how your body stores and uses energy. Glucose, you may recall, is simply a molecule of sugar produced from the carbohydrate foods you eat and break down during the digestion process. It is your body's preferred energy source. When we eat and digest a meal with carbohydrates, blood glucose levels rise and the pancreas secretes insulin. Insulin allows the glucose to be taken up into the muscle, forming muscle glycogen. Glycogen is how your body stores glucose to use as fuel when you need energy, such as during an Alpha Wave Basic Training workout. When you run out of glycogen, you will feel exhausted. When this happens, you need to replenish glycogen stores with proper nutrition—more glucose—along with rest.

During the Spartan Diet, our objective is to radically limit foods that contain carbohydrates so that your body switches away from a stored glucose–burning metabolism and uses alternative sources as fuel. When your body adapts to a very low-carb diet, you will be using very little glucose for your fuel source. With lowered carbohydrate consumption, your insulin levels will go down. Your liver converts fats into fatty acids and ketones. Your body begins to use ketones, protein, and its own stored body fat as fuel. You are said to then be in "ketosis." If you want to be absolutely sure you're in a state of ketosis, there is a tool that will tell you instantly. Most pharmacies carry ketogenic strips, which are often used by diabetics who are monitoring their blood glucose levels.

Some people may wonder whether you can reach a ketogenic state by not eating at all—a starvation diet. The answer is yes, you'll deplete your glucose and glycogen stores. But your body needs a small amount of glucose to function, and it will make it from the protein you eat. Without dietary protein intake, your body will extract the protein necessary from your hard-earned muscle tissue. No guy wants that!

Over the 2 weeks of the Spartan Diet, you will be taking in very few carbohydrates. Your diet will primarily be made up of protein and fats.

With restricted carb intake, your body will switch over into ketosis in about 48 hours. It will then be burning your stored body fat at a higher rate than ever before. If you're looking to melt the fat off your belly or love handles, the Spartan Diet is made for you! *Note:* You will still be entitled to a Feast Meal on each of the two Spartan Diet weeks, with the usual rules: If your chest-to-waist differential is still less than 6 inches or your waist circumference is more than 38 inches, you limit your Feast Meal to *either* one appetizer, one main course, or one dessert—but just one of the three.

THE FACTS ON CREATINE

Creatine (methylguanidine-acetic acid) is a naturally occurring amino acid–based substance that was first identified in 1832 as a constituent of meat. Creatine occurs naturally in your body, synthesized in the liver and pancreas from the amino acids arginine, glycine, and methionine. About 95 percent of your body's creatine is stored in your muscles. Serious research into creatine's effects on muscle growth and performance began in the 1990s. Creatine monohydrate is now popular among many resistance trainers, with sales estimated to be more than $100 million per year. Creatine plays a vital role in the ATP-PC (adenosine 5'-triphosphate and phosphocreatine) system, which involves providing energy to cells. The effects of supplementing with creatine monohydrate have been reported to be increased muscle mass, decreased muscular fatigue, decreased time needed for recovery, and improved performance.

The mass media regularly bash creatine. The claims include that all weight gained during supplementation is due to water retention; creatine supplementation causes renal distress; and creatine supplementation causes cramping, dehydration, and/or altered electrolyte status.

According to our experts, that's *not* what the science says. In 2007, our friends over at the International Society of Sports Nutrition (ISSN) put creatine to the test. Their research committee issued a Position Statement of the Society after an exhaustive review of the body of evidence on creatine. Here are their most relevant findings:

⊙ Creatine monohydrate is the most effective performance-enhancing nutritional supplement currently available to athletes for increasing high-intensity exercise capacity and lean body mass during training.

⊙ There is no scientific evidence that the short- or long-term use of creatine monohydrate has any detrimental effects on otherwise healthy individuals.

⊙ Creatine monohydrate supplementation is not only safe, but also may be beneficial for preventing injury when taken within recommended guidelines.

So, it's safe and it works according to the experts who've reviewed the science to date. It might even help ward off injuries. The ISSN found that the best way to increase your body's creatine stores appears to be by taking a daily amount of about 0.3 grams of creatine per kilogram of body weight (about 30 grams for a 220-pound guy) for at least 3 days, followed by 3 to 5 grams a day after that to maintain elevated stores. They also suggested that taking smaller amounts of creatine monohydrate, such as 2 or 3 grams a day, will increase muscle creatine stores over a 3- to 4-week period (however, the performance effects of this method are less supported). As for the newer variations of creatine, they allowed that "the addition of carbohydrate or carbohydrate and protein to a creatine supplement appears to increase muscular retention of creatine, although the effect on performance measures may not be greater than using creatine monohydrate alone."

If you want to add creatine to the Alpha Fuel Solution, choose a trustworthy manufacturer. Take the product right after your workout to help optimize its effects, although studies suggest that splitting it up so as to take it both before and after training has shown substantial benefits. On days you don't hit the weights, take it with a meal or just before bed. Questions on creatine? Visit us online at www.alphamalechallenge.com.

DIETARY SUPPLEMENTS: THE EXTRAS

Our primitive Stone Age ancestors certainly weren't popping vitamin pills or downing protein shakes. They got all the nutrients they needed from the nutritious foods they ate; the popular category of dietary supplements known as "sports nutrition" products, such as creatine monohydrate, wouldn't be invented for many thousands of years. But times have changed. Ancient hunter-gatherers didn't consume cupcakes, ice cream, potato chips, soda pop, doughnuts, jelly beans, french fries, or any of the other processed foodstuffs on the typical American menu. Many of the foods available today are pesticide-ridden and contain fewer nutrients than the foods from our ancestral food supply. Food additives are loaded into most of the staple foods you eat to prevent bacteria from growing and to add pretty colors and tasty artificial flavoring to the mix. Whatever nutritional value may have existed in the raw natural materials from which these foods were made has been compromised or outright "processed out."

Multivitamins

According to Dr. Jose Antonio of the International Society of Sports Nutrition (ISSN), "The fact that most individuals in the United States are overweight and out of shape indicates to me that eating clean and taking a multivitamin is not on their top 10 list of things they should do. Everyone should take a daily multivitamin just to ensure that they get sufficient amounts of micronutrients." Taking a multivitamin provides partial protection from our dietary lapses, but it should never be viewed as a substitute for a healthy diet.

Our friend Doug Kalman, PhD, RD, FACN, director of Nutrition Research at Miami Research Associates and the author of nutrition texts, recommends looking for a multivitamin that contains levels that are between 75 and 100 percent of the recommended daily intake (RDI), and he notes that studies suggest that three-times-per-day dosing is better than one-a-days. He says that both the water-soluble vitamins (the Bs, C, biotin, pantothenic acid, and folate) and the fat-soluble vitamins (A, D, E, and K) are better absorbed when taken with food. He stresses that *more* does not always mean *better* and that vitamins and minerals at high doses (two to five times the RDI) can cause negative reactions between the nutrients in the body, thus leading to poorer—not better—nutrition and health.

Most guys are probably not meeting their daily nutrient requirements. The rigors of Alpha Wave Basic Training place even greater demands for vitamins and minerals on your body, as well as a need for more protein. You wouldn't want a body that only meets the minimum standards, so neither should your nutrition. By exercising with great intensity, you're automatically placing yourself in a different category from the average couch potato. Men who exercise intensely put their bodies under a significant amount of physical stress. If you're doing Alpha Wave Basic Training, you're most likely sweating. (If not, you're simply not working out hard enough!) You need to replace the vital nutrients lost in sweat to allow adequate recovery and maintenance of your lean muscle tissue. A multivitamin with minerals is a perfect insurance policy for optimal nutritional intake.

EFAs

We've already discussed the importance of more omega-3s in your diet. For those who don't like fish or who want extra omega-3's, daily fish oil supplementation is the way to go. Fish oil contains both docosahexaenoic acid (DHA) and eicosapentaenoic acid (EPA). Evidence from several studies has suggested that amounts of DHA and EPA in the form of fish or fish oil supplements lowers triglycerides, slows the buildup of atherosclerotic plaques ('hardening of the arteries'), lowers blood pressure slightly, as well as reduces the risk of death, heart attack, dangerous abnormal heart rhythms, and strokes in people with known heart disease.

According to the National Institutes of Health, omega-3 fatty acids can have adverse interactions with certain herbs and other supplements or drugs. They may:

- theoretically increase the risk of bleeding when taken with herbs and supplements that are believed to increase the risk of bleeding.
- lower blood pressure, and theoretically may add to the effects of agents that may also affect blood pressure.
- slightly lower blood sugar levels.
- lower triglyceride levels, but may slightly increase LDL ("bad cholesterol") levels by a small amount.
- may over extended periods cause a deficiency of vitamin E

So, guys taking any supplements regularly or in high doses should discuss risks with their health-care practitioners.

What should you look for in a fish oil supplement? Choose a brand you trust, and look for a high potency of DHA and EPA. Some cheaper fish oil supplements can repeat on you—the dreaded fish burps—so it's best to sample small bottles of a few brands to find one you like. A study was conducted looking at the reliability and label claims of more than 40 fish oil products on the market. The results suggest that most products are in fact very reliable with less mercury and other toxins on a parts per billion basis than even most whole food fish on the market. As for dosing, the National Institutes of Health advocate discussing doses with a qualified health care provider before starting fish oil supplementation but offer the following guidelines:

For adults (18 years and older), the average dietary intake of omega-3/omega-6 fatty acids: Average Americans consume approximately 1.6 grams of omega-3 fatty acids each day, of which about 1.4 grams (about 90 percent) comes from alpha-linolenic acid, and only 0.1 to 0.2 grams (about 10 percent) from EPA and DHA. In Western diets, people consume roughly 10 times more omega-6 fatty acids than omega-3 fatty acids. These large amounts of omega-6 fatty acids come from the common use of vegetable oils containing linoleic acid (for example, corn oil, evening primrose oil, pumpkin oil, safflower oil, sesame oil, soybean oil, sunflower oil, walnut oil, and wheat-germ oil). Because omega-6 and omega-3 fatty acids compete with each other to be converted into active metabolites in the body, benefits can be reached either by decreasing intake of omega-6 fatty acids or by increasing omega-3 fatty acids.

So, there you have it! If you want the latest information on EFAs, visit us at www.alphamale challenge.com.

WRAPPING IT ALL UP

Conventional diets, aimed exclusively at *weight loss,* miss the target. Bad move. You want fat loss and muscle gain. More muscle means not only a bigger, stronger, more masculine body, but also a leaner, sharper, harder, and more defined body, too. Muscle places a metabolic demand on your body, ordering it to *burn more fat.* Even if you don't aspire to look like a competitive bodybuilder, the proper diet, combined with training and a good attitude, will improve your personal look more than you ever imagined.

The Alpha Fuel Solution is a lifelong way to enjoy delicious foods, optimize your health, and give you all the nutrients needed for masculine excellence. For anyone undergoing the extreme rigors of a program like the 10-week Challenge, the Handshake Diet will provide the extra nutrition needed without adding extra body fat, and the Spartan Diet will blast through any fat loss plateaus to make sure you keep shedding the soft stuff hiding your precious abdominal six-pack. Ready to put these awesome dietary rules and tools to use? We'll walk you through the process every step of the way, week by week, starting on the next page. Get ready to be your best!

ALPHA MALE CHALLENGE CLIENT:
TOMAS JONES, AGE 42

TOMAS, A GRAPHIC DESIGNER, started to feel the beginnings of physical decline prior to age 30 due to poor lifestyle choices so common among American men today. He yo-yoed on the health front over the years. At age 42, he had hit some hard times in his personal life and it was wearing on him heavily. He felt that he needed to get back on track toward health and happiness. Tomas only weighed 168 pounds when he began, but he felt out of shape and knew that he needed to get back to optimum health. He desperately wanted more energy and stamina to keep up with his young son.

Original Alpha Factor: 35.

Tomas accepted the Challenge at 168 pounds.

He weighed 149 at Week 10.

He lost 19 pounds in only 10 weeks!

He dropped 7 inches of fat from his waist while adding size to his biceps. He reduced his time on the 300-yard shuttle run by a full 21 seconds, and added a whopping 3 inches to his vertical jump. His maximum bench press increased by nearly 20 pounds, with an improvement in bench press to body weight ratio of nearly 28 percent.

His Alpha Attitude soared through the roof. He tripled his score on willpower, boosted his courage by 200 percent, and increased his physical confidence by a spectacular 350 percent. He now has "the confidence and clarity that comes from being in shape not only physically, but mentally." Tomas enjoys the attention that his new body gets from women, "but the most important change is that people have noticed that I am a lot more relaxed and positive."

Overall, physically and mentally Tomas is a new man with a mind-blowing increase of 41 points on the MaleScale™.

His New Alpha Factor: 76.

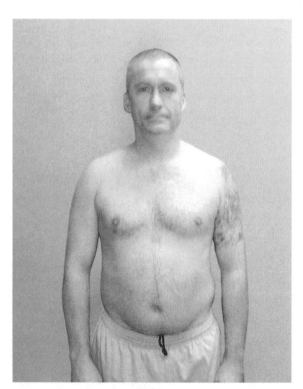

Before

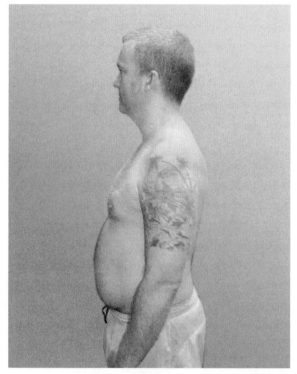

Before

Testimonial:

"The Alpha Male Challenge was a perfect match for my personal and fitness goals at the time I was introduced to it. The combination of a well-thought-out exercise program, excellent nutritional guidelines, and a very thoughtful approach to the psychology of reclaiming your 'power' was something I had not encountered before and dovetailed perfectly with my personal needs.

"The changes I witnessed not only physically, but just as importantly in terms of attitude and positivity, totally floored me. This was not just a quick fix/aesthetically-oriented program. The foundations for a sustainable lifestyle change are given to you, and the tools to empower you and to control your own life are made very explicit and clear. I would most definitely recommend this program to anyone who really wants to have a thorough understanding of the elements of true fitness laid out in a very simple, approachable, and doable program."

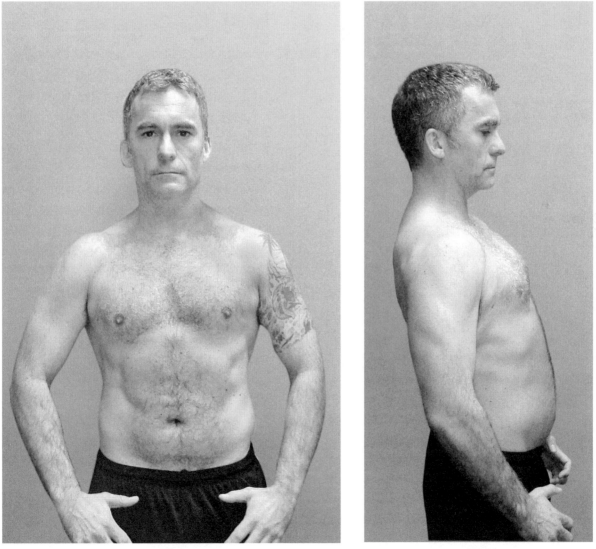

After   After

CHAPTER SIX

THE 10-WEEK ALPHA MALE CHALLENGE

WEEK 1

Alpha Attitude Drill

The Challenge starts with *commitment,* the first of the foundational four Cs of Alpha Attitude. To prepare for your first Alpha Attitude drill—the "Alpha Bet"—you'll need to set your goals. Go back to the lists you made to determine your Destination, and remind yourself why you accepted the Challenge and what you want to accomplish before D-Day (the last day of the 10-week Challenge). Now make your benchmarks specific and tangible (but realistic and achievable).

- Set Your Long-Term Goals = The Big Picture Outcomes
  - Example: "I will complete every planned workout each week of the Challenge."
- Set Your Midterm Goals = Name a Date
  - Example: "On the 30th of next month, I will not have missed a single workout."
- Set Your Short-Term Goals = Plan Your Actions

  - Example: "Tomorrow I will make my workout a priority by doing it early in the day."

Revise these statements *daily* to account for detours and roadblocks .

You can write out your commitment goals using pen and paper, or go to www.alphamalechallenge.com for easy online options and support. Now, make your "Alpha Bet" on success—but bet on performance (what you'll do) rather than on a specific outcome or result:

- Choose the long-term or midterm goal that's most important to you, and place a $40 (or more!) performance-based wager on it with a friend or family member. Now you've got your skin in the game!
- Be specific about what you are betting on. Here are some more examples.
  - Long-term example: "I will perform all 27 workouts by D-Day."
  - Long-term example: "I will eat no fast food at all until D-Day."
  - Midterm example: "I will eat no bread,

pasta, rice, or cereal during Weeks 8 and 9 of the Challenge."

 ○ Midterm example: "I will take five kickboxing classes over the next 3 weeks."

- Don't forget to target short-term action goals, too (e.g., "Tomorrow I will eat no junk food, but I will eat enough protein to sustain lean muscle growth and fat torching because I am a true Alpha Male."). And feel free to *reward* yourself frequently for adhering to your short-term goals—these little payoffs will keep you on track.

Be sure to place the $40 (or more) where you can see it every day, such as taped to the refrigerator or bathroom mirror. It makes it public, and every time you see it you can recommit yourself to your goals and Destination. If you can afford it, go ahead and make the same bet with somebody you will be exercising with. Or, better yet, get a buddy to join the *Alpha Male Challenge* with you. One of your training partner's responsibilities is to encourage you and continually remind you of your promise to yourself. And, of course, you will have made a promise to yourself in public to take those actions necessary to succeed—and someone will be watching. Unless you meet your goals, you don't get your money back. You have to want it, it has to be a way you define yourself . . . but a little bit of external motivation never hurts to get that ball rolling.

Congratulations on setting your goals! You've made a 100 percent commitment to the Challenge. Honor your Pledge, and full speed ahead!

Alpha Architecture Program

ALPHA WAVE BASIC TRAINING (WORKOUTS 1–3)

Over the next 4 weeks, Alpha Wave Basic Training will focus on two things:

primary target—torching excess body fat and building up lean muscle

secondary target—boosting power and maximizing strength

These 4 weeks will target the Muscle Up segment of each workout. For the first 2 weeks, you will be training your *whole body* during each of the three weekly workouts. Always rest at least 1 day between workouts. Your level—A, B, or C—will always determine your total number of sets. Remember: A key to the system is keeping close watch on rest intervals. *You must bring a watch with a second hand or a stopwatch to every workout!* Also, bring a bottle of water and a towel.

Here is the overview for Week 1:

Reps

- Power Boost movements: 4 reps
- Strength Max movements: 10 reps
- Muscle Up movements: 20 reps

Tempo

- Standard rep tempo of 1-0-1-0 (see page 60), other than on Power Boost moves (and the bicycle maneuver for abs). That means a fluid, natural tempo with 1 second for the lowering of the weight and 1 second for raising it, with no pauses at the top or bottom.

Rest Intervals

- Rest between sets is timed to maximize results.
- Rest intervals during the Power Boost segments of the workouts are 1.5 minutes.
- Rest intervals during the Strength Max segments of the workouts are 2 minutes.
- During the Muscle Up segments of the workouts, the rest intervals are only 1 minute—just long enough to permit a partner to complete his set, change weights if necessary, and position yourself for the next set.

If you've never done explosive Power Boost movements, this week's training will introduce a whole new style of exercise. The movements are performed as quickly as you possibly can (at a tempo of 0-0-0-0). Go easy at first if you haven't hit the gym in a while, or even if your training has been exclusively traditional strength or bodybuilding training. Before you begin your Power Boost movements, take a minute or two to become acquainted with these new movements. On all jumps and body weight exercises, perform a practice set and perfect your form. For Power Boost movements that require the use of resistance, begin with a practice set, using a very light weight, and go through the motions for 5 reps or so. Men who weigh more than 220 pounds must use extra caution when performing Power Boost movements. Begin with limited range of motion half jump squats and half lunge jumps, as well as power pushups executed on your knees instead of from the standard full-body pushup position. If you are concerned about performing Power Boost movements because of your lack of conditioning or perhaps are worried that you'll be embarrassed to perform them, please reconsider this. Virtually all pro athletes use these plyometric (Power Boost) movements in their training and do so because they work brilliantly!

Abdominal and/or core movements finish off each workout. The number of reps will be as many as you can do, up to 20. The last repetition should be difficult and intense. If you can perform 20 repetitions, add resistance. Note that some core movements are performed as quickly as possible, denoted by a tempo of 0-0-0-0.

WORKOUT 1
Target: Muscle Up

Dynamic Warmup—All Levels

MOVEMENT	SETS Level A	SETS Level B	SETS Level C	REPS	REST	TEMPO
Squat Jump	3	2	2	4	1.5	0-0-0-0
Power Row	3	2	2	4	1.5	0-0-0-0
Dumbbell Squat	3	2	1	10	2	1-0-1-0
Flat Barbell Bench Press	3	2	1	10	2	1-0-1-0
Machine Row (Neutral Grip)	2	2	1	20	1	1-0-1-0
Close-Grip Bench Press	2	2	1	20	1	1-0-1-0
Standing Dumbbell Curl	2	2	1	20	1	1-0-1-0
Dumbbell Lateral Raise (Standing)	2	2	1	20	1	1-0-1-0
Stiff-Legged Deadlift	2	2	1	20	1	1-0-1-0
Donkey Calf Raise	2	2	1	20	1	1-0-1-0
Bench Leg Lift	3	2	2	≤20*	1	1-0-1-0
Standard Crunch on Floor	3	2	2	≤20*	1	1-0-1-0
Total	30	24	16			

*Add resistance if too easy.

WORKOUT 2
Target: Muscle Up

Dynamic Warmup—All Levels

MOVEMENT	SETS Level A	SETS Level B	SETS Level C	REPS	REST	TEMPO
Speed Skater	3	2	2	4	1.5	0-0-0-0
Power Pushup	3	2	2	4	1.5	0-0-0-0
Standing Barbell Shoulder Press	3	2	1	10	2	1-0-1-0
Dumbbell Shrug (Seated)	3	2	1	10	2	1-0-1-0
Barbell Squat*	2	2	1	20	1	1-0-1-0
Lying Leg Curl	2	2	1	20	1	1-0-1-0
Lat Pullup or Pulldown	2	2	1	20	1	1-0-1-0
Rear Deltoid Machine	2	2	1	20	1	1-0-1-0
Dumbbell Skull Crusher	2	2	1	20	1	1-0-1-0
Barbell Curl (Shoulder-Width Stance)	2	2	1	20	1	1-0-1-0
Oblique Crunch	3	2	2	≤20 each side	1	0-0-0-0
Superman Back Extension	3	2	2	≤15	1	1-0-1-0
Total	30	24	16			

Substitute hip-width leg press for barbell squats for those with knee or back problems.

WORKOUT 3
Target: Muscle Up

Dynamic Warmup—All Levels

MOVEMENT	SETS Level A	SETS Level B	SETS Level C	REPS	REST	TEMPO
Lunge Jump	3	2	2	4	1.5	0-0-0-0
Full-Body Resisted Cable or Tubing Extension	3	2	2	4	1.5	0-0-0-0
Incline Dumbbell Bench Press	3	2	1	10	2	1-0-1-0
Romanian Deadlift	3	2	1	10	2	1-0-1-0
Leg Press (Hip Width)	2	2	1	20	1	1-0-1-0
Triceps Pushdowns (Rope Attachment or V-bar)	2	2	1	20	1	1-0-1-0
Preacher Curl Machine	2	2	1	20	1	1-0-1-0
Arnold Press	2	2	1	20	1	1-0-1-0
Seated Leg Curl	2	2	1	20	1	1-0-1-0
Seated Calf Raise	2	2	1	20	1	1-0-1-0
Bench Leg Lift	3	2	2	≤20	1	1-0-1-0
Swiss Ball Crunch	3	2	2	≤20	1	1-0-1-0
Total	30	24	16			

WORK HEART SYSTEM

Remember, true Alpha Males "work hard, play hard!" (hence, the name of our cardio system). To introduce you to the fat-torching Work Heart system (see page 74), you'll be making new choices this week to weave your commitment to fitness into your daily activities. You need to make choices each weekday that will total roughly 10 purposeful effort minutes that haven't previously been part of your day. Always use a watch to keep track of your time, although exact time is not nearly as important here as it is with your Alpha Wave Basic Training. Here's your Work Heart overview for Week 1.

- During each workday (5 days weekly), your objective is to collect 10 points (10 minutes' worth of Work Heart).
- Focus not on the exact time, but rather on making the best use of each activity.
- Fail to collect all 10 points and you lose all credit for that day.
- You need **50 points** by week's end to meet the Challenge.

Remember, one of the best Work Heart opportunities for most guys is getting to and from work (see page 75).

- If you drive to work, park far enough away to add a brisk 5-minute walk. Don't just focus on the walk from the car, but work on the walk back, too. This will add up to the 10 total minutes of Work Heart effort that you need for the day. Also, focus on the effort you put into the walk and not as much the time.
- Whenever you can, choose the stairs over the elevator. If you live or work in a high-rise building, take the stairs for 5 minutes, then take the elevator up for the remainder. Challenge yourself: If you carry a briefcase, switch hands halfway through to balance out the effort.

If your circumstances absolutely prevent you from adding Work Heart effort to your daily trip to work, try integrating your Work Heart activity into your work hours.

- Take a brisk 10-minute walk at lunchtime or during a meal break.
- Take two brisk 5-minute walks or climb stairs during short work breaks.

Do whatever it takes to get those **50 points** by the end of the week, and you'll be on your way to the Work Heart 1,000!

PLAY HEART ACTIVITIES

Your approach to the Play Heart component (see page 76) of your Alpha Architecture program will vary by your current fitness condition.

Level C trainers and those who have been "on hiatus" from exercise in general, you're about to embark on something new. This week is all about your commitment to the Challenge!

- You'll only do a minimum of one Play Heart activity *once* this week, for a minimum of 30 continuous minutes.*
- We suggest you schedule it in for this weekend.
- You can do it with your training partner, with your family, or on your own. Working with a group of buddies is inspirational. The key, though, is to just do it.

If losing body fat is your main goal, you should aim for three sessions of Play Heart this week, with two of the sessions (20 minutes each) performed in the gym right after your Alpha Wave Basic Training session. The third (30 minutes) should be on one of your days off.

Level A and B trainers, and those who are already involved in a regularly scheduled competitive Play Heart activity (such as tennis or racquetball), should continue that routine this week. So, if you already play racquetball twice a week, just keep going with it this week. If you are already doing gym-based cardio, such as running on the treadmill or pedaling on the stationary bicycle, and you enjoy it, feel free to continue it. But substitute one session for something different—preferably a Play Heart activity that's new to you. It must be at least once this week, for a minimum of 30 continuous minutes, and we urge you to do it with a training partner or with family members.

If the weather is fair this week, we suggest one or two outdoor activities such as Hill Hiking or Bleacher Runs.

- Hill Hiking
  - Alternate between walking, jogging, and running (sprinting), for at least 30 minutes.
- Bleacher Runs
  - Start at the bottom and ascend the bleacher stairs as quickly as you can to the top, then walk across the top to the nearest adjacent set of stairs and walk briskly down. Repeat 10 times, then briskly walk the track for 15 minutes, followed by 10 more bleacher ascents. The intensity should be based on your current fitness level.

  At level C, you should try walking, rather than running.

  At level A or B, take each ascent as vigorously and quickly as possible, pumping your arms and driving your knees upward to your chest with each bound, then walk or jog across the top to another set of stairs and walk briskly down. Repeat 15 to 20 times, then briskly walk the track for 10 minutes, followed by 15 to 20 more bleacher ascents.

  Remember to stay focused, and play it safe!

If the weather isn't suitable for outdoor activity this week, we suggest trying a new approach to indoor training treadmill work: the Kilimanjaro Walking Climb (see page 283). Due to the intensity of this activity, 20 minutes will satisfy your 30-minute Play Heart commitment this week.

Keep in mind throughout the Challenge that your Play Heart activities are best scheduled for days when you are *not* doing your Alpha Wave Basic Training. The exception is any gym-based Play Heart activity. If you're already in the gym for your resistance training, you may economize your time and follow it up with your Play Heart activity. Making the most efficient use of your time is a key to adhering to any exercise regimen and building a true masterpiece of Alpha Architecture.

Alpha Fuel Solution

You'll begin your first week of the Alpha Fuel Solution by proving your commitment to a healthy new way of eating. This week we want you to focus on choosing the right Fuel Foods.

Start with a Mission Mine Sweep (see page 99) in your kitchen for any "enemy" foodstuffs—the highly refined and processed, heavily sweetened stuff that'll sabotage your strength, health, and appearance. Remember, if you share your home with others, recruit their help on your Mission Mine Sweep!

Breakfast Suggestions

- Blender smoothie with two scoops of whey protein, water, mixed berries, one banana, and ice
- Instant unsweetened/unflavored oatmeal with shredded coconut, cashews, fresh mixed berries, and skim milk

Lunch Suggestions

- Deli-sliced turkey breast, low-fat Swiss cheese, sun-dried tomatoes, and lettuce on a whole grain wrap
- Chick'n Wrapper (see page 311)

Dinner Suggestions

- Lean steak (see "Eat Meat!" list on page 106 and "Simplest Meat Preparation" on page 303), steamed broccoli with garlic, and a mixed garden salad with oil and flavored vinegar

- Baked chicken with mozzarella cheese and marinara sauce, and grilled asparagus with slivered almonds and macadamia nut oil

Snacking choices are many and varied, and will apply throughout the 10-week Challenge. Keep healthy snacking choices out where you can see them at home. And be prepared for snack attacks away from home: Always keep a few small bags of almonds or other nuts in your glove box and office desk drawer. For a list of snack options, see page 101.

If you're already on a sensible supplement program, feel free to continue it this week. If you'd like to start, consider purchasing a good multivitamin and a product containing EFAs (see page 104).

Don't forget to drink plenty of water and other calorie-free fluids, especially before and after exercise. Don't wait until you're thirsty to drink! It's vital to stay properly hydrated. Review our drinking advice (see page 113).

Results

You're now invested in the Challenge!

Certainly, this has been a week of new and different experiences. You may not be used to regular resistance training sessions, and you may experience some muscle soreness. That's okay. Integrating aerobic activity into your workday and recreational time may also be a shock to your system, but stick with it and it will pay big dividends soon enough.

Consider keeping a log of your workout results: How much weight did you lift for each exercise? How many reps did you execute? How was your form? This will allow you to see how you did the last time you did the exercise/workout and will arm you with the motivation to beat your previous numbers. You would greatly benefit from a log of *all* aspects of the program—Work Heart/Play Heart, and diet as well. Writing things down strengthens your commitment to them.

One purpose of your first week was to exercise your goal-setting commitment muscles and to

prepare you for the rigors ahead. At the week's end, look back and reflect.

If you hit your goals this week:

- What helped you do so?
- What obstacles did you overcome?

If you didn't hit your goals:

- What could you have done better to achieve your goals?
- What got in the way; did you fail to plan well or did you fail to anticipate obstacles?
- Were your goals unrealistic?

Next week, you'll do even better. For now, you've set definite goals and you've made an Alpha Bet on your success. You've gotten three hard Alpha Wave Basic Training workouts under your belt, keeping careful track of time. These full-body workouts are awesome for making sure that you're adequately training all of your major muscle groups. You've also collected 50 Work Heart points and performed at least 30 continuous minutes of Play Heart activity. You've swept your house and office of land mines and you've stuck to the Fuel Rules, including drinking adequate water. You're invested now. On to Week 2!

WEEK 2

Alpha Attitude Drill

This week's Alpha Attitude drill will make you flex your *confidence* muscles. The "Walk Tall" drill focuses on your sense of masculine presence. Here's a refresher on presence.

Many guys take their posture and body language for granted. Big mistake. You're going to practice consciously comporting yourself in a way that reflects the way you want to feel: confident and in control. Commit to doing the following drill one day this week:

- Spend 1 hour walking briskly and purposefully around a retail or commercial area.

- Pay careful attention to your posture, body language, gait, and facial expressions.
- Walk tall, keeping your shoulders back, chin up, and arms relaxed comfortably at your sides.
- Go into establishments and ask questions of the merchants.
- Stand tall but relaxed, without leaning, slouching, or putting your hands in your pockets.
- Greet those around you with a strong voice and clear intention, maintaining a warm and respectful tone.
- Keep eye contact and handshake strength appropriate.
- Make a mental note of how you acted, how people responded to you, and how it felt to you.

Remember, this is about being the best *you*, not impersonating the Duke. And it's not an endorsement of the exaggerated flared-lats-with-arms-stiffly-out look that some aspiring weight lifters affect. That sort of posturing is as sure a sign of weakness and lack of confidence as slouching. Don't ever do it! Stand, walk, talk, and act as if you are relaxed and supremely confident, and your own feedback system will relay it to the brain . . . and adjust your attitude accordingly.

Later, once the drill is over, spend some time reviewing your experiences. Take special note of how much better you feel when you are mindful of posture and positive body language. The review itself can change your future actions, thoughts, and feelings. So ask:

- What went right in your interactions?
- Were there times when it was difficult to maintain your presence? If so, what kinds of thoughts were involved in the difficult times?
- What solutions did you use to remind yourself to stay on task and how might you better approach such interactions in the future?

Remember, you are creating experiences that can change your future actions; attend to the details.

Each time you practice this presence drill, try to connect more meaningfully with those you encounter within a shorter and shorter time span. Like all the other drills, the more times you try this, the more you'll develop the skill set. And, of course, you'll intersperse your shop visits with plenty of brisk, fat-burning walking.

Alpha Architecture Program

ALPHA WAVE BASIC TRAINING (WORKOUTS 4–6)

As you did in Week 1, you will be training the whole body during each of the three weekly workouts, targeting the Muscle Up training segment. Always rest at least 1 day between workouts. Your level—A, B, or C—will always determine your total number of sets. Level C trainers will increase their total sets from 16 to 18.

Reps

- Power Boost movements: 5 reps
  - Try to do the reps faster than last week.
- Strength Max movements: 8 reps
  - Add weight over last week's poundages.
- Muscle Up movements: 15 reps
  - Add weight over last week's poundages.

Tempo

- Power Boost movements and some abdominal or core exercises are performed as quickly as you possibly can (0-0-0-0).
- For most movements, you'll emphasize the negative (lowering) portion of each repetition—the tempo is a slower lowering of the weight: 2-0-1-0 (see page 60). That's a fluid, natural tempo with a deliberately more focused and controlled lowering of the weight and 1 second raising it, with no pauses at the top or bottom.

Rest Intervals

- Rest intervals during the Power Boost segments of the workouts are 1.5 minutes.
- Rest intervals during the Strength Max segments of the workouts are 2 minutes.
- In the Muscle Up segments of the workouts, the rest intervals are only 1 minute—just long enough to permit a partner to complete his set, change weights if necessary, and position yourself for the next set.

During each workout, be sure to challenge yourself. Remember, you're not working out to simply go through the motions; you're there to work, hence the term *workout*. Ways to make your workouts more challenging include giving each exercise your complete all and concentration, adding weight when you can, sticking to rest times between sets, maintaining great form, putting your mind in the muscle, and sticking to the plan. Concentrate on trying to increase the speed of your Power Boost movements this week and add weight to your Strength Max and Muscle Up exercises. *Note:* If your workouts are going way over the 70-minute mark, it usually means that you're not sticking to your rest periods.

This week includes several partner-assisted exercises, as will subsequent weeks of the program. We highly recommend these movements; however, the exercise descriptions include alternatives for those who may be training alone.

Abdominal and/or core exercises are done with fewer reps and shorter rests than last week. The last repetition of a set should be difficult to execute and should be performed with maximum intensity.

Also, this week will introduce an exciting new test of strength and endurance: the Power Pushup Challenge (see page 197).

- Level C trainers will perform one set only. Levels A and B will do two sets, separated by a 1-minute rest interval. It takes confidence to get down on the floor and meet the Pushup Challenge, but don't back down! Keep going until you can't do one more. Try your hardest to do as many reps as you can. You'll revisit this challenge later on in the program.

WORKOUT 4
Target: Muscle Up

Dynamic Warmup—All Levels

MOVEMENT	SETS Level A	SETS Level B	SETS Level C	REPS	REST	TEMPO
Pushup Challenge*	2	2	1	Max	1.5	0-0-0-0
Forward Backward Cone Hop (each leg)	3	2	2	5	1.5	0-0-0-0
Smith Machine Hack Squat	3	2	2	8	2	2-0-1-0
Lying Leg Curl	3	2	2	8	2	2-0-1-0
Chest Dumbbell Pullover	2	2	1	15	1	2-0-1-0
T-Bar Row	2	2	1	15	1	2-0-1-0
Lateral Raise (Cable)	2	2	1	15	1	2-0-1-0
Triceps X-tensions	2	2	1	15	1	2-0-1-0
Barbell Curl (Wide Grip)	2	2	1	15	1	2-0-1-0
Leg Press Calf Press	2	2	1	15	1	2-0-1-0
Samurai Swing (Cable or Tubing)	3	2	2	10	1	0-0-0-0
Partner-Assisted Leg Throw+	3	2	2	10	1	1-0-1-0
Total	29	24	17			

*The goal is to continue until muscular failure, with full reps and no pauses. In martial arts, testing for black belts requires 75 repetitions to pass.
+If training without a partner, do the captain's chair.

WORKOUT 5
Target: Muscle Up

Dynamic Warmup—All Levels

MOVEMENT	SETS Level A	SETS Level B	SETS Level C	REPS	REST	TEMPO
Situp and Pike	3	2	2	5	1.5	0-0-0-0
Long Jump	3	2	2	5	1.5	0-0-0-0
Flat Barbell Bench Press	3	2	2	8	2	2-0-1-0
Dumbbell Shoulder Press Seated	3	2	2	8	2	2-0-1-0
Chinup or Chindown	2	2	1	15	1	2-0-1-0
Triceps Dip	2	2	1	15	1	2-0-1-0
Incline Dumbbell Curl	2	2	1	15	1	2-0-1-0
Cross the River (each leg)	2	2	1	15	1	2-0-1-0
Stiff-Legged Deadlift	2	2	1	15	1	2-0-1-0
Donkey Calf Raise	2	2	1	15	1	2-0-1-0
Swiss Ball Throw*	3	2	2	10	1	0-0-0-0
Superman Back Extension	3	2	2	10	1	1-0-1-0
Total	30	24	18			

*If training without a partner, perform the Swiss ball crunch with weight.

WORKOUT 6
Target: Muscle Up

Dynamic Warmup—All Levels

MOVEMENT	SETS Level A	SETS Level B	SETS Level C	REPS	REST	TEMPO
Lateral Push-Off Jump (each leg)	3	2	2	5	1.5	0-0-0-0
Power Pushup*	3	2	2	5	1.5	0-0-0-0
Deep Deadlift	3	2	2	8	2	2-0-1-0
One-Arm Dumbbell Row (each arm)	3	2	2	8	2	2-0-1-0
Weighted Stepup (each leg)	2	2	1	15	1	2-0-1-0
Seated Leg Curl	2	2	1	15	1	2-0-1-0
Incline Dumbbell Bench Press	2	2	1	15	1	2-0-1-0
Preacher Curl Machine	2	2	1	15	1	2-0-1-0
Dumbbell Skull Crusher	2	2	1	15	1	2-0-1-0
Standing Calf Raise	2	2	1	15	1	2-0-1-0
Grand Slam (Cable or Tubing)	3	2	2	10	1	0-0-0-0
Captain's Chair Leg Lift	3	2	2	≤20	1	1-0-1-0
Total	30	24	18			

*Levels A and B only: Clap hands between each repetition.

WORK HEART SYSTEM

Here's your Work Heart overview for Week 2.

- During each workday (5 days weekly), your objective is to collect 10 points (10 minutes' worth of Work Heart).
- The level of your effort this week—the heart in your Work Heart—must be greater than last week.
- Fail to collect all 10 points and you lose all credit for that day.
- You need **50 points** by week's end to meet the Challenge.
- If you particularly enjoy brisk walking during work breaks, perform all 10 minutes of Work Heart effort at one time.
- The 1-hour Walk Tall drill counts, but it can only be used to meet 25 points, so you still need to pick up the other 25 points for the week.

Do what it takes to get those **50 points** by the end of the week!

PLAY HEART ACTIVITIES

This week, we ratchet up your Play Heart activity time.

- You'll do one Play Heart activity this week, for a minimum of 40 minutes.*
- We favor one 40-minute outdoor Play Heart bout, typically over the weekend and as part of a family or group experience. But you have a choice of doing it all at once or dividing it into two sessions of 20 minutes each. Whichever option works best with your individual schedule is fine—the critical thing is to do it!

*If losing body fat is your main goal, you should aim for three sessions of Play Heart this week, with two of the sessions (20 minutes each) performed in the gym right after your Alpha Wave Basic Training session. The third, 40-minute session, should be on one of your days off.

Some guys are loyal to their gym-based treadmill or stationary bicycle sessions. If that's the case, you should continue as long as you engage in at least 40 minutes of the activity. You can go with the Kilimanjaro 20-Minute Walking Climb this week (see alphamalechallenge.com) or move on up to interval training with the Savage Mountain (K2) Sprint Training (see page 298). Interval training is an awesome way to maximize your conditioning. If you have a training partner, do your interval Play Heart training together and push each other in a competitive (but supportive) way. And if you're a level A or B trainer and/or are already involved in a regularly scheduled competitive Play Heart activity, keep doing what you have been doing this week.

Alpha Fuel Solution

Your shopping list will be the same as last week, although if you bought in bulk you'll likely have plenty of the nonperishables left. So you'll mostly need to get fresh meat, fish, fruits, and vegetables. (And don't forget that many of these items can be frozen to reduce trips to the market.)

You've been choosing the right foods. Now it's time to make sure you're eating them in the appropriate amounts. Remember to follow the Handshake Diet (see page 117) and the Man-Hand method of determining portion size (see page 96).

Remember, the Handshake Diet means eating three or four meals and one or two snacks each day consisting of the healthy food choices we discussed last week. But you may substitute whey protein shakes for one meal (typically breakfast) and one snack, or for two snacks, each day. (See page 117 for the skinny on whey protein, including timing your shakes for maximum effect.)

Breakfast Suggestions

- Alpha Artichoke Scramble (see page 304)
- Smoked salmon with fat-free cream cheese on bran crisp bread and an apple or a pear

Lunch Suggestions

- True Tuna Salad (see page 306) and raw vegetables
- Lean hamburger (no bun) with sautéed onions and mushrooms on a plate with mixed vegetables

Dinner Suggestions

- Manly meat loaf (sirloin, turkey, or ground chicken), spinach sautéed in garlic, and fresh raspberries with slivered almonds
- Simplest Fish Preparation (see page 303) and sautéed kale or spinach with garlic and macadamia nut oil

Results

You've now gotten 2 full weeks of whole body workouts under your belt and you've mustered the confidence to meet the Push-Up Challenge for the first (but not the last!) time. Have you found a training partner or partners? Having a committed gym buddy can keep you on track. When choosing a training partner, try to find someone who has similar goals as you. You want to find partners that communicate well with you and are as concerned with your results as they are with their own. Check out www.alphamalechallenge.com for ideas.

Make sure you kept close tabs on your tempo this week. It's easy to forget about how fast you should be lifting and lowering the weight. Trust us, the more you keep to the prescribed tempo times, the more challenge you'll bring to your workouts and muscles—and challenge equals better results. Also, you're likely getting more confident with Alpha Wave Basic Training, but don't skip the Dynamic Warmup! Muscles that are warmed and prepared for the work ahead are more pliable and allow you to work harder than muscles that are trained cold. A proper warmup will also help prevent injuries.

The Walk Tall drill has more deeply connected you to your sense of manly presence, you've collected your full 50 Work Heart points, and you've performed at least 40 minutes of Play Heart activity. You've gotten familiar with the two crucial components of the Alpha Fuel Solution: the Handshake Diet and the Man-Hand portion. It's time to face Week 3—and an even more intensive training system—with newfound levels of confidence.

WEEK 3

Alpha Attitude Drill

This week we target the *courage* it takes to stand up for what you want or believe in. Your Alpha Attitude drill is intended to help build the assertive courage you need to get what you deserve without disrespecting or bullying others, or being bullied.

Your drill is called "Straight Talk." List several ongoing interpersonal situations you've neglected to deal with for a while. They could be problems you're having with a co-worker, a neighbor, a local merchant you deal with, or a family member. Decide which is the most important to address now that also has a reasonable chance of a satisfactory resolution. Sit down and think through the following:

- What is the other party's specific behavior?
- What effect is it having on you?
- What is the solution or remedy you want?

Having these sorts of exchanges can be extremely stressful for many people. However, allowing the situation to fester can be worse. When you're straight and clear on these points, address the other party by asking whether you could have a few minutes to talk about something that's important to you. Maintain a calm demeanor and be direct in your approach.

1) State the facts: "When you _____."
(Specifically describe the behavior.)

2) State your feelings: "I feel _____."
(Honestly describe how the behavior makes you feel.)

3) State your requirement: "I would like _____." (Say what you want in a direct manner, respecting the rights of the other person.)

Congratulations! Hopefully, you resolved the situation amicably and to your satisfaction. Regardless of the outcome, take time to think about what happened (writing down your thoughts is best).

- Think about how you approached the conversation, how you felt, what you thought, how you acted, and how it felt afterward.
- Consider what the other party did and said. Were you surprised at the reaction? How?
- How did it go? What could you have done better, and how can you improve your approach to these conversations in the future?

Alpha Architecture Program

ALPHA WAVE BASIC TRAINING (WORKOUTS 7–9)

This week we take a whole new approach to training! We will continue to target the Muscle Up segment of training, but we will now split up the training for the various muscle groups over the 3 training days. This more intensive strategy will be employed over the remainder of the 10-week Challenge. Dividing the workouts in this way will enable you to devote a greater variety of exercises and a larger volume of work to each muscle group within the course of a workout. The physical demands on the individual muscle groups will increase. As always, rest at least 1 day between workouts. The total number of training sets for all levels increases this week.

We introduce an intense new strategy for levels A and B: the drop set (see page 60). Don't worry, level C trainers: You will experience the drop set soon enough. The total reps per set in this week's drop sets are 30. The drop set is only performed for one set (the last set for levels A and B). Rest for 2 minutes after a drop set (this will afford an interval for your partner to perform his drop set) before starting the next exercise. Make sure you don't jump the gun and choose a weight that's too heavy. You want to focus on hitting the 30-rep mark, so the weight you choose is critical in making sure that you reach your training goal.

Reps (Other Than Drop Sets)

- Power Boost movements: 5 reps
  - Try to do the reps faster than last week.
- Strength Max movements: 6 reps
  - Add weight over last week's poundages.
- Muscle Up movements: 12 reps
  - Add weight over last week's poundages.

Tempo

- Power Boost movements and some abdominal/core movements are performed as quickly as you possibly can (0-0-0-0).
- For most movements, the tempo of all repetitions this week involves an even slower lowering of the weight: 3-0-1-0. That still means a fluid tempo, but with a much longer and more controlled lowering of the weight, and then 1 second raising it, with no pauses at the top or bottom (see page 60).

Rest Intervals

- Rest intervals during the Power Boost segments of the workout are 1.5 minutes.
- Rest intervals during the Strength Max segments of the workouts are 2 minutes.
- Rest intervals in the Muscle Up segments of the workouts are 1 minute—just long enough to permit a partner to complete his set, change

weights if necessary, and position yourself for the next set.

Always be fully aware of what each movement's training objective is. Is the upcoming movement a Power Boost movement, where the goal is to shoot for lower reps with maximum explosiveness? Is it a Strength Max exercise, where you're going for a mid-range rep count using the most weight you can handle? Or is it a Muscle Up exercise, where you are shooting for many more reps and need to consciously choose a weight that you can manage for the higher number of repetitions?

Your Strength Max reps and Muscle Up reps are lower this week, so you should absolutely add more weight to those exercises. If you don't, you're only taking a step backward. Step it up and meet this week's challenge! Your number of training sets increases this week, so be ready for a bit more work, and pace yourself accordingly.

The Power Boost segments of the workouts this week will be more challenging. Try to perform them quicker than ever this week. This will help you develop even more explosive power.

WORKOUT 7
Target: Muscle Up

Dynamic Warmup—All Levels

MOVEMENT	SETS Level A	SETS Level B	SETS Level C	REPS	REST	TEMPO
Lateral Long Jump (each side)	3	2	2	5	1.5	0-0-0-0
Power Row (each arm)	3	2	2	5	1.5	0-0-0-0
Incline Barbell Bench Press	3	3	3	6	2	3-0-1-0
Flat Dumbbell Bench Press	3	3	3	6	2	3-0-1-0
Pec Deck	2*	2*	1	12	1	3-0-1-0
Close-Grip Bench Press	3	2	1	12	1	3-0-1-0
Overhead Single Arm Dumbbell Extension (each arm)	2*	2*	1	12	1	3-0-1-0
Leg Extension	2	2	1	12	1	3-0-1-0
Donkey Calf Raise	2	2	1	12	1	3-0-1-0
Seated Calf Raise	3	2	1	12	1	3-0-1-0
Bicycle Maneuver	3	2	2	≤25 each side	1	0-0-0-0
The Plank	3	2	2	>1 min	1	N/A
Total	32	26	20			

*Levels A and B only: Drop set! On your last set only, hit 12 reps, drop 20 percent, hit 10 reps, drop 20 percent, and hit 8 reps. This is a 30-rep total set and the key is to start slightly lighter. Your first set should be a standard 12-rep set, with a 1-minute rest. Rest for 2 minutes after a drop set (This will afford an interval for your partner to perform his drop set.)

WORKOUT 8
Target: Muscle Up

Dynamic Warmup—All Levels

MOVEMENT	SETS Level A	SETS Level B	SETS Level C	REPS	REST	TEMPO
Squat Jump	3	2	2	5	1.5	0-0-0-0
Situp and Pike	3	2	2	5	1.5	0-0-0-0
Romanian Deadlift	3	3	3	6	2	3-0-1-0
Lat Pullup or Pulldown	3	3	3	6	2	3-0-1-0
Seated Cable Row (Underhand Grip)	2*	2*	1	12	1	3-0-1-0
Lat Dumbbell Pullover	2	2	1	12	1	3-0-1-0
Barbell Shrug	3	2	1	12	1	3-0-1-0
Dumbbell Curl (Standing)	3*	2*	1	12	1	3-0-1-0
Incline Dumbbell Curl	2	2	1	12	1	3-0-1-0
Reverse EZ-bar Curl	2	2	1	12	1	3-0-1-0
Swiss Ball Crunch	3	2	2	≤20	1	1-0-1-0
Bench Leg Lift	3	2	2	≤25	1	1-0-1-0
Total	32	26	20			

*Levels A and B only: Drop set! On your last set only, hit 12 reps, drop 20 percent, hit 10 reps, drop 20 percent, and hit 8 reps. This is a 30-rep total set and the key is to start slightly lighter. Your first set should be a standard 12-rep set with a 1-minute rest. (Level A will do two standard 12-rep sets before the drop set. Rest for 2 minutes after the drop set. (This will afford an interval for your partner to perform his drop set.)

WORKOUT 9
Target: Muscle Up

Dynamic Warmup—All Levels

MOVEMENT	SETS Level A	SETS Level B	SETS Level C	REPS	REST	TEMPO
Jump to Box/Bench	3	2	2	5	1.5	0-0-0-0
Barbell Upright Power Row	3	2	2	5	1.5	0-0-0-0
Barbell Squat*	3	3	3	6	2	3-0-1-0
Barbell Lunge (each leg)	3	3	3	6	2	3-0-1-0
Lying Leg Curl	3+	2+	1	12	1	3-0-1-0
Stiff-Legged Deadlift	2	2	1	12	1	3-0-1-0
Leg Press Calf Press	2	2	1	12	1	3-0-1-0
Shoulder Press Machine	3+	2+	1	12	1	3-0-1-0
Dumbbell Lateral Raise	2	2	1	12	1	3-0-1-0
Rear Deltoid Machine	2	2	1	12	1	3-0-1-0
Partner-Assisted Twisting Leg Throws++	3	2	2	8 each side	1	1-0-1-0
Superman Back Extension	3	2	2	≤20	1	1-0-1-0
Total	32	26	20			

*Substitute hip-width leg press if you have knee or back problems.

+Levels A and B only: Drop set! On your last set only, hit 12 reps, drop 20 percent, hit 10 reps, drop 20 percent, and hit 8 reps. This is a 30-rep total set and the key is to start slightly lighter. Your first set should be a standard 12-rep set with a 1-minute rest. (Level A will do two standard 12-rep sets before the drop set. Rest for 2 minutes after the drop set. (This will afford an interval for your partner to perform his drop set.)

++Substitute bicycle if training alone.

WORK HEART SYSTEM

This week we kick our Work Heart system up a notch. Here's your Work Heart overview for Week 3.

- During each workday (5 days weekly), your objective is to collect 15 points (15 minutes' worth of Work Heart).
- Your level of effort this week—the heart in your Work Heart—must be equal to or greater than last week.
- Fail to collect all 15 points and you lose all credit for that day.
- You need **75 points** by week's end to meet the Challenge.

So, you need 5 extra minutes each day. How do you collect this week's added points? Choose from these activities, and remember that it's not so much the exact time that matters, but the effort you put into it.

- Add about 2½ minutes to your time walking to and from work. This may mean rerouting your walk just a bit.
- Add the extra 5 minutes at lunchtime or during a break, especially if you can get outside the office. Take a co-worker with you and make it a daily occurrence. Challenge yourselves to increase the distance covered each day.
- Alternatively, you can choose to do all 15 minutes of Work Heart effort at one time instead of breaking it up.

Now, here's a surprise for you—a little twist we call "Redemption" offered right when some of you may need it! If you lost credit on any day over the past 2 weeks, now's your chance to make it up. How many points are you short—10, 15, or even 20? Here's your one and only chance to square up.

- Choose a task, even a long-neglected one, you need to do around the house that requires some

physical effort. It should preferably involve machinery or tools—a hammer or a drill.

- If it involves lifting and carrying, pulling or pushing, or works up a sweat, then so much the better. Maybe it's putting up a shelf, assembling a piece of furniture, fixing a leaky sink, organizing the shed, taking down a tree, planting a tree, cleaning out the gutters, mowing the lawn with a push mower, or cleaning out the garage.
- If you can't think of anything, ask around the house—you may be surprised at the number of suggestions!
- Whatever it is that you do, make sure you do it for the full duration needed to make up the fat-incinerating points you lost.

You'll start Week 4 of the Challenge with a clean slate. But don't count on any more chances like this one, guys! If you want to play with the big boys, you'd better bring your A game from this day on!

PLAY HEART ACTIVITIES

This week, we boost your Play Heart cardio activity time to a minimum of 60 minutes, which can be done either in one time block or broken into two 30-minute sessions or three 20-minute sessions. The best option is the one that will work within *your* schedule.

If you especially liked any of last week's outdoor activities, go for it again, or revisit the "Play Heart Activity Menu" on page 80. If you still can't give up your gym-based treadmill or stationary bicycle sessions, we suggest you compromise this week. Do at least one 30-minute gym-based cardio equipment session (preferably the Kilimanjaro Climb on page 283 or an interval-style session), and do one 30-minute outdoor Play Heart activity you haven't done in a long time.

We have another cool suggestion for this week: jumping rope. Ask any boxer—jumping rope is a terrific way to get in shape. All you need is a jump rope and some clear space above you, such as a high-ceilinged gym or the great outdoors. Jumping rope is very intense, so get ready for an awesome Play Heart session. Our friend Buddy Lee, U.S. Olympic wrestler and jump rope training expert, has offered the following 10-minute jump rope plan. (See The Boxer's Workout Quick Tips below.)

1st minute: basic bounce
2nd minute: alternate foot step
3rd minute: combine basic bounce and alternate foot step (4 of each)
4th minute: combine basic bounce and alternate foot step (8 of each)
5th minute: sprint with alternate foot step (180 to 240 rpm)
6th–10th minutes: repeat

If you have trouble jumping rope but still like the idea of training like a boxer, try the Boxer's Workout below. It's an awesome fast-paced and high-intensity sample workout featuring a combination of shadowboxing, heavy bag, and speed bag training. Get yourself some wrist wraps and boxing gloves, and go to work.

Do a Boxer's Workout after two of your Alpha Wave Basic Training workouts this week, and also do one 30-minute outdoor Play Heart activity. Our boxing expert, Ross Enamait, offers the fol-

lowing sample workout, but feel free to change things up from week to week:

- 2 rounds of shadowboxing
- 2 rounds on the heavy bag
- 2 rounds on the speed bag
- 2 rounds of jumping rope

Each round should last between 2 and 3 minutes, with 1 minute of rest between rounds.

Always make sure you wrap your hands and wrists before punching the bag—you could do serious damage without it.

Alpha Fuel Solution

This week you'll continue your Handshake Diet with Man-Hand portions, and you'll generally stick with the Fuel Rules (see page 108). By now you understand why white bread, pasta, and most cereals shouldn't be a main part of your daily diet. But that doesn't mean that the right carbohydrates shouldn't be a part of your diet. They were good for our prehistoric ancestors, and they absolutely will be good for you, too. Here's a refresher on why fruits and vegetables are such an important part of the Alpha Fuel Solution. They have a variety of vitamins, minerals, and antioxidants and help you get the recommended 30 or more grams of daily dietary fiber you need.

Start each day by washing some fruit and leaving it in a bowl on the table or counter for snack-

THE BOXER'S WORKOUT QUICK TIPS

- ◉ Aggressively shadowbox for 2 to 3 minutes, punching with jabs, crosses, hooks, and uppercuts. Keep those knees bent and keep your feet moving during each round.
- ◉ Even if you don't know perfect form, the act of moving your hands and feet will provide a heart-pounding activity.
- ◉ You can always ask a qualified trainer or boxing coach for some boxing basics.
- ◉ Expect muscle soreness in your shoulders—don't go too crazy with the speed of these moves, especially if you have shoulder problems. We guarantee you'll feel these burning!

ing. Always keep some fruit in plain sight! Seedless grapes make a great snack—leave them where you (and others in the household) can readily see them rather than hiding them in a refrigerator drawer. You'll find that they become your first snacking choice.

You can try these or any of the other samples suggested for the weeks that follow. The emphasis is on the fiber-filled, nutritional power of fruits and vegetables.

Breakfast Suggestions

- Nonfat Greek yogurt with berries, pecans, and a teaspoon of 100 percent fresh fruit preserves
- 3 slices of Canadian bacon with 2 poached eggs and a sliced banana with shredded coconut and walnuts

Lunch Suggestions

- Spinach omelet with turkey, spinach, and low-fat cheese
- 5 roll-ups (no bread) consisting of deli-sliced turkey or roast beef and sliced low-fat cheese, plus one piece of fresh fruit

Dinner Suggestions

- Great Buffalo Chili (see page 303) and frozen grapes

- Simplest Chicken Preparation (see page 299) and mixed green salad with choice of dressing (see pages 307–308)

Okay, you're eating lots of fruits and vegetables like you should. So this week we introduce a new bonus: the Feast Meal (see page 118). The Feast Meal is a delicious hero's reward for your efforts this week. However, it's also a test of your mettle—eating the forbidden food for only one meal as allowed but then going right back to the regimen takes commitment and courage.

For *one* meal this week (Sunday dinner, for instance), go ahead and have whatever you want to eat. Whether it's pizza or pasta and a sweet dessert, go ahead and have a feast fit for a hero!

- Just remember, it's just one meal—one appetizer, one entrée, and one dessert. If you deviate from the Alpha Fuel Solution more than once a week, you will slip backward.
- A single "mortal" meal will help you adhere to the Handshake Diet by reducing your sense of self-deprivation.

Crucial caveat: Remember, if your chest-to-waist differential is less than 6 inches or your waist circumference is more than 38 inches, you must limit your Feast Meal to *either* one appetizer,

CREATINE MONOHYDRATE FOR EXTRA MUSCLE

If you want to take it to the max, this week you can add creatine monohydrate to your Alpha Fuel Solution. While this is an optional part of the program and you can get amazing results without it, studies support giving creatine a try if you're looking for maximum muscle-building results (see page 121). Here's the protocol.

- ◎ Buy a creatine monohydrate product, such as a bulk powder, from a reputable manufacturer.
- ◎ Take 20 grams of creatine per serving each day for 5 days straight. After that, take 5 grams per day.
- ◎ Mix creatine powder in a shaker with ½ cup of grape or pomegranate juice and 2 cups of water.
- ◎ Drink it 15 to 30 minutes before your Alpha Wave Basic Training workout, or just before bed on rest days.
- ◎ Take creatine for 6 weeks.

one main course, or one dessert—but only one of the three. If you think you'll have a difficult time getting immediately back on track, you should avoid the Feast Meal until you are ready for the challenge of climbing right back on the wagon (see page 118).

Results

You should be feeling a little more heroic by the end of this week. You have faced the challenges of this week in your Alpha Attitude drill, your Alpha Wave Basic Training, your Work Heart and Play Heart efforts, and in all aspects of the Handshake Diet. You have conquered each with your new sense of courage! On the physical side, you'll likely have some muscle soreness as a result of the switch to a split body part routine and more sets per muscle group. Make sure you've been sticking to the prescribed rest intervals. This is perhaps the most important element to follow to get the greatest results possible.

You're adhering to the terms of your Alpha Bet. You've collected your full 75 Work Heart points, and you've performed at least 60 minutes of Play Heart activity—maybe including some shadowboxing or jumping rope. You've consciously added more fruits and vegetables to your diet—could you ever go back to a toxic diet of junk food? If you are supplementing with creatine to speed up the muscle-building process, you may have begun seeing some increased strength gains. Regardless, you may notice your clothes starting to fit a little looser in the right spots, especially in the waist, and possibly a little more snug in the chest and arms. Just wait: The best is yet to come!

WEEK 4

Alpha Attitude Drill

What separates the true Alpha Male from selfish posers and egotistical wannabes is *conscience,* and empathy is its basis (see pages 46 to 51).

The Native Americans had a saying often translated as, "Judge no man until you walk a mile in his moccasins." The "Moccasin Mile" drill isn't a cardio exercise, so you won't be walking a mile. But you will be putting yourself in another person's shoes for a while. How? By listening. *Really* listening. Here's how it works:

- Engage in a conversation with a person you would not normally talk to, or who you think is boring, off-putting, or even a little scary.
- As you chat with this person, let him be in charge of the conversation.
- Accept what the other person says without judging him. You won't criticize or correct him at all; remember, this doesn't mean you agree with him, only that you are allowing him to have an opinion or point of view that is different from your own, and you are trying to understand it.
- Really listen to what the person is saying. Maintain eye contact and express interest by rephrasing what you hear using your own words, letting him know what you understand his message to be. Try your best to imagine how the other person feels.

Afterward, review how really listening made you feel and think. How did the other person react to it? Rate the quality of the interaction—did you learn something that you may not have known about the other person? One of the most prevalent weaknesses in guys today is a failure to listen. It's a weakness you need to address to be the best man you can be. Learn to enjoy hearing another person's perspective without feeling the need to validate yourself by correcting him or her. Make others feel safe enough to talk about what's really going on in their lives, without fear of being judged or criticized. Being a true Alpha Male isn't about always dominating; it isn't always a battle to see who is right or wrong. Listen and you may learn something important. You'll begin to become the kind of leader that's most respected and admired.

Alpha Architecture Program

ALPHA WAVE BASIC TRAINING (WORKOUTS 10–12)

This is your last week targeting the Muscle Up segment of your training; next week you move on to maximizing strength. We introduce two new strategies this week: the circuit set (see page 60) and an exercise called 21 curls (see page 270). As always, rest at least 1 day between workouts. The total number of sets increases only for level A this week.

Reps (Other Than 21 Curls)
- Power Boost movements: 5 reps
  - Try to do the reps faster than last week.
- Strength Max movements: 5 reps
  - Add weight over last week's poundages.
- Muscle Up movements: 10 reps
  - Add weight over last week's poundages.

Tempo
- Power Boost movements and some abdominal/core movements are performed as quickly as you possibly can (0-0-0-0).
- For most movements, the tempo of all repetitions this week involves an even slower lowering of the weight: 3-0-3-0. These "super-slow" reps will be fluid, but performed very slowly: a highly controlled lowering over 3 seconds and a very controlled lifting of the weight over 3 seconds, with no pauses at the top or bottom. These sets will be up to a full minute long, so the rest between them will be 2 minutes, to permit your training partner to complete his set.

Rest Intervals
- Rest intervals during the Power Boost segments of the workouts are 1.5 minutes.
- Rest intervals during the Strength Max segments of the workouts are 3 minutes.
- Rest intervals during the Muscle Up segments of the workouts are 2 minutes, except:
  - Rest only 1 minute between the first two sets of the circuit set, then 2 minutes after the third.

Here's a tip: At the top of each repetition, always try to achieve a maximum muscle contraction. Outside the gym, occasionally practice isometric contractions (squeezing and flexing) your muscles without moving at your joints. By practicing this static contraction exercise outside the gym or even between sets of exercise, you'll gain a better sense of how a maximum muscle contraction should feel during your exercises.

The circuit sets will be a tough test of your commitment and courage. You will use relatively light weights on the 21 curls, but the high reps combined with the super-slow tempo will produce an intense burn that will test you as never before. But don't surrender, and don't let your training partner surrender! Exercise your empathy—feel his pain—but push him through to the very last rep. As you fatigue, you may have a tendency to close your eyes. Keep those eyes open and bring awareness and focus to yourself. That's why it's helpful to train in front of a mirror, so that you can assess your form and motivate yourself to get the most out of every movement, set, and rep.

Abdominal and/or core exercises finish off each workout; the last repetition should be difficult and intense.

WORKOUT 10
Target: Muscle Up

Dynamic Warmup—All Levels

MOVEMENT	SETS Level A	SETS Level B	SETS Level C	REPS	REST	TEMPO
Speed Skater (each side)	2	2	1	5	1.5	0-0-0-0
Power Row (each arm)	2	2	1	5	1.5	0-0-0-0
Leg Press (Wide Stance)	3	2	1	5	3	3-0-3-0
One Arm Dumbbell Row (each arm)	3	2	1	5	3	3-0-3-0
Flat Barbell Bench Press*	3	3	2	10	2	3-0-3-0
Incline Dumbbell Bench Press*	3	3	2	10	2	3-0-3-0
Flat Dumbbell Fly*	3	2	2	10	2	3-0-3-0
Close-Grip Bench Press	3	2	2	10	2	3-0-3-0
Triceps Pushdown (Rope Attachment)	3	2	2	10	2	3-0-3-0
Standing Calf Raise	3	2	2	10	2	3-0-3-0
Oblique Crunch (each side)	3	2	2	≤15	1	1-0-1-0
Captain's Chair Leg Lift	3	2	2	≤20	1	1-0-1-0
Total	34	26	20			

These three exercises are performed in a consecutive sequence as one circuit set. Rest for 1 minute after the first two exercises and for 2 minutes after completing the whole circuit set.

WORKOUT 11
Target: Muscle Up

Dynamic Warmup—All Levels

MOVEMENT	SETS Level A	SETS Level B	SETS Level C	REPS	REST	TEMPO
Clean and Power Press (Alternate: Push Press)	2	2	1	5	1.5	0-0-0-0
Full-Body Resisted Cable or Tubing Extension	2	2	1	5	1.5	0-0-0-0
Chest Dips with Weights	3	2	1	5	3	3-0-3-0
Stiff-Legged Deadlifts	3	2	1	5	3	3-0-3-0
Chinups or Chindowns*	3	3	2	10	2	3-0-3-0
Machine Row* (Neutral Grip)	3	3	2	10	2	3-0-3-0
Lat Dumbbell Pullovers*	3	3	2	10	2	3-0-3-0
Dumbbell Shrug (Seated)	3	3	2	10	2	3-0-3-0
Barbell Curl (Narrow Grip)	3	3	2	10	2	3-0-3-0
21 Curls	3	3	2	21	2	3-0-3-0
Samurai Swing (Cable or Tube)	3	2	2	10	1	0-0-0-0
The Plank	3	2	2	>1.5 min	1	N/A
Total	34	30	20			

These three exercises are performed in a consecutive sequence as one circuit set. Rest for 1 minute after the first two exercises and for 2 minutes after completing the whole circuit set.

WORKOUT 12
Target: Muscle Up

Dynamic Warmup—All Levels

MOVEMENT	SETS Level A	SETS Level B	SETS Level C	REPS	REST	TEMPO
Power Pushup	2	2	1	5	1.5	0-0-0-0
Barbell Upright Power Row	2	2	1	5	1.5	0-0-0-0
Barbell Squat	3	2	1	5	3	3-0-3-0
Lying Leg Curl	3	2	1	5	3	3-0-3-0
Barbell Lunge (each leg)	3	3	2	10	2	3-0-3-0
Leg Extension	3	3	2	10	2	3-0-3-0
Seated Calf Raise	3	3	2	10	2	3-0-3-0
Dumbbell Shoulder Press*	3	3	2	10	2	3-0-3-0
Lateral Raise (Cable)*	3	3	2	10	2	3-0-3-0
Bent-Over Dumbbell Lateral Raise*	3	3	2	10	2	3-0-3-0
Swiss Ball Throw+	3	2	2	10	1	0-0-0-0
Bicycle Maneuver (each side)	3	2	2	≤25	1	0-0-0-0
Total	34	30	20			

*These three exercises are performed in a consecutive sequence as one circuit set. Rest for 1 minute after the first two exercises and for 2 minutes after completing the whole circuit set.
+If training without a partner, perform the Swiss ball crunch with weight.

WORK HEART SYSTEM

This week we only ask you to maintain the same Work Heart time commitment as last week. However, it's crucial that even though there's no increase in time commitment, you kicked up the intensity level yet another notch. Whether you're briskly walking or doing any other type of Work Heart activity, put more heart into the work than ever before.

- During each workday (5 days weekly), your objective is to collect 15 points (15 minutes' worth of Work Heart).
- Focus not on the exact time but rather on making the best use of each activity.
- Your level of effort this week—the heart in your Work Heart—must be greater than last week's.
- Fail to collect all 15 points and you lose all credit for that day.
- You need **75 points** by week's end to meet the Challenge.

PLAY HEART ACTIVITIES

We didn't add a single second to your Work Heart investment this week, but that's not true for your Play Heart requirement. This week, we boost your Play Heart activity time to a minimum of 75 minutes, which can be broken into two 35- to 40-minute sessions or three 25-minute sessions. As always, the best option is the one that works within your schedule.

You can choose any one of the options presented in the "Play Heart Activity Menu" (under "Alpha Active" and "Alpha Action" only) on page 79.

Alpha Fuel Solution

Continue your Handshake Diet and Man-Hand portion control. Maintain your creatine supplementation, if applicable. Don't forget to drink plenty of water, leave some fruit out each day for snacking, and make a dozen hard-boiled eggs to snack on through the week.

A strict Stone Age diet would make any dairy

product off-limits, but we think that the high levels of protein, calcium, and vitamin D in these items—and their relatively low cost—make them worthy of a role in the Alpha Fuel Solution. The key is to consume them in modest amounts and avoid full-fat varieties. Try some of this week's suggested meals highlighting healthy dairy choices.

Breakfast Suggestions

- Nonfat cottage cheese with sliced apples, banana, and walnuts (optional: add a packet of calorie-free sweetener to taste)
- Blender smoothie with two scoops (we prefer chocolate) whey protein, skim milk, nonfat Greek yogurt, peanut or almond butter, and ice

Lunch Suggestions

- Three-cheese egg-white omelet with spinach and sun-dried tomatoes
- Warm sliced grilled chicken cutlet with lettuce, salsa, and low-fat cheese in a whole grain wrap

Dinner Suggestions

- Shrimp stir-fry in reduced-sodium soy sauce and macadamia nut oil with water chestnuts, fresh ginger, and Chinese vegetables (add hot red pepper to taste), and fresh papaya
- Lean pork tenderloin, mixed salad with Gorgonzola cheese and walnuts, and one medium orange or pear

You can have one Feast Meal (see page 118) this week. If your chest-to-waist differential is still less than 6 inches or your waist circumference is more than 38 inches, you must again limit your Feast Meal to *either* one appetizer, one main course, or one dessert—but only one of the three. Pretty good incentive to get that belly off fast!

Results

You should be settling into the routine of Alpha Wave Basic Training, hopefully with a buddy or two. Your body has gotten stronger; the limits of your physical capabilities have stretched and expanded. However, no single workout is perfect for everybody. If you find that certain exercises hurt you or that you feel decidedly more comfortable with some exercises than others, by all means follow your instincts—as long as you're not just letting yourself off easy! Just make sure that the alternative exercise that you choose focuses on the same muscle group, and always use proper form. You'll find a list of alternatives in "Alpha Wave Home Body/Substitutes" in Chapter 4 for tips on other exercises.

We know how hard you're pushing yourself; we also know that rest is not usually part of a man's vocabulary. It is essential that you get enough rest if you expect the greatest results to occur. Adequate rest in between workouts and the prescribed rest intervals between sets must both be kept to, to ensure your greatest workout results.

You've collected your full 75 Work Heart points, and you've performed at least 75 minutes of Play Heart activity—maybe you took our suggestion and tried a martial arts or white collar boxing class. You're eating healthier than ever before. If you've opted to use creatine monohydrate, you may notice a little added strength boost from the creatine supplementation—just in time for next week's switch to targeted Strength Max training.

Take a moment to think about how far you've come. You're rapidly approaching the halfway point of the Challenge. Yes, there's heightened intensity ahead and a few surprises, but you're likely getting more overall exercise than you have in years. And much of it is being woven into the fabric of your daily life—the key to making the changes permanent. You've now begun to put your new attitude to good use toward both fulfilling your own needs and goals and becoming more effective in your caring and concern for those around you. That is the essence of the true Alpha Male. Each week, you come closer to that ideal.

WEEK 5

Alpha Attitude Drill

You've spent 4 weeks exploring the four Cs of Alpha Attitude one by one. But the drills are only a mechanism to start you thinking about how you can incorporate Alpha Attitude into your everyday life. This week you'll look for one single but memorable opportunity to exercise any or all of your four Cs. Here are some suggestions:

- Exercise your commitment muscles by working one extra Play Heart activity into this week's schedule. How about 30 minutes of hill sprints or a run on the beach? Or treadmill work—either the Kilimanjaro or Savage Mountain (K2) Sprint Training.
- Exercise your confidence muscles by tackling a long-neglected task. All of us have some things that we have wanted to get to, that we see every day and know need doing, but have always put off. This is the time to put that newfound attitude to work.
- Exercise your courage muscles by daring to surpass your previous efforts in the gym in this, your first week of Strength Max training. You'll face the Punisher this week—a fearsome test of your fortitude. Conquer it by attaining an unprecedented level of ferocious intensity.
- Exercise your conscience muscles by playing the "Random Acts of Kindness" game. Spend 1 day this week committing random acts of kindness for those around you. You have 1 hour from leaving your house that day to commit your first one. It could be offering help to someone who needs it. It could be buying a surprise gift for someone who deserves it. It could be giving a homeless man a sandwich. It could be simply letting the other guy go first at the checkout counter or in traffic. A true Alpha Male isn't always looking out for

numero uno. He's developing higher order social skills to be respected and admired. Let the other guy go first, and instead establish your dominance when you get to the gym and face the challenge of your next Alpha Wave Basic Training workout.

Alpha Architecture Program

ALPHA WAVE BASIC TRAINING (WORKOUTS 13–15)

You now switch your primary focus to maximizing strength, while continuing to advance the gains made over the past 4 weeks of muscle building and laying the groundwork for boosting power. You'll be focusing on the Strength Max movements in each workout. As always, rest at least 1 day between workouts. The total number of sets for all levels increases this week.

This week we introduce to all levels an innovative and extremely intense strategy: the Punisher (see page 60). The Punisher is a savage test of your commitment, courage, and endurance. You'll do 100 reps of an exercise, pausing only as needed. You will perform the Punisher on three muscle groups this week: calves, biceps, and hamstrings.

Reps (Other Than The Punisher)

- Power Boost movements: 4 reps
  - ⓘ Try to do the reps faster than last week.
- Strength Max movements: 6 reps
  - ⓘ Maintain last week's poundages.
- Muscle Up movements: 15 reps
  - ⓘ Try to maintain last week's poundages.

Tempo

- Power Boost movements and some abdominal/core movements are performed as quickly as you possibly can (0-0-0-0).
- For most movements, the tempo of all repetitions this week is 2-0-1-0. That means a fluid,

natural tempo but with a decidedly emphasized lowering of the weight and 1 second raising it, with no pauses at the top or bottom. The Punisher movements, however, will be performed at 1-0-1-0.

Rest Intervals

- Rest intervals during the Power Boost segments of the workouts are 1.5 minutes.
- Rest intervals during the Strength Max segments of the workouts are 2.5 minutes.
- Rest intervals during the Muscle Up segments of the workouts are 1 minute—just long enough to permit a partner to complete his set, change weights if necessary, and position yourself for the next set.
- For the Punisher, each partner will complete all 100 reps before the other does his 100 reps.

Note that your Power Boost movement reps are lower than they were last week. Because you'll have fewer reps to perform, you should either add weight for resistance-based Power Boost movements or increase the speed of the movement whenever you can.

Abdominal and/or core exercises finish off each workout. The last repetition should be difficult and intense.

WORKOUT 13
Target: Strength Max

Dynamic Warmup—All Levels

MOVEMENT	SETS Level A	SETS Level B	SETS Level C	REPS	REST	TEMPO
Lunge Jump (each leg)	2	2	1	4	1.5	0-0-0-0
Multidirectional Hop	2	2	1	4	1.5	0-0-0-0
Flat Barbell Bench Press	3	2	2	6	2.5	2-0-1-0
Incline Dumbbell Bench Press	3	2	2	6	2.5	2-0-1-0
Incline Dumbbell Fly	3	2	2	6	2.5	2-0-1-0
Chest Dumbbell Pullover	3	2	2	6	2.5	2-0-1-0
Triceps Dip	3	2	2	6	2.5	2-0-1-0
Dumbbell Skull Crusher	3	2	2	6	2.5	2-0-1-0
Weighted Stepup (each leg)	2	2	1	15	1	2-0-1-0
Leg Press Calf Press Punisher*	>1	>1	>1	100	Minimum	1-0-1-0
Grand Slam (Cable or Tubing)	3	2	2	12	1	0-0-0-0
Bench Leg Lift	3	2	2	≤25	1	1-0-1-0
Total	>31	>23	>20			

*All levels: Do 100 reps in as short a time as possible using a weight with which you can do 30 to 50 reps without stopping.

WORKOUT 14
Target: Strength Max

Dynamic Warmup—All Levels

MOVEMENT	SETS Level A	SETS Level B	SETS Level C	REPS	REST	TEMPO
Tuck Jump	2	2	1	4	1.5	0-0-0-0
Push Jump to Bench	2	2	1	4	1.5	0-0-0-0
Lat Pullup or Pulldown	3	2	2	6	2.5	2-0-1-0
T-Bar Row	3	2	2	6	2.5	2-0-1-0
Seated Cable Row	3	2	2	6	2.5	2-0-1-0
Lat Dumbbell Pullover	3	2	2	6	2.5	2-0-1-0
Barbell Shrug	3	2	2	6	2.5	2-0-1-0
Preacher Curl Machine	3	2	2	6	2.5	2-0-1-0
Incline Dumbbell Curl	3	2	2	15	1	2-0-1-0
Reverse EZ-Bar Curl Punisher*	>1	>1	>1	100	Minimum	1-0-1-0
Captain's Chair Leg Lift	3	2	2	≤25	1	1-0-1-0
Partner-Assisted Twisting Leg Throw**	3	2	2	8 each side	1	1-0-1-0
Total	>32	>23	21			

*All levels: Do 100 reps in as short a time as possible using a weight with which you can do 30 to 40 reps without stopping.
**If training without a partner, perform the Swiss ball crunch with weight.

WORKOUT 15
Target: Strength Max

Dynamic Warmup—All Levels

MOVEMENT	SETS Level A	SETS Level B	SETS Level C	REPS	REST	TEMPO
Barbell Upright Power Row	2	2	1	4	1.5	0-0-0-0
Power Pushup	2	2	1	4	1.5	0-0-0-0
Leg Press (Wide-Stance)	3	2	2	6	2.5	2-0-1-0
Smith Machine Hack Squat	3	2	2	6	2.5	2-0-1-0
Dumbbell Squat	3	2	2	6	2.5	2-0-1-0
Standing Barbell Shoulder Press	3	2	2	6	2.5	2-0-1-0
Dumbbell Lateral Raise (Standing)	3	2	2	6	2.5	2-0-1-0
Rear Deltoid Machine	3	2	2	6	2.5	2-0-1-0
Donkey Calf Raise	2	2	1	15	1	2-0-1-0
Seated Leg Curl Punisher*	>1	>1	>1	100	Minimum	1-0-1-0
Swiss Ball Crunch	3	2	2	≤25	1	1-0-1-0
Samurai Swing (Cable or Tubing)	3	2	2	10	1	0-0-0-0
Total	>31	>23	>20			

*All levels: Do 100 reps in as short a time as possible using a weight with which you can do 30 to 40 reps without stopping.

WORK HEART SYSTEM

This week we ratchet up your Work Heart time commitment a bit higher than last week. Here's your Work Heart overview for Week 5.

- During each workday (5 days weekly), your objective is to collect 20 points (20 minutes' worth of Work Heart).
- Focus not on the exact time, but rather on making the best use of each activity.
- Your level of effort this week—the heart in your Work Heart—must be equal to or greater than last week's.
- Fail to collect all 20 points and you lose all credit for that day.
- You need **100 points** by week's end to meet the Challenge.

If you need fresh ideas on how to best fit the Work Heart system into your day, check out www.alphamalechallenge.com. Some guys like to book-end each workday with 10 minutes of Work Heart effort. That certainly doesn't seem like much extra effort, does it? If you already have a co-worker committed to Work Heart efforts with you, by all means continue, even if it means a solid block of 20 minutes during the workday. Recognize that by getting all 100 points, you'll now be adding more than 1½ hours of fat-burning Work Heart effort to your week as compared to your days before the Challenge! Watch that belly fat melt away and those rock-hard abdominals start showing through!

PLAY HEART ACTIVITIES

This week, we hold steady on your Play Heart activity time, keeping it to a minimum of 75 minutes. Again, the time can be broken into two 35- to 40-minute sessions or three 25-minute sessions, with the best option being the one that works within your schedule.

This week, however, we're going to impose a different restriction: You should do *no* gym-based treadmill or stationary bicycle sessions. That means no gym-based machine cardio, period! The treadmill will survive without you.

- If your two or three Play Heart sessions take place at your gym or health club, they must *not* be based on equipment (treadmill, stair-climber, or bicycle); they can, however, be composed of jumping rope, shadowboxing, or punching the speed bag or heavy bag
- Better yet, refer to the "Play Heart Activity Menu" on page 79, choosing from the "Alpha Active" or "Alpha Action" lists. How about pickup basketball? It may have been a while since you played hoops, but basketball is a great cardiovascular exercise. Some of the bigger health club chains have courts where you can get involved, or you can find a game in your area at many online sports networking sites.
- How about racquetball or squash? The pace can be brutal, so this highly competitive sport can be quite an intense workout. Why not challenge your training partner to a game? Or challenge a family member or friend to a game of tennis or handball on an outside court? Fresh air is terrific, and competition is awesome for your Alpha Factor.

Want to grab 25 minutes of Play Heart credit for less than half that time? Here's the deal: You can shave 25 minutes off your Play Heart minute minimum this week by taking the following special but simple challenge: Run 1 mile.

- Measure out 1 mile, either on a local track, at a park, or in a suitable neighborhood area.
- Warm up thoroughly—you don't want to run with cold knees, hips, and back.
- Pace yourself! If you're not a runner, a good starting goal is a pace of 2 minutes per ¼ mile (an 8-minute mile).

If you're a level-C trainer or you haven't tried a mile run in years, be careful. It's okay if a mile run takes longer than 9 minutes. Level B trainers should seek to meet or break that 8-minute mile marker, and the top dogs and level-A trainers should try to beat a 7-minute mile.

When you've caught your breath, write down your time here: _____.

Alpha Fuel Solution

Stick with the Handshake Diet and Man-Hand portions, and your creatine plan, if applicable. However, this week we make a minor adjustment. Your diet this week is even closer to what preagricultural folks ate, except for the dairy. We know you've greatly limited the bread, pasta, and cereal, but this week we cut it out completely—including whole wheat products and oatmeal. Go ahead and shop for all your favorite fresh meats, chicken, fish, fruits, and vegetables. But this week's Challenge is not one single piece of bread or cereal, and not one bit of pasta or rice. (Use cauliflower in place of rice beneath stir-fries and in place of pasta under homemade meat sauce.) You can go back to eating healthy grain and rice products in limited quantities next week. But this week we test your willpower with this simple challenge. Get creative—you'll be surprised at the delicious non-starchy concoctions you can come up with!

For many guys, the toughest meal is lunch. Having a wrap or sandwich is quick and easy. But sandwiches and wraps are out this week. However, there's an easy solution. Rather than a grilled chicken breast wrap, have grilled chicken breast on a bed of salad greens. You can do the same with ½ pound of lean deli roast beef and mustard. Virtually any diner or deli will take the meat-and-vegetable ingredients of your average wrap and put them in a fresh lettuce wrap with some balsamic vinegar and olive oil, instead. Of course, omelet dishes are always an acceptable lunch alternative, as long as you tell your server to hold the toast and hash browns. Or how about a mean (and delicious!) chili with a jar of salsa, two cans

of no-sodium tomatoes, and a pound of lean ground beef with a healthy dose of red pepper flakes and fresh cilantro?

You fully know the importance of protein in the Alpha Fuel Solution (see page 101), and this week we want to highlight the value of both chicken and turkey as terrific low-fat sources of great taste and enough protein to kick-start your Alpha Factor with absolutely *no* bread, pasta, rice, or cereal.

Breakfast Suggestions

- Diced grilled chicken scrambled into packaged egg whites with low-fat cheese, spicy salsa, spinach, and fresh cilantro
- Low-fat turkey bacon or sausage and mixed fresh fruit chunks (prepared the night before)

Lunch Suggestions

- No-bun turkey burger with low-fat cheese and mixed green salad with oil and flavored vinegar
- Hot grilled chicken cutlet with balsamic vinegar, plus olives, raw carrots, cucumber, and celery sticks

Dinner Suggestions

- Kebabs with grilled chicken, onion, tomato, pineapple chunks, red pepper, and reduced-sodium soy sauce, plus an apple with peanut butter
- Fresh turkey breast, romaine lettuce, and radishes with Dijon balsamic dressing

Of course, feel free to mix in some mouthwatering fish, shellfish, lean pork, and red meat choices as well. And yes, you can have your Feast Meal this week with the crucial caveat (page 118).

Results

How do you feel? Week 5 is a great time to take stock. By now you've tested yourself in ways you never thought you would, and as you approach the halfway point of your Challenge you have new information about how to do things differently and what happens when you do. Have you been true to your Alpha Bet? Look back, see what worked and what didn't, and plot your course for success over the next 5 weeks. And if you fell short in any regard, it's time to bounce back for the weeks to come. That's what we call resiliency—our capacity to take a risk, learn from it, and then use that new knowledge to do better next time. What can you do better? Are you sticking to the training and following all of the training variables, such as your rest intervals between sets? Are you following the Handshake Diet just as we've laid it out for you? Are you working on your true Alpha Attitude by performing your weekly drills? The more committed and confident you are, the more power you give yourself to excel in all things. Again, take inventory and make sure that you are covering all areas of the program. If you do slip at any point, do not delay and immediately get back in the saddle.

This may have been a tough week for some bread and pasta lovers, but take solace in the fact that you're stronger for having survived this week. With only 3 days of Alpha Wave Basic Training each week, you should have plenty of time to get your workouts in.

Collecting your Work Heart points should be getting even easier by now, as you become more and more habituated to the system. And getting in your Play Heart activities shouldn't be a problem, especially if you've incorporated your family into the activities or are doing them with a training partner or buddies. If you're making challenging and athletic Play Heart choices, you will no doubt be noticing the dividends from your Power Boost training. When it comes to improving your athletic performance in sports or on functional activities—jumping, running, twisting, throwing—nothing

beats Power Boost movements. That's why they're such an essential part of your program.

Of course, if you hit any snags, visit us at www.alphamalechallenge.com for our tips on getting the very most out of your 10-week Challenge. Now take a deep breath and prepare for Week 6—you're going to strengthen and deepen your commitment to being your best!

WEEK 6
Alpha Attitude Drill

It's time to make your commitment to the Challenge even stronger. You've come this far and you're already stronger for it. This week you'll be putting your *willpower* to the test by putting your head in the "Lion's Mouth." Remember the more you exercise your willpower, the stronger it will get.

Here's what you'll do 1 non-gym day this week:

- Write down your favorite fast food or take-out junk food. Is it burgers, pizza, fries, shakes, ice cream, or frozen coffee drinks?
- Pick a place where you've indulged in this food many times.
- Find a healthy alternative served there, such as a chicken salad or a low-fat, low-sugar product.
- Instead of letting the automatic pilot program run, you're going to take charge. That's right: You're going to walk into the gladiator pit, stick your head into the lion's mouth, and accept the challenge. You're going to order that healthy alternative instead of your favorite fast food.

Prepare yourself right now. Think about the sights and smells you will encounter. Acknowledge the fact that when you walk up to the counter you will be tempted to jettison the plan and order your favorite. In fact, the person behind the counter might very well push your oversized favorites on you. Don't give in! This is your opportunity to build your willpower muscle, to change the way things usually go. Do what most ordinary guys won't—stick to your true Alpha Male guns and eat healthy; you'll create a new experience and challenge those old ways of doing things.

Afterward, take a few moments to reflect on what just happened:

- *You* made the choice; how did you do it?
- *You* took control; what did you say to yourself to stay on track if the old plan started to emerge, if temptation reared its ugly head?
- *You* proved that you can master temptation; it doesn't control you. You mastered the challenge.

Now what?

- Avoid putting yourself back into another tough situation for the rest of the day.
- Allow your willpower muscle to rest and recover.
- With proper rest, the science says you will be even stronger tomorrow.

And remember, you now have the evidence that you control what you do. No more automatic thoughts like "I can't resist this, I have to have this." Now you know you are in charge! Doesn't it feel good to be *in control*? Take the bull by the horns and make your commitment to lasting change in all areas of your life.

Alpha Architecture Program

ALPHA WAVE BASIC TRAINING (WORKOUTS 16–18)

This week we again focus on maximizing strength, but we also throw a new strategy into the mix: the superset (see page 60). The superset consists of two exercises performed without any rest in between, other than the time it takes to move from one station to another. Supersets *burn*. When it starts burning, you or your training partner is going to want to give up. That's natural. But don't do it. You now have the commitment to see it through to the end. Don't surrender!

Reps (Other Than Supersets)
- Power Boost movements: 3 reps
  - Try to do the reps faster than last week.
- Strength Max movements: 4 reps
  - Add weight to last week's poundages.
- Muscle Up movements: 15 reps
  - Try to maintain last week's poundages.

Tempo
- Power Boost movements and some abdominal/core movements are performed as quickly as you possibly can (0-0-0-0).
- For most movements, the tempo of all repetitions this week involves a slow lowering of the weight: 3-0-1-0. That still means a fluid tempo, but with a much longer and more controlled lowering of the weight and then 1 second raising it, with no pauses at the top or bottom (see page 60).

Rest Intervals
- Rest intervals during the Power Boost segments of the workouts are 1.5 minutes.
- Rest intervals during the Strength Max segments of the workouts are 2.5 minutes.
- Rest intervals during the Muscle Up segments of the workouts are 2 minutes.
- There's no rest between the two superset exercises, but rest for 3 minutes between supersets.

Abdominal and/or core exercises finish off each workout. The number of reps will be as many as you can do, up to 20. The last repetition should be difficult and intense.

WORKOUT 16
Target: Strength Max

Dynamic Warmup—All Levels

MOVEMENT	SETS Level A	SETS Level B	SETS Level C	REPS	REST	TEMPO
Squat Jump	2	2	1	3	1.5	0-0-0-0
Lateral Bench/Box Push-Off Jump (each leg)	2	2	1	3	1.5	0-0-0-0
Incline Barbell Bench Press	3	2	2	4	2.5	3-0-1-0
Flat Dumbbell Bench Press	3	2	2	4	2.5	3-0-1-0
Pec Deck Fly	3	2	2	4	2.5	3-0-1-0
Chest Dip	3	2	2	4	2.5	3-0-1-0
Close-Grip Bench Press *Supersetted with* *	3	2	2	4	2.5	3-0-1-0
Triceps Pushdown* (V-Bar Attachment)	3	2	2	4	2.5	3-0-1-0
Triceps X-Tension	2	2	1	15	1.5	3-0-1-0
Standing Calf Raise	2	2	1	15	1.5	3-0-1-0
Floor Crunch	3	2	2	≤15	1	1-0-1-0
Superman Back Extension	3	2	2	≤20	1	1-0-1-0
Total	32	24	20			

These supersets are very difficult. Set the weight so you barely get your reps. Take only enough time to change exercise stations between the two exercises, but be sure to rest for the full 3 minutes in between supersets.

WORKOUT 17
Target: Strength Max

Dynamic Warmup—All Levels

MOVEMENT	SETS Level A	SETS Level B	SETS Level C	REPS	REST	TEMPO
Situp and Pike	2	2	1	3	1.5	0-0-0-0
Forward-Backward Cone Hop	2	2	1	3	1.5	0-0-0-0
Romanian Deadlift	3	2	2	4	2.5	3-0-1-0
Chinup or Chindown (Weighted)	3	2	2	4	2.5	3-0-1-0
One Arm Dumbbell Row (each arm)	3	2	2	4	2.5	3-0-1-0
Lat Dumbbell Pullover *Supersetted with* *	3	2	2	4	2.5	3-0-1-0
Machine Row (Neutral Grip)*	3	2	2	4	2.5	3-0-1-0
Dumbbell Curl (Standing)	3	2	2	4	2.5	3-0-1-0
Barbell Curl (Wide Grip)	2	2	1	15	1.5	3-0-1-0
Reverse EZ-Bar Curl	2	2	1	15	1.5	3-0-1-0
Bicycle Maneuver	3	2	2	≤25	1	0-0-0-0
Bench Leg Lift	3	2	2	≤25	1	1-0-1-0
Total	32	24	20			

These supersets are very difficult. Set the weight so you barely get your reps. Take only enough time to change exercise stations between the two exercises, but be sure to rest for the full 3 minutes in between supersets.

WORKOUT 18
Target: Strength Max

Dynamic Warmup—All Levels

MOVEMENT	SETS Level A	SETS Level B	SETS Level C	REPS	REST	TEMPO
Power Pushup	2	2	1	3	1.5	0-0-0-0
Power Row (each arm)	2	2	1	3	1.5	0-0-0-0
Barbell Squat	3	2	2	4	2.5	3-0-1-0
Weighted Stepup (each leg)	3	2	2	4	2.5	3-0-1-0
Cross the River (each leg)	3	2	2	4	2.5	3-0-1-0
Lying Leg Curl	3	2	2	4	2.5	3-0-1-0
Stiff-Legged Deadlift	3	2	2	4	2.5	3-0-1-0
Dumbbell Shoulder Press	3	2	2	4	2.5	3-0-1-0
Lateral Raise (Cable) *Supersetted with**	2	2	1	15	1.5	3-0-1-0
Rear Deltoid Machine*	2	2	1	15	1.5	3-0-1-0
Grand Slam (Cable or Tubing)	3	2	2	15	1	0-0-0-0
Swiss Ball Throw**	3	2	2	15	1	0-0-0-0
Total	32	24	20			

*These supersets are very difficult. Set the weight so you barely get your reps. Take only enough time to change exercise stations between the two exercises, but be sure to rest for the full 3 minutes in between supersets.
**If training without a partner, perform the Swiss ball crunch with weight.

WORK HEART SYSTEM

By now you've likely developed a personalized approach to your Work Heart system. Keep it going! Your Work Heart time commitment this week is increased from Week 5.

- During each workday (5 days weekly), your objective is to collect 25 points (25 minutes' worth of Work Heart).
- Focus not on the exact time, but rather on making the best use of each activity.
- Your level of effort this week—the heart in your Work Heart—must be equal to or greater than last week's.
- Fail to collect all 25 points and you lose all credit for that day.
- You need **125 points** by week's end to meet the Challenge.

Now, here's the new twist for Week 6:

- If you've been doing your Work Heart efforts empty-handed, it's time to add a load, such as a weighted backpack. If you've been carrying a briefcase, make it heavier (and always switch hands for balanced effort). If you have a pre-existing back problem, either skip adding weight or be sure to start out with a light load and gradually build up over the next few weeks.
- If you have a co-worker committed to Work Heart efforts with you, encourage him or her to add a load, as well. After all, you're in this together!

PLAY HEART ACTIVITIES

This week, we ratchet up your Play Heart activity time to a minimum of 90 minutes, which can be broken into two 45-minute sessions or three 30-minute sessions. The best option is the one that works within your schedule.

You can do *one* gym-based treadmill or stationary bicycle session this week (preferably the Kilimanjaro 20-Minute Walking Climb or the Savage Mountain (K2) Sprint Training), but no more. The balance of your Play Heart activity may *not* be based on equipment (treadmill, stair-climber, or bicycle); if they occur at the gym, they must either be shadowboxing, jumping rope, or punching the speed bag or heavy bag, or else a competitive game such as pickup hoops or racquetball. Why? Because we want you to test and develop your confidence by facing new and different challenges, especially competitive ones! Again, visit the "Play Heart Activity Menu" on page 79. Only choose from the "Alpha Active" or "Alpha Action" lists.

Alpha Fuel Solution

Stick with the Handshake Diet and Man-Hand portions, and your creatine plan, if applicable. Last week you tested yourself by eliminating all grain products from your diet—and you survived. You've proven you have a warrior's heart! And this week you have the Lion's Mouth drill—a tough exercise for many guys. But now there's good news and bad news. The good news is that this week we're suggesting the most delicious red meat dishes you can devise. What guy doesn't love a juicy charbroiled steak? The bad news:

- *No* Feast Meal this week!

No matter how lean you are, there's no Feast Meal this week. After all, this is a week focusing on commitment. Are you committed, or not? We know you are! But don't worry: You may not even notice the lack of a Feast Meal, given all the mouthwatering red meat selections you can savor.

We recommend that you treat yourself to a few gourmet meat meals this week. Remember eating red meats is a great way to naturally boost your testosterone levels. Lean beef provides a combination of protein, zinc, magnesium, iron, and B vitamins (especially B_{12}), all good stuff for your Alpha Factor. Other meats, including lean pork loin, also provide a hearty helping of muscle-building protein.

Now, before you start bingeing nightly at the local steakhouse, note that we said lean meats. All red meats are not created equal (see page 105). Choose cuts that are low in saturated fat. Here are general rules on making meat healthier and lower in saturated fat:

- Buy meat from a store and cook it yourself.
- Choose grass-fed beef, if possible.
- Trim off all visible fat.
- Don't add butter, as some restaurants do.
- Grill or marinate; never deep-fry.
- Always marinate before cooking (see page 107).

Although you can't have a Feast Meal, you can enjoy a first-class gourmet menu all week.

Breakfast Suggestions

- Ham and low-fat cheese packaged egg white omelet with mushrooms and diced peppers, plus mixed citrus fruits (grapefruit and orange chunks) with shredded coconut and slivered almonds
- Steak and egg platter and bran crisps with nonfat cream cheese

Lunch Suggestions

- Omelet with 2 whole eggs, 3 egg whites, tomato, peppers, and feta cheese
- Deli-sliced roast beef with lettuce and sun-dried tomatoes and horseradish on Ezekiel bread, mixed greens, and one piece of fresh fruit

Dinner Suggestions

- Broiled veal sirloin and mixed salad with Pepper-Based Vina-great (see page 308)
- Shrimp and steak mixed with spicy lime salsa and spread over reduced-sodium canned beans, plus mixed mango and papaya chunks

Why not treat yourself to a bowl of fresh raspberries and blackberries? How about some strawberries and kiwis? If you like shrimp, thaw some frozen tail-on shrimp, add a little dab of cocktail sauce, and have a mouthwatering snack.

Results

Without a Feast Meal this week, you were forced to dig deep into your commitment resources to get through. They will be stronger than ever now, and next week your Feast Meal will be all the more delicious. You should be feeling more committed than ever to the Challenge. The more time you've invested—6 full weeks now—the more foolish it would be to surrender to weakness or laziness. You are strong enough to see it through to the end.

If you really enjoyed the gourmet red meat options this week, you may have hardly noticed the lack of a Feast Meal. Start thinking about simple, natural foods—shrimp, berries, and macadamia nuts, for example—as the true gourmet treats they are. Do you really miss all that salt and sugar and high-fructose corn syrup? Doesn't it feel good to be free and clear of all the junk food and heavily processed foods that so many people put into their bodies?

It should be even easier now to stick to your Alpha Bet, as the various facets of the Challenge become woven into the fabric of your everyday life. You've collected your full 125 Work Heart points, and you've performed at least 90 minutes of Play Heart activity. If you're choosing competitive Play Heart options, you'll find that Alpha Wave Basic Training—especially the Power Boost movements—is dramatically improving your performance. And by now you should be seeing some major changes in the way you look and feel. Your Alpha Factor is rising. Others are probably noticing!

WEEK 7

Alpha Attitude Drill

Most guys would say that the single most important ingredient in masculine mojo is raw confidence. That confidence often comes out of a sense that you can competently handle yourself in whatever circumstances life throws at you.

You can drive the highways searching for a distressed maiden in need of a fixed flat tire, but these days, that might not be the best of ideas. Perhaps you can just go out and do things that you can improve at, and even master. *Be* the taskmaster. There's an endless variety of activities and tasks that will build competence—check out the suggestions on page 41.

Be sure to get proper instruction if it's something you've never tried before. After all, the point is to build a sense of competence, not to undermine it. The idea here is to get your hands dirty doing things that most guys now just "call a man" to do. Even if it's something as simple as washing and waxing the family car, those with an aversion to manual labor will derive a nice shot of competence. Nothing needed around the hacienda this week? Well, then why not offer to help a friend or neighbor? You can ask your training partner whether he needs a hand with anything over the weekend.

If you work with your hands all the time, then try taking a different tack.

- How about taking an online or local adult education course?
- How about learning a new language or new computer skills?
- Look into that side business that you never made the time to research—it could be more than worth your while.

The possibilities are endless. You may find that becoming a student again brings with it an excitement you may not have felt back in your full-time student days. Meanwhile, you can also find recreational activities that will build your sense of competence in your physical abilities. These may be things you have always wanted to do but have never had the time for.

- Have you ever tried horseback riding, skiing, snowboarding, surfing, triathlon sports, rock climbing, hiking the forest, mountain biking, kayaking, sport fishing, Frisbee, or golf? Check out the list of "Alpha Active" and "Alpha Action" activities on page 79, and go for it!

- How about a brainstorming session with your workout partners? It doesn't just have to be about fitness. You'll be surprised at what you will collectively come up with, especially with like-minded friends.

Remember, it is always good to get off the couch and being active is great, but the goal here is to build competence and change the way you see yourself. Even playing chess or poker is a terrific way to build a sense of competence—and winning can boost your testosterone levels! Of course, competition doesn't need to be against anyone else. Competing against your own past personal best is a fantastic method of building competence, and doing it outdoors is even better. You can measure factors such as time or distance and seeking to improve them for a variety of pursuits, including sprinting, swimming, skiing, rock climbing, or hiking. Other great options are the many new opportunities for "adventure travel" or "extreme travel" expeditions. Post your experiences on the forum at www.alphamalechallenge.com.

Alpha Architecture Program

ALPHA WAVE BASIC TRAINING (WORKOUTS 19–21)

This week is the last of our 3 weeks targeting the Strength Max movements. We also return to our old friend the drop set (see page 60). Only this time, *all* levels will be incorporating drop sets. The same 20 percent drops will apply, but the repetition ranges will be lower than before: Do 5 reps, drop weight and do another 5 reps, then drop again and do 4 or 5 more reps (for a total of 14 or 15). The weights used will be comparatively heavier than before. This advanced technique will

push your physical limits; if you train with a partner, push him as hard as possible, but be mindful—and empathic—as to his physical limits so that he's in "good pain," not "bad pain." Strive hard to make each workout this week better than any previous sessions.

Reps (Other Than Drop Sets)
- Power Boost movements: 6 reps
  - Try to do the reps faster than last week.
- Strength Max movements: 6 reps
  - Add weight to last week's poundages.
- Muscle Up movements: 20 reps
  - Try to maintain last week's poundages.

Tempo
- Power Boost movements and some abdominal/core movements are performed as quickly as you possibly can (0-0-0-0).
- For most movements, the tempo of all repetitions this week involves a slow lowering of the weight: 2-0-1-0. That still means a fluid tempo but with a much longer and more controlled lowering of the weight and then 1 second raising it, with no pauses at the top or bottom (see pages 161–162).

Rest Intervals
- Rest intervals during the Power Boost segments of the workouts are 1.5 minutes.
- Rest intervals during the Strength Max segments of the workouts are 1.5 minutes.
- Rest intervals during the Muscle Up segments of the workouts are 2 minutes.
- On drop sets, all reps are performed with only enough of an interval to switch weights before continuing. At the end of all reps, take a 2-minute rest.

Abdominal and/or core exercises finish off each workout. The number of reps will be as many as you can do, up to 25 on some movements. The last repetition should be difficult and intense.

WORKOUT 19
Target: Strength Max

Dynamic Warmup—All Levels

MOVEMENT	SETS Level A	SETS Level B	SETS Level C	REPS	REST	TEMPO
Jump to Box/Bench	3	2	2	6	1.5	0-0-0-0
Speed Skater (each side)	3	2	2	6	1.5	0-0-0-0
Flat Barbell Bench Press	3	2	2	6	2	2-0-1-0
Incline Dumbbell Bench Press	3	2	2	6	2	2-0-1-0
Chest Dumbbell Pullover	3	2	2	6	2	2-0-1-0
Flat Dumbbell Fly Drop Set	3*	2*	2*	6	2	2-0-1-0
Triceps Dip	3	2	1	6	2	2-0-1-0
Triceps Pushdown (Rope Attachment) Drop Set	3*	2*	1*	6	2	2-0-1-0
Overhead One Arm Dumbbell Extension (each arm)	3	2	1	20	2	2-0-1-0
Leg Press Calf Press	3	2	1	20	2	2-0-1-0
Captain's Chair Leg Lift	3	2	2	≤25	1	1-0-1-0
Swiss Ball Crunch	3	2	2	≤25	1	1-0-1-0
Total	36	24	20			

*On the last set only, hit 5 reps, drop 20 percent, hit 5 reps, drop 20 percent, and hit 4 or 5 more reps. (This is a 14- or 15-rep total set and the key is to start slightly lighter. Your first set should be a standard rep set. Rest for 2 minutes after all sets, including the drop set. This will afford an interval for your partner to perform his drop set.)

WORKOUT 20
Target: Strength Max

Dynamic Warmup—All Levels

MOVEMENT	SETS Level A	SETS Level B	SETS Level C	REPS	REST	TEMPO
Lateral Long Jump (each side)	3	2	2	6	1.5	0-0-0-0
Clean and Power Press	3	2	2	6	1.5	0-0-0-0
Deep Deadlift	3	2	2	6	2	2-0-1-0
Lat Pulldown	3	2	2	6	2	2-0-1-0
T-Bar Row	3	2	2	6	2	2-0-1-0
Seated Cable Row (Underhand) Drop Set	3*	2*	2*	6	2	2-0-1-0
Incline Dumbbell Curl	3	2	1	6	2	2-0-1-0
Preacher Curl Machine Drop Set	3*	2*	1*	6	2	2-0-1-0
Stiff-Legged Deadlift	3	2	1	20	2	2-0-1-0
Seated Leg Curl	3	2	1	20	2	2-0-1-0
Samurai Swing (Cable or Tubing)	3	2	2	15	1	0-0-0-0
Superman Back Extension	3	2	2	15	1	1-0-1-0
Total	36	24	20			

*On the last set only, hit 5 reps, drop 20 percent, hit 5 reps, drop 20 percent, and hit 4 or 5 more reps. This is a 14- or 15-rep total set and the key is to start slightly lighter. Your first set should be a standard rep set. Rest for 2 minutes after all sets, including the drop set. (This will afford an interval for your partner to perform his drop set.)

WORKOUT 21
Target: Strength Max

Dynamic Warmup—All Levels

MOVEMENT	SETS Level A	SETS Level B	SETS Level C	REPS	REST	TEMPO
Lunge Jump (each leg)	3	2	2	6	1.5	0-0-0-0
Full-Body Resisted Cable or Tubing Extension	3	2	2	6	1.5	0-0-0-0
Shoulder Press Machine Drop Set	3*	2*	2*	6	2	2-0-1-0
Rear Deltoid Machine	3	2	2	6	2	2-0-1-0
Dumbbell Lateral Raise	3	2	2	6	2	2-0-1-0
Dumbbell Shrugs	3	2	2	6	2	2-0-1-0
Leg Press (Wide Stance)	3	2	1	6	2	2-0-1-0
Smith Machine Hack Squat Drop Set	3*	2*	1*	6	2	2-0-1-0
Barbell Lunge (each leg)	3	2	1	20	2	2-0-1-0
Seated Calf Raise	3	2	1	20	2	2-0-1-0
Partner-Assisted Twisting Leg Throw+	3	2	2	10 each side	1	1-0-1-0
Bench Leg Lift	3	2	2	≤25	1	1-0-1-0
Total	36	24	20			

*On the last set only, hit 5 reps, drop 20 percent, hit 5 reps, drop 20 percent, and hit 4 or 5 more reps. This is a 14- or 15-rep total set and the key is to start slightly lighter. Your first set should be a standard rep set. Rest for 2 minutes after all sets, including the drop set. (This will afford an interval for your partner to perform his drop set.)

+If training without a partner, perform the Swiss ball crunch with weight.

WORK HEART SYSTEM

This week your Work Heart time commitment will be even greater than last week.

- During each workday (5 days weekly), your objective is to collect 30 points (30 minutes' worth of Work Heart).
- Focus not on the exact time, but rather on making the best use of each activity.
- Your level of effort this week—the heart in your Work Heart—must be greater than last week's.
- If you're using a backpack or briefcase, make it heavier (and always switch hands for balanced effort).
- If you have a co-worker committed to Work Heart efforts with you, encourage him or her to add to their load, as well.

- Fail to collect all 30 points and you lose all credit for that day.
- You need **150 points** by week's end to meet the Challenge.

PLAY HEART ACTIVITIES

While we increased your Work Heart investment this week, we hold your Play Heart investment steady: Your Play Heart activity requirement is a minimum of 90 minutes, which can be broken into two 45-minute sessions or three 30-minute sessions. The best option is the one that works within your schedule.

This week will be the most competitive Play Heart week in the entire Challenge. You will have many options, but whatever the activity, we urge you to make it a competition with somebody else. Exercise your empathic conscience to help him or her get the most out of the activity, but strive hard to win, as well. After all, remember that the winner of a competition experiences a boost in testosterone—that most manly of hormones.

- You should do *no* gym-based treadmill or stationary bicycle sessions this week.
- If your two or three Play Heart sessions take place at your gym or health club, they must *not* be based on equipment (treadmill, stairclimber, or bicycle).
- They can, however, be composed of a competitive game such as pickup hoops or racquetball. Refer to the "Play Heart Activity Menu" on page 79 for activity choices.

If you want to do your Play Heart sessions outside the gym, how about arranging a group sport this week? You're bound to have enough friends who would love to engage in a healthy game of football or basketball. Why not exercise your assertive courage and be the leader here? Put up a flyer at your gym and arrange some weekly group sports. People will love you for taking the stand; they need this stuff. If you can't put together a team, what about a 30-minute one-on-one game of basketball, tennis, handball, or racquetball?

Alpha Fuel Solution

The Handshake Diet continues and you're eating Man-Hand portions. Last week we highlighted the benefits of lean red meats. This week we're highlighting the awesome nutritional value of fish. If you love fish, you'll love this week. If you weren't raised to eat fish as a kid, you may have never acquired a taste for it. We're going to see whether we can change your mind. Fish is a great source of both protein and heart-healthy omega-3s and is lower in saturated fat than meat and poultry. Here are the week's suggestions, with an emphasis on tasty dishes from the sea.

Breakfast Suggestions
- Liquid egg white omelet with low-fat cheese, avocado, imitation crabmeat, and shrimp; mixed berries
- Smoked salmon with reduced-sodium soy sauce and wasabi

Lunch Suggestions
- True Tuna Salad on bran crisp bread (see page 308)
- Combination of sashimi and sushi (at about a 3-to-1 ratio) and miso soup

Dinner Suggestions
- Broiled filet of sole with mashed sweet potato
- Grilled mahi mahi with reduced-sodium soy sauce; tossed salad with Tomato Vina-great (see page 312)

And a bit of great news: the Feast Meal is back on the menu, boys! But remember the rules: If your chest-to-waist differential is still less than 6 inches or your waist circumference is more than 38 inches, you limit your Feast Meal to *either* one appetizer, one main course, or one dessert—but just one of the three.

Results

Right about now you should be feeling more confident than ever before. You are starting to get used to testing yourself with new and different activities because you now know you can handle more than you ever thought. Expanding your comfort zone is a great feeling, isn't it? Stretching the boundaries of what you can do stretches the boundaries of who you are. You may be thinking that your potential is greater than you ever thought. We think you're right about that.

This was a tough week of physical challenges, but you have proven yourself a true warrior. You should be beyond doubts now about your ability to persevere and triumph. This week you've collected your full 150 Work Heart points, and you've performed at least 90 minutes of Play Heart activity, engaging in competitive activities that can cause spikes in your manly hormone.

If you enjoyed this week's seafood-weighted menu, we're delighted! From this day forward, we want you to include more fish in your diet than ever before—not only for the remainder of the Challenge, but also far beyond. If you need to be reminded why, go back to page 103 and you'll recall that more seafood is a fantastic way to improve the way you feel and look.

You are strong. You don't quit. Take that sense of peak-level confidence with you into the next 2 weeks. You'll need it. Prepare to test yourself as never before.

WEEK 8

Alpha Attitude Drill

This is the week you've trained for; this is your big test . . . and triumph! This is the week you bring your Alpha Attitude game to a new level. You'll test your mental toughness to the max. Conveniently, your Alpha Attitude drill this week is combined with your Play Heart activity.

The drill is simple: Check out the third column of the activity menu on page 79. That's the column we've told you to avoid for the past 7 weeks. The time has now come to choose one of these "Alpha Extreme" activities, challenge yourself, and declare victory over fear and hesitation! We call this drill the "Alpha Extreme Triumph." Choose something on the list that you've thought you might enjoy doing but never tried because, on some level, you feared doing it. Make arrangements right now to do the activity as soon as possible.

Everyone's "Alpha Extreme Triumph" is different. Some are more formidable than others. The

point is that it must be *you*. It must make your heart pound and your adrenaline rush. It must be something you ordinarily wouldn't do, something that you've avoided doing. While we offer plenty of rugged suggestions, the list is far from all-inclusive. You should feel free to create your own drill based on what scares you.

Be realistic—don't start out with skydiving if you're deathly afraid of heights. But don't let yourself off easy, either—push yourself as hard as you dare. Remember, tasks are not going to do you any good if you do not pick things that force you to go beyond actions that you would usually take.

Afterward, try to enjoy the richness of the experience. Make some notes on it. What was it like? How did it feel? What were your thoughts before you did it? After you did it? How did you tell yourself to go for it? How did you make it happen this time? What will you tell yourself in the future to get over that hump again? You have done it, so now you have a model for how to approach tasks that have some fear associated with them.

The "Alpha Extreme Triumph" doesn't have to be a solitary experience. In fact, we advocate that you involve friends or family, either as participants or as spectators. If you have a training partner, do it together. If his "Alpha Extreme Triumph" is different from yours, why not join him on his triumph and have him join you on yours?

Next week you'll return to a somewhat more traditional Alpha Attitude Drill, but not this week. "The Alpha Extreme Triumph" *is* your Play Heart activity this week!

So go out and face your demons. You already have nearly 2 months of Alpha Wave Basic Training under your belt, and you've likely pushed your Play Heart activities beyond your previous limits. You're ready. The "Alpha Extreme Triumph" is your only Play Heart requirement this week—there's no treadmill work, no hill hiking, nothing you're used to doing or have already done. Only this, so that you can target it with ultimate intensity. By your Destination Day only 2 weeks from now, you will be blown away by how courageous you've grown over the course of this Challenge; you may also be shocked and even embarrassed by some of the things that once made you fearful.

Alpha Architecture Program

ALPHA WAVE BASIC TRAINING (WORKOUTS 22–24)

This week we switch our primary target from strength to power. We will concentrate on the Power Boost movements of the workouts, while also maintaining strength and muscularity. Be prepared to also hit both 30-rep drops sets (see page 60) and the Punisher (see page 60). The total number of sets for levels B and C increases this week.

As you'll remember, the Punisher involves the execution of 100 repetitions of a given exercise, pausing only as needed. There are few resistance-training tests of your courage that exceed this grueling exercise. It's also a great conscience trainer—it requires your total focus on your *training partner's* workout for the full span of all 100 reps. Choose a weight or resistance that is about 50 percent of what you would use for a set of 8 to 10 repetitions. You should perform between 30 and 50 reps without stopping. Rest *no more than* 20 seconds, then launch into more reps—likely between 15 and 25 more. Rest again for no more than 20 seconds, and then continue. Your last sequence of reps may only be 10, but do not stop until 100 reps are completed. You will perform

the Punisher on four muscle groups this week: triceps, back, shoulders, and quadriceps.

Reps (Other Than Drop Sets and the Punisher)

- Power Boost movements: 5 reps
  - Try to do the reps faster than last week.
- Strength Max movements: 8 reps
  - Add weight to last week's poundages.
- Muscle Up movements: 12 reps
  - Try to maintain last week's poundages.

Tempo

- Power Boost movements and some abdominal/core movements are performed as quickly as you possibly can (0-0-0-0).
- For most movements, the tempo of repetitions this week is a standard 1-0-1-0.

Rest Intervals

- Rest intervals during the Power Boost segments of the workouts are 1.5 minutes.
- Rest intervals during the Strength Max segments of the workouts are 2 minutes.
- Rest intervals on the Muscle Up segments of the workouts are 1 minute.
- On drop sets, all reps are performed with only enough of an interval to switch weights before continuing. At the end of all reps, take a 2-minute rest.

Abdominal and/or core exercises finish off each workout. The number of reps will be as many as you can do, up to 35 on some movements. The last repetition should be difficult and intense.

WORKOUT 22
Target: Power Boost

Dynamic Warmup—All Levels

MOVEMENT	SETS Level A	SETS Level B	SETS Level C	REPS	REST	TEMPO
Power Pushup	3	2	2	5	1.5	0-0-0-0
Push Jump to Bench	3	2	2	5	1.5	0-0-0-0
Barbell Upright Power Row	3	2	2	5	1.5	0-0-0-0
Long Jump	3	2	2	5	1.5	0-0-0-0
Situp and Pike	3	2	2	5	1.5	0-0-0-0
Grand Slam (Cable or Tubing)	3	2	2	5	1.5	0-0-0-0
Flat Barbell Bench Press	3	3	2	8	2	1-0-1-0
Incline Barbell Bench Press	3	3	2	8	2	1-0-1-0
Pec Deck Fly Drop Set	3*	2*	1*	12	1	1-0-1-0
Triceps Pushdown (Rope Attachment) Punisher+	>1	>1	>1	100	Minimum	1-0-1-0
Bicycle Maneuver (each side)	3	2	2	≤35	1	0-0-0-0
Superman Back Extension	3	2	2	≤20	1	1-0-1-0
Total	34	25	22			

*On the last set only, hit 12 reps, drop 20 percent, hit 10 reps, drop 20 percent, and hit 8 reps. This is a 30-rep total set and the key is to start slightly lighter. Your first set should be a standard rep set. Rest for 2 minutes after all sets, including the drop set. (This will afford an interval for your partner to perform his drop set.)

+All levels: Do 100 reps in as short a time as possible using a weight with which you can do 30 to 40 reps without stopping.

WORKOUT 23
Target: Power Boost

Dynamic Warmup—All Levels

MOVEMENT	SETS Level A	SETS Level B	SETS Level C	REPS	REST	TEMPO
Power Row (each arm)	3	2	2	5	1.5	0-0-0-0
Full-Body Resisted Cable or Tubing Extension	3	2	2	5	1.5	0-0-0-0
Jump to Box/Bench	3	2	2	5	1.5	0-0-0-0
Squat Jump	3	2	2	5	1.5	0-0-0-0
Box Landing Two Step Sprint	3	2	2	5	1.5	0-0-0-0
Multidirectional Hop	3	2	2	5	1.5	0-0-0-0
Chinup or Chindown	3	3	2	8	2	1-0-1-0
One Arm Machine Row (each arm)	3	3	2	8	2	1-0-1-0
Machine Row Punisher*	>1	>1	>1	100	Minimum	1-0-1-0
Barbell Curl (Narrow) Drop Set	3+	2+	1+	12	1	1-0-1-0
Captain's Chair Leg Lift	3	2	2	≤20	1	1-0-1-0
Swiss Ball Toss‡	3	2	2	15	1	0-0-0-0
Total	36	26	22			

*All levels: Do 100 reps in as short a time as possible using a weight with which you can do 30 to 40 reps without stopping.

+On the last set only, hit 12 reps, drop 20 percent, hit 10 reps, drop 20 percent, and hit 8 reps. This is a 30-rep total set and the key is to start slightly lighter. Your first set should be a standard rep set. Rest for 2 minutes after all sets, including the drop set. (This will afford an interval for your partner to perform his drop set.)

‡If training without a partner, perform the Swiss ball crunch with weight.

WORKOUT 24
Target: Power Boost

Dynamic Warmup—All Levels

MOVEMENT	SETS Level A	SETS Level B	SETS Level C	REPS	REST	TEMPO
Speed Skater	3	2	2	5	1.5	0-0-0-0
Side-To-Side Cone Hop	3	2	2	5	1.5	0-0-0-0
Lateral Long Jump	3	2	2	5	1.5	0-0-0-0
Lunge Jump (Switch Legs)	3	2	2	5	1.5	0-0-0-0
Clean and Power Press (Alternate Push Press)	3	2	2	5	1.5	0-0-0-0
Samurai Swing (Cable or Tubing)	3	2	2	5	1.5	0-0-0-0
Dumbbell Shoulder Press	3	3	2	8	2	1-0-1-0
Dumbbell Squat	3	3	2	8	2	1-0-1-0
Lateral Raise (Cable) Punisher*	>1	>1	>1	100	Minimum	1-0-1-0
Cross the River (50 each leg)	>1	>1	>1	100	Minimum	1-0-1-0
Swiss Ball Crunch	3	2	2	≤20	1	1-0-1-0
Bench Leg Lift	3	2	2	≤35	1	1-0-1-0
Total	36	26	22			

*All levels: Do 100 reps in as short a time as possible using a weight with which you can do 30 to 40 reps without stopping.

WORK HEART SYSTEM

Your Work Heart commitment this week will be the same as last week—but you will get a bonus, as follows: If you are following a new variation of the Alpha Fuel Solution that we call the Spartan Diet (see page 120), you'll be eating a lot fewer carbohydrates. It will last for only the next 14 days, but it will work like a blowtorch to burn your most stubborn body fat stores. You get 50 bonus points for adhering to the Spartan Diet this week! Accordingly, the "heart," or effort, in your Work Heart should be scaled back. In other words, you'll be doing both less duration and less intensity in your Work Heart, which will maximize your strength and muscle while following the Spartan Diet.

- During each workday (5 days weekly), your objective is to collect 20 points (20 minutes' worth of Work Heart).

- Focus not on the exact time, but rather on making the best use of each activity.
- Your level of effort this week—the heart in your Work Heart—should be *less* than last week.
- Don't carry a backpack or briefcase because we want you to conserve some energy during this energy-taxing diet period.
- As always, fail to collect all 20 points and you lose all credit for that day.
- You will automatically be awarded 50 bonus points for the Spartan Diet, so you only need 100 additional points by week's end to meet the Challenge of **150 points** total.

Note: If you are not seeking the more intense fat-burning effects of the Spartan Diet and are instead following the Handshake Diet this week, you do not get 50 bonus points and should stick to the Work Heart recommendations of Week 7 (30 points a day, 150 points for the week).

PLAY HEART ACTIVITIES

For those following the Spartan Diet this week, your Alpha Fuel plan is changing, dropping your carbohydrate intake. You'll be burning fat like never before, but we want you to hold on to every single ounce of muscle you've built. Therefore, we don't want you doing any high-intensity Play Heart activities. Next week you'll return to a somewhat more traditional Play Heart activity requirement, but not this week. This week you will combine your Alpha Attitude drill with your Play Heart activity requirement and face and conquer something that truly scares you in the "Alpha Extreme Triumph" (see page 70). Remember, everyone's triumph is different. Some are bigger than others. The point is that it must be the right choice for *you*. It must make your heart pound and your adrenaline rush. It must be something you ordinarily wouldn't do, or even something that you've avoided doing. How about fire walking? Skydiving? A near-vertical roller coaster? Only you know. It's *your* triumph. Earn it!

Note: If you are not seeking the more intense fat-burning effects of the Spartan Diet and are instead following the Handshake Diet this week, you may follow the same Play Heart recommendations as for Week 6 (see page 157). However, you *must* perform the "Alpha Extreme Triumph"—no excuses—as one of the sessions!

Alpha Fuel Solution

This is a week of surprises. Just as we surprised you with the "Alpha Extreme Triumph" in your "Alpha Attitude" drill, we have an Alpha Fuel surprise, as well. For the next 2 weeks, you'll be dining on what we call our Spartan Diet. It's a much stricter regimen than the Handshake Diet, but it's designed to shed lingering fat . . . fast! Is that your goal? Then have the confidence to step up! This is going to take extreme commitment and courage.

The Spartan Diet isn't applicable to you men who are primarily looking to build muscle and not burn fat. It's for any guy who's looking to torch that excess and stubborn body fat. If you're looking to add muscle and not drop body fat, you should just stick to the standard Handshake Diet you've been following.

You'll be shopping for and eating all the same meats, fish, chicken, and turkey, and you can even enjoy carb-free string cheese. You'll also be able to eat some nuts in moderation, some salad greens, and a small serving of a vegetable each day. Those will provide you with enough carbohydrates. You will not take in any other carbohydrates for this week. That means no fruit or skim milk, and of course no breads or cereals. The net effect will limit your carb intake to fewer than 50 grams.

Of course, you can eat eggs. And you shouldn't worry about the yolks—so have a few whole egg omelets this week. At the start of the week, make a dozen hard-boiled eggs for snacking. Boil another dozen halfway through the week. Only eat one whole egg out of every four—throw away the other yolks. Add cayenne pepper and just a dash of salt.

Note that the Spartan Diet can have a dehydrating effect, so you should drink *extra* water while following it. We suggest at least 10 cups a day for smaller guys, and up to 15 for larger guys. Take this advice seriously, because even mildly insufficient fluid intake can have a serious negative effect on your performance. You can't risk that now!

Also, constipation can be an issue for many people when following ketogenic diets for extended periods. Although you'll only be following it for 2 weeks, we nevertheless suggest you take a powdered fiber supplement with an extremely low-carbohydrate content, such as UniFiber.

Here are the week's meal suggestions.

Breakfast Suggestions
- Omelet with broccoli, asparagus, and turkey breast
- Two eggs over easy with 4 slices of Canadian bacon

Lunch Suggestions
- Roasted chicken with string beans drizzled with olive oil and slivered almonds
- A Mean Egg Salad (see page 301)

Dinner Suggestions
- Lean steak with Steak Dip (see page 309) and mushrooms, and macadamia nuts and cashews
- Catfish sprinkled with crushed pecans and macadamia nut oil and steamed cauliflower with red and green peppers

The Feast Meal is still on the menu this week, with the usual crucial caveat (page 118).

This week, guys taking creatine will end the use of the product.

Results

Remember that courage is like a muscle—the more you exercise it, the stronger it grows. If you met the Alpha Extreme Triumph this week, you should be beaming with pride. You have willfully put yourself to the test and have come out on top. We can't think of a bigger boost to your Alpha Factor than that! Of course, what's really important isn't the fact that you conquered your fear in this specific drill. It's that you have reaffirmed to yourself that you are capable of conquering fear and that your true Alpha Male potential is beyond what you may have ever expected. Knowing that gives you an immeasurable advantage in the real world. Take your courage and apply it to all the things in life that truly matter.

Next week will be less taxing on your Alpha Attitude muscles, and you have only 7 more days of the Spartan Diet. You shall overcome!

WEEK 9

Alpha Attitude Drill

This week we return to conscience as the focus of our drill. However, this time it's not our capacity for empathy we seek to build, but our capacity for *altruism*.

Heroic altruism was a knightly virtue in medieval times. We call this drill "The Good Knight." It should help you connect with the hero inside you. It isn't about looking good, but about *doing* good. There are homeless veterans, kids in need of mentors, and hospitals filled with sick children. There are countless worthy causes in need of *your* help. If you are waiting for someone else to care for the world around you, think again—that is not what the true Alpha Male does. He acts. No one truly leads without caring.

- Choose one specific volunteer activity you can engage in *this week*, even if only for an hour or two.
- Start by contacting any of the following:
  - www.volunteermatch.org
  - www.bethechangeinc.org
  - www.voa.org
  - www.onebrick.org
  - www.serve.gov

Schedule a volunteer activity for this week. No objections. No excuses. Just do it. A better country, a better world starts with little things that each of us can do, so on a daily basis be on the lookout for opportunities; they really do come up all the time. Certainly you cannot help in every situation, but there are likely many small opportunities each day to use your mental or physical strength to aid others, times when you could step out of your comfort zone and make a difference. Not only will this aid others, but it will also set an excellent example for those around you. And you may be surprised at how it improves your mood, your day, and your confidence and even your health when you choose to use your abilities to help others.

Alpha Architecture Program

ALPHA WAVE BASIC TRAINING (WORKOUTS 25–27)

This is our last training week before the Breaking Wave. You have only three Alpha Wave Basic Training workouts left to complete the Challenge! This week your primary focus is on Power Boost. But you'd better brace yourself: You'll also be doing drop sets (see page 60), supersets (see page 60), the Punisher (see page 60), and the Power Pushup (see page 197). Yikes! On the Pushup Challenge, your goal is to beat your previous result by at least 10 pushups. You'll also return to the plank for core strength. This time, you'll shoot to double your time on every set from Workout 7 (see page 139). If you lasted 1 minute on each set then, you'll shoot for 2 minutes in Workout 25. If you lasted for 2 minutes on the first set and 1 minute on the second, you'll shoot for 4 minutes on the first set and 2 minutes on the second.

Note that if you are following the Spartan Diet this week, the combination of extreme physical challenges will push you to the brink. Even if you're following the Handshake Diet, we won't kid you: It won't be easy. However, it's not quite as taxing on the recuperative system as it may look. Most of the exercises are Power Boost movements, so the reps are low (only 5). Also, note that your Work Heart and Play Heart demands are reduced if you are eating Spartan-style. Look, we think that just 9 weeks ago you likely would not have been able to endure the dreaded Week 9. But now, we know that you will conquer it decisively!

Reps (Other Than Supersets)
- Power Boost movements: 5 reps
  - Try to do the reps faster than last week.
- Strength Max movements: 8 reps
  - Add weight to last week's poundages.
- Muscle Up movements: 12 reps
  - Try to maintain last week's poundages.

Tempo
- Power Boost movements and some abdominal/core movements are performed as quickly as you possibly can (0-0-0-0).
- For other movements, the tempo of repetitions this week is 1-1-1-1. That means there will be a 1-second pause at both the top and the bottom of each repetition. The pause is not to rest, but to hold the top contracted position and the bottom stretched position for 1 second before continuing with the rep. The key is to never let the tension off the muscle being worked.

Rest Intervals
- Rest intervals during the Power Boost segments of the workout are 1.5 minutes.
- Rest intervals during the Strength Max segments of the workouts are 2 minutes.
- Rest intervals during the Muscle Up segments of the workouts are 2 minutes.
- On drop sets, all reps are performed with only enough of an interval to switch weights before continuing. At the end of all reps, take a 2-minute rest.

Abdominal and/or core exercises finish off each workout. The number of reps will be as many as you can do, up to 30 or, on the bicycle maneuver, even 40 on each side. The last repetition should be difficult and intense.

WORKOUT 25
Target: Power Boost

Dynamic Warmup—All Levels

MOVEMENT	SETS Level A	SETS Level B	SETS Level C	REPS	REST	TEMPO
Multidirectional Hop	3	2	2	5	1.5	0-0-0-0
Push Jump to Bench	3	2	2	5	1.5	0-0-0-0
Barbell Upright Power Row	3	2	2	5	1.5	0-0-0-0
Full-Body Resisted Cable or Tubing Extension	3	2	2	5	1.5	0-0-0-0
Grand Slam (Cable or Tubing)	3	2	2	5	1.5	0-0-0-0
Lateral Push Off Jump (each leg)	3	2	2	5	1.5	0-0-0-0
Incline Dumbbell Fly	3	3	2	8	2	1-1-1-1
Pec Deck Fly	3	3	2	8	2	1-1-1-1
Close-Grip Bench Press	3	2	1	12	2	1-1-1-1
Dumbbell Skull Crusher Punisher*	>1	>1	>1	100	Minimum	1-1-1-1
Partner-Assisted Leg Throw+	3	2	2	15	1	1-0-1-0
The Plank	3	2	2	>2 min	1	N/A
Total	>36	>26	>22			

*All levels: Do 100 reps in as short a time as possible using a weight with which you can do 30 to 40 reps without stopping.
+If training without a partner, perform the captain's chair.

WORKOUT 26
Target: Power Boost

Dynamic Warmup—All Levels

MOVEMENT	SETS Level A	SETS Level B	SETS Level C	REPS	REST	TEMPO
Squat Jump	3	2	2	5	1.5	0-0-0-0
Clean and Power Press (Alternate Push Press)	3	2	2	5	1.5	0-0-0-0
Long Jump	3	2	2	5	1.5	0-0-0-0
Lunge Jump (each leg)	3	2	2	5	1.5	0-0-0-0
Speed Skater (each side)	3	2	2	5	1.5	0-0-0-0
Situp and Pike	3	2	2	5	1.5	0-0-0-0
Deep Deadlift	3	3	2	8	2	1-1-1-1
T-Bar Row	3	3	2	8	2	1-1-1-1
Seated Cable Row Drop Set	3*	2*	1*	12	2	1-1-1-1
21 Curls	3	2	1	21	2	1-1-1-1
Superman Back Extension	3	2	2	15	1	1-0-1-0
Bicycle Maneuver	3	2	2	≤40 each side	1	0-0-0-0
Total	36	26	22			

*On the last set only, hit 12 reps, drop 20 percent, hit 10 reps, drop 20 percent, and hit 8 reps. This is a 30-rep total set and the key is to start slightly lighter. Your first set should be a standard rep set. Rest for 2 minutes after all sets, including the drop set. (This will afford an interval for your partner to perform his drop set.)

WORKOUT 27
Target: Power Boost

Dynamic Warmup—All Levels

MOVEMENT	SETS Level A	SETS Level B	SETS Level C	REPS	REST	TEMPO
Pushup Challenge	3	2	2	max	1.5	0-0-0-0
Jump to Box/Bench	3	2	2	5	1.5	0-0-0-0
Power Row (each arm)	3	2	2	5	1.5	0-0-0-0
Samurai Swing (Cable or Tubing)	3	2	2	5	1.5	0-0-0-0
Lateral Long Jump (each side)	3	2	2	5	1.5	0-0-0-0
Side-to-Side Cone Hop (each leg)	3	2	2	5	1.5	0-0-0-0
Barbell Squat	3	3	2	8	2	1-1-1-1
Weighted Stepup (Dumbbell or Barbell)—each leg	3	3	2	8	2	1-1-1-1
Stiff-Legged Deadlift	3	2	1	12	2	1-1-1-1
Arnold Press Drop Set	3*	2*	1*	12	2	1-1-1-1
Captain's Chair Leg Lift	3	2	2	≤30	1	1-0-1-0
Swiss Ball Throw+	3	2	2	≤30	1	0-0-0-0
Total	36	26	22			

*On the last set only, hit 12 reps, drop 20 percent, hit 10 reps, drop 20 percent, and hit 8 reps. This is a 30-rep total set and the key is to start slightly lighter. Your first set should be a standard rep set. Rest for 2 minutes after all sets, including the drop set. (This will afford an interval for your partner to perform his drop set.)

+If training without a partner, perform the Swiss ball crunch with weight.

WORK HEART SYSTEM

If you are on the second and final week of the Spartan Diet, you may be running a bit lower on energy than usual. But you will automatically get 50 bonus points for sticking to the Spartan Diet. Here's your Work Heart overview for Week 9.

- During each workday (5 days weekly), your objective is to collect 20 points (20 minutes' worth of Work Heart).
- Focus not on the exact time, but rather on making the best use of each activity.
- Your level of effort this week—the heart in your Work Heart—should be *less* than last week's.
- Don't carry a backpack or briefcase because we want you to conserve some energy during this energy-taxing diet period.
- As always, fail to collect all 20 points and you lose all credit for that day.
- You will automatically be awarded 50 bonus points for the Spartan Diet, so you only need

100 additional points by week's end to meet the Challenge of **150 points** total.

Note: If you are not seeking the more intense fat-burning effects of the Spartan Diet and are instead following the Handshake Diet this week, you do not get 50 bonus points and should stick to the Work Heart recommendations of Week 7 (30 points a day, 150 points for the week).

Now here's our final surprise for you—redemption again, just when you may need it! We know, we know—we said there'd be no more second chances (so please don't tell anybody, especially new recruits to the Challenge!). But this is a program all about second chances, so we couldn't resist. We recognize that no matter how diligently you've followed the program, life sometimes gets in the way. So, if you lost credit on any day over the past 2 months, now's your final chance to make it up. However many points you are short, this really is your last chance to square up. Choose a household or other local task that requires physical effort. But here's the twist: It can't be at *your* house. It has to be at somebody else's. That's right: You have to find a way to help a neighbor, a friend, an extended family member, or a co-worker with a physical task. It should be a random act of kindness that involves lifting and carrying, pulling or pushing, but not necessarily working up a sweat. Consider this an extension of this week's Good Knight drill—and something that should make you feel even better about yourself!

PLAY HEART ACTIVITIES

This week you go back to traditional Play Heart activities, with a requirement of only 90 minutes, which can be broken into two 45-minute sessions or three 30-minute sessions.

If you are on the Spartan Diet, you can do the activities you want, including going for a hike or shooting some hoops, but we strongly suggest that you keep the intensity levels low. You can do gym-based treadmill or stationary bicycle sessions this week, but at low speeds. We don't want you to do any intense interval or Kilimanjaro training. Our goal is to shock your body into scalding off any remaining excess body fat while preserving every ounce of hard-earned muscle. Again, we want you to do *low-intensity* activities. Nothing that makes your heart pound—just activities that will keep you in a nice fat-burning, muscle-sparing mode.

If you are not seeking the more intense fat-burning effects of the Spartan Diet and are instead following the Handshake Diet this week, you should stick to the Play Heart recommendations from Week 6.

Alpha Fuel Solution

Hopefully you enjoyed the Feast Meal that ended Week 8. This is the final week of your Spartan Diet and the true test of your resolve. Again, you'll also be able to eat some nuts in moderation,

some salad greens, and a small serving of a vegetable each day. Those will provide you with enough carbohydrates. You will not take in any other carbohydrates for this week. That means no fruit or skim milk, and of course no breads or cereals.

Remember to drink *extra* water while following the Spartan Diet. We suggest at least 10 cups a day for smaller guys and up to 15 for larger guys. Also, we suggest you take a powdered fiber supplement, such as UniFiber, to avoid constipation.

Let's mix it up with a few special meals: Pick one steak, one bison burger, one fish, two chicken, and one turkey meal. Lunches can be cold cuts (roast beef, etc.).

Breakfast Suggestions
- Omelet with broccoli
- Turkey scramble with packaged egg whites and roasted mushrooms, plus ½ cup roasted zucchini (3 g carbs)

Lunch Suggestions
- Warm grilled chicken on a bed of romaine lettuce with oil and flavored vinegar, sprinkled with Parmesan cheese
- Chicken, Nuts, and Spinach (see page 307)

Dinner Suggestions
- Sizzlin' Pepper Steak (see page 309)
- Wild Dijon Salmon (see page 309) and ½ sliced cucumber

The Feast Meal is still on the menu this week, and it's okay to have even more carbs than usual during your Week 9 Feast Meal. You'll notice a dramatic increase in muscle fullness a day or two after your Feast Meal this week! However, once again, be mindful of the crucial caveat regarding your waist (page 119).

Results

The combined exercise and diet regimen this week was truly punishing, yet you survived it and will be forever stronger for it. But you are more than merely stronger; you are better. The heroic altruism exercised in the Good Knight drill is at the heart of what the true Alpha Male is all about. You faced this Challenge because you wanted to be a better man, inside and out. There can be no doubt—you are.

You are approaching your Destination. It is on the horizon. You are nearing the end of a journey that started with a single step, as every journey does. You now know how little changes, little steps, setting daily goals, and doing small things can add up to big changes. You have moved yourself from where you were to a new place, taking one step at a time.

WEEK 10

Alpha Attitude Drill

This is the Breaking Wave—your week for rest and recovery. You have no specific obligations for Alpha Attitude drills, but be on the lookout for opportunities to flex your commitment, confidence, courage, and conscience muscles this week. Remember, these muscles grow when you exercise them. Let then languish, and they will atrophy.

So here's a little game you might want to play; we call it "Reversal of Fortune." In a famous episode of the *Seinfeld* television series, the character called George Costanza—a self-described "short, stocky, slow-witted, bald man" known for his negative attitude—visits the beach and has the revelation that every decision that he has made in life has been wrong. He resolves to improve his life by doing the exact opposite of everything he normally would have done. The result is great success. He even gets a job with the Yankees.

It's natural to feel discouraged when bad things happen. Your mission, for an entire day this week, is to approach every negative experience that befalls you by taking the opposite approach from discouragement. Every setback, every slight, every bump in the road, large or small, you will respond

to with a positive spirit of hope, optimism, and opportunity. Traffic jam? Take the time to listen to music or call a friend (use your earpiece!) whom you haven't connected with in a long time. Trouble on the job? Take control of your responses. Don't give up, don't get discouraged, and don't blame anyone else. Take it as an opportunity for problem solving and coming back tomorrow even stronger and better. Stay totally focused for 1 full day on responding positively to every problem, no matter how big or small. At the end of the day, reflect back. Sure, it may have felt weird at times, but we'll make you a bet: The more you approach life like this, beyond the scope of this exercise, the better you'll be at distinguishing the big problems from the little ones, and not sweating the small stuff. And the lower your testosterone-crushing stress levels will be. This is the real-world culmination or manifestation of living a life in accord with the four Cs of Alpha Attitude.

Go to www.alphamalechallenge.com and join the community of men who've completed the Challenge, just like you.

Alpha Architecture Program

ALPHA WAVE BASIC TRAINING

Remember the importance of rest and recovery? This is the week for you to recharge your batteries! There are no Alpha Wave Basic Training sessions this week, and you can use the break. Although it's not mandatory, we suggest that you do some light whole-body training to pump a little blood into your muscles, but only twice this week. And keep the poundages light—about half the weights you would use for sets of 8 to 10 repetitions. Because you'll be spending less time in the gym this week, you'll have some time to spare. Spend it with your friends or family.

You won't be subjecting your body to the demands of Alpha Wave Basic Training, so the end of this week, when your body is well rested, is the perfect time to donate blood. Blood banks often report dangerously low supplies. Donating blood is a heroically altruistic thing to do and could actually save someone's life!

Giving blood will make you feel great about yourself and just might do even more for you. How? Each time you donate, you remove some of the excess iron in your blood. There's evidence that high blood iron levels can increase the risk of heart disease. A study of 2,682 men in Finland reported in the *American Journal of Epidemiology* found that those who donated blood at least once a year had an 88 percent lower risk of heart attacks. Another study published in *Heart* found that men who gave blood were less likely to show signs of cardiovascular disease. So donating blood is a win-win proposition.

You'll be retaking the MaleScale this week on the day most convenient to you. You can retake the MaleScale in the early or middle part of the week and arrange to donate blood afterward, because some (but not all) guys feel slightly weaker right after giving blood. Or you can give blood early in the week, and take the MaleScale closer to the end of the week. What's most important, of course, is that you do both—no excuses! You can arrange a donation through www.givelife.org, or call the Red Cross at 1-800-GIVELIFE (1-800-448-3543).

WORK HEART SYSTEM

By now, Work Heart should be woven into your daily life. It should actually feel awkward not to do it. You should *want* to do it. You've already invested 9 intense weeks into revamping your body. You've collected 925 points so far in your Work Heart efforts—proof that you've integrated functional fitness into your daily life. You need only 75 more points to reach 1,000. Go for it!

- During each workday (5 days weekly), your objective is to collect 15 points (15 minutes' worth of Work Heart).

- Focus not on the exact time, but rather on making the best use of each activity.
- Fail to collect all 15 points and you lose all credit for that day.
- You need 75 points by week's end to meet the Challenge.

Your total Work Heart points for the 10 weeks of the Challenge will be 1,000 points!

PLAY HEART ACTIVITIES

This week you go back to traditional Play Heart activities, with a minimum requirement of 90 minutes, which can be broken into two 45-minute sessions or three 30-minute sessions. The best option is the one that works within your schedule. You can do any activities you want, including gym-based treadmill or stationary bicycle sessions. You can do shadowboxing, jumping rope, or punching the speed bag or heavy bag. You can take classes in parkour, martial arts, kickboxing, or white collar boxing, or play basketball, tennis, handball, or racquetball. Go crazy! Visit the "Play Heart Activity Menu" on page 79 for a list of choices.

Want to grab 30 minutes of Play Heart credit for less than half that time? Here's the deal: You can shave 30 minutes off your Play Heart minute minimum this week by revisiting the 1-mile run (see page 152) that you did in Week 5. Remember:

- Measure out 1 mile, either on a local track, at a park, or in a suitable neighborhood area.
- Warm up thoroughly—you don't want to run with cold knees, hips, and back.
- Pace yourself! If you're not a runner, a good starting goal is a pace of 2 minutes per ¼ mile (8-minute mile).

Alpha Fuel Solution

Hopefully you enjoyed the Feast Meal that ended Week 9. The Spartan Diet is behind you! It's back to the standard Handshake Diet. Anyone who endured the Spartan Diet for the past 2 weeks should find it pretty easy to stick to now.

Breakfast Suggestions
- Power Pancakes (see page 304)
- Man Made Quiche (see page 305)

Lunch Suggestions
- Tough Guy Turkey Burger (see page 306)
- Deli-sliced roast beef with lettuce and sun-dried tomatoes in a whole grain wrap with horseradish over mixed salad greens; one piece of fresh fruit

Dinner Suggestions
- Manly Meat Loaf (see page 310); mixed salad with choice of dressings (see pages 311–312)
- Texan Shrimp (see page 310); mixed fruit salad with shredded coconut

You can treat yourself to a glass of red wine this week to celebrate! But what happens after this week ends? Will you return to your old ways of eating? Will you let your body settle back down onto the couch? The Alpha Fuel Solution is a way of eating for the rest of your life—simple, nutritious, and friendly to maintaining the lean, strong, and muscular body you've invested so much time and effort working on.

Results

You have braved the Challenge and survived. It didn't kill you; you are stronger. You are also a better man.

Look back on the past 10 weeks. Did things go as you expected? Did you meet all of your goals? Did you reach your Destination? We expect that the changes you've made in your life have improved the way you look and feel. But we also expect that it has been hard to make these changes, and that you may have had times when you wanted to give up and lie down on the couch. Take a moment to look back at those times when things got hard, when you had a choice to make, to go on . . . or to go back. How did you deal with the roadblocks? How did you make the decision to keep pushing, how did you get past those hard times, how were you the resilient, true Alpha Male that you needed to be? How were you able to tap into those motivations as a resource? And what have you learned about yourself?

As you look forward toward your goals for the next 10 weeks, or for the rest of your life, remember those times and how you overcame the obstacles, how you developed your resiliency, how you found a reason and a way to push forward. The new habits and thoughts you have worked hard to develop, including resiliency and the four Cs, will serve you well as you continue to grow. Exercising commitment, living with confidence and courage, and acting true to your conscience are not always easy in today's world; many forces can stand against you. But true Alpha Males don't quit; they regroup, learn from their misadventures, and come back stronger for having been an active member of their community and not a passive observer of events around them. They turn to face the new challenge with the strength they accrued from facing those in the past. The *Alpha Male Challenge* is at your disposal—it's here for you if you dare to renew your commitment and restart the program all over again. Why not take a friend, colleague, or family member through the Challenge with you this time, and be his experienced, empathic, and altruistic guide to his Destination? You have conquered the Challenge, and that is motivating and inspiring to those around you seeking to improve themselves.

Now the moment of truth has arrived. Your primary and most important obligation this week is to revisit the MaleScale. That's right: The time has come to see how you measure up against the man you used to be (see page 17).

CHAPTER SEVEN

TRUE ALPHA FOREVER

It was 10 weeks ago that you made a pledge to yourself. Remember your promise? You vowed as follows:

> Having decided that I am ready to improve myself physically and psychologically for the benefit of myself and those I love, I pledge to commit myself wholly to the *Alpha Male Challenge*. I understand that my level of commitment is commensurate with the level of benefit to be gained through this program. For at least the next 10 weeks, I pledge to forgo excuses in favor of accountability. I pledge to sacrifice the comfort of old habits in favor of a new style of living that maximizes my inner and outer potential as one of a new breed of *true* Alpha Males.

Did you honor the Pledge? If so, you stand at the other end of the 10-week gauntlet. Do you feel any different than you did 10 weeks ago? We suspect you do. You have been tested, you have struggled, you have undergone the fiery hardships of the Challenge, but you did not surrender and you are forever stronger for it. We salute you! You committed yourself with diligence and passion and you survived the Challenge. Whatever you do and wherever you go, nobody can ever take that away from you.

If you were truly motivated to change—to improve your health, your body, your attitude—then you've seen and felt changes in yourself. Others have probably seen those changes, too. How much have you changed? Let's put a number on it. It's time for you to revisit the MaleScale and put yourself to the test. Once again, you'll need a bathroom scale, a pencil, a calculator, a cloth or vinyl tape measure, a watch with a second hand, a piece of chalk, a standard weight bench, and a barbell. You'll also need an area for your 300 Run and a helper to ensure that the five assessments of Alpha Architecture are accurate.

Now pick up your pencil and get to it, being just as honest now as you were when you first took it!

Note to those who've read up to this part without having begun the Challenge:

It's now time for you to begin your journey! We're excited for you, as you should be for yourself. In only 10 weeks' time, you will once again come to this part of the book, but at that time, you will be forever changed. For now, stop reading and start applying!

THE MALESCALE REVISITED!

Enter your new weight here: _____ pounds

10 MEASURES OF ALPHA ATTITUDE

1) Over the past week, I set concrete and specific goals for myself to get where I want to be.

1	2	3	4	5	6	7	8	9	10

Not true   Somewhat true   Mostly true   Absolutely true

2) I can resist eating my favorite junk food even when others are eating it in front of me.

1	2	3	4	5	6	7	8	9	10

Never   Rarely   Mostly   Always

3) I am satisfied with my current physique. (Answer now in light of your *progress* over the past 10 weeks; how satisfied are you with your body as compared to 10 weeks ago?)

1	2	3	4	5	6	7	8	9	10

Not satisfied   Somewhat satisfied   Mostly satisfied   Absolutely satisfied

4) I am able to handle whatever obstacles life throws in my way.

1	2	3	4	5	6	7	8	9	10

Never   Rarely   Mostly   Always

5) I am ready right now to stand up and take charge of a group that needs a leader.

1	2	3	4	5	6	7	8	9	10

No   Unlikely   Likely   Absolutely

6) When I'm faced with a tough yet safe challenge that's within my physical capabilities, I face my fear and do it.

1	2	3	4	5	6	7	8	9	10

No way   Unlikely   Likely   Absolutely

7) I am very good at looking at things from the viewpoint of other people.

1	2	3	4	5	6	7	8	9	10

No   Somewhat   Mostly   Absolutely

8) I tried my hardest over the past week to help people in need, without being rewarded or expecting anything in return.

1	2	3	4	5	6	7	8	9	10

No   Somewhat   Mostly   Absolutely

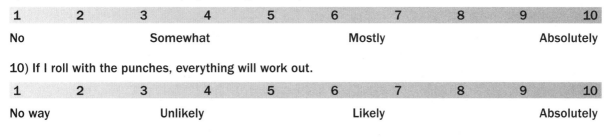

9) I bounce back from hardship by learning from my mistakes.

1	2	3	4	5	6	7	8	9	10
No		Somewhat			Mostly				Absolutely

10) If I roll with the punches, everything will work out.

1	2	3	4	5	6	7	8	9	10
No way		Unlikely			Likely				Absolutely

How did you score? Add up all your new scores and enter your subtotal (between 10 and 100) here:

_____

Divide by 2 and round to the nearest whole number (between 5 and 50): _____

Now move on to the physical assessments. You'll measure the circumference of your flexed biceps and the differential between your chest and your waist. You'll assess your vertical jump, your bench-press to body-weight ratio, and your speed on the 300 Run. Mark down all your measurements and scores. (See pages 14–16 to review all instructions.)

5 ASSESSMENTS OF ALPHA ARCHITECTURE

1) Flexed Biceps Circumference

My flexed biceps circumference is _____ inches.

2) Chest-to-Waist Differential

My expanded chest circumference is _____ inches.

My waist circumference is _____ inches.

3) Vertical Jump

My vertical jump height is _____ inches.

4) Maximum Bench-Press to Body-Weight Ratio

The number of repetitions (10 or fewer) performed is_____ reps.

The weight on the barbell is _____ pounds.

5) The 300 Run

My 300 run time is _____ seconds.

Use the charts on pages 20 and 21 to determine your new Alpha Architecture subtotal (between 5 and 50) and write it here: _____

What's your new Alpha Factor? Add up the Alpha Attitude and Alpha Architecture subtotals for a number between 10 and 100.

Write it here: _____

Congratulations!

This is your *new* Alpha Factor.

We'll make *you* an Alpha Bet that you've increased your score! You should be proud of what you've accomplished in only 10 weeks. You are living, breathing proof that true Alpha Males are made, not just born.

Assess your Alpha Attitude and see how far you've come. You should be setting goals more than you ever did in your pre-Challenge days, as well as exercising willpower and discipline like never before. You should feel more confident about your abilities and much better about your body. Your courage to assert leadership and to tackle physical challenges despite fears or hesitations should be measurably stronger. And you will likely be paying more attention to being a better person in everyday life—more empathic toward others and more likely to put yourself out just to help others. As you move forward from here, you will be more likely to stay positive despite life's changes and to learn from your failures and move on. You should feel more *manly*—more rugged and powerful—and yet you should understand more than ever that true power is never having to exert it over others.

What about your body? Go ahead. Take off your clothes. You may be tempted to leave the shades up this time! Stand in front of the mirror in your underwear. Take a long look. We suspect you're smiling. You should be. You should be feeling absolutely great about yourself. If you have been working hard on your Alpha Architecture and rigorously following the principles of Alpha Wave Basic Training and the Work Heart/Play Heart system, you should see dramatic changes in your physique. Your arms look harder and more muscular and your chest-to-waist ratio is improved. Your bench-press to body-weight ratio is better, your vertical jump higher, your 300 run faster. All good stuff, not to mention that you're feeling better and healthier because you're eating like you were meant to. The Alpha Fuel Solution isn't a quick fix; it's the way to eat for the long haul. Without excessive grains, sweets, and highly processed foods, and with optimal testosterone-boosting fats and muscle-building protein, your body is energized and stronger than ever.

YOUR RESILIENT FUTURE

"What doesn't kill me, makes me stronger," wrote the German philosopher Friedrich Wilhelm Nietzsche in *Twilight of the Idols*. Besides being a monumentally manly thing to say, there's a great deal of support for the idea, even if Nietzsche himself was a little crazy. "Strength does not come from winning," said a famous Austrian who went from bricklayer to bodybuilding champion to California governor. "Your struggles develop your strengths. When you go through hardships and decide not to surrender, that is strength." One of the most prominent American psychology theorists of the last century, Abraham Maslow, called it a "continental divide": a struggle that can break people who are initially too weak to handle it will make those already strong enough to survive it even stronger.

There are both triumphs and defeats ahead. Sooner or later, you will miss a workout or slip up on your diet. You will fail in some way, and it may not even be your fault. So much in the world today is outside your control, and nothing stays the same. The skills that matter most going into battle must sometimes give way to the most essential quality at the other end of the fight: *resilience*. Resilience is the ability to bounce back and adapt to life's rough patches and outright calamities, and come out stronger and with your optimism for the future undimmed. Resilience is a hallmark of true Alpha Attitude. Resilient guys have a perspective that life's many changes are something they can cope with, learn from, and adapt to.

Learning from Failure

Everyone makes mistakes. Not everything we do works out as planned or as we hoped. Sometimes our mistakes have dreadful consequences for ourselves or those around us. But we need to move forward—to allow ourselves to "fail forward." In *The Power of Failure*, Charles Manz, PhD, says that to really succeed meaningfully in life you *must* fail. History is filled with examples of individuals who suffered devastating defeats in war, sports, or business but bounced back to succeed in future endeavors. Why did these guys succeed?

They relied on their commitment, their confidence, their courage, and their conscience. They avoided falling into the trap of mental myostatin—those defeatist beliefs that limit true Alpha Attitude.

Even if it's just succumbing to the temptations of wolfing down 2 pints of Häagen-Dazs or hitting the couch instead of the gym, you need to accept that you slipped, put it behind you, and quickly move forward with a plan to do things differently. A single lapse is best overcome *before* it becomes a major relapse, before it becomes a long-term pattern. But often, when people "fall off the wagon," mental myostatin kicks in and says, "If I have given in to one bowl I might as well eat all of it—in for a pint, in for a gallon." No matter how badly you mess up, there is always time to go back and start over again. It's not too late for second chances. A theme in the 2001 psychological thriller *Vanilla Sky* is represented in the film's recurring line: "Every passing moment is another chance to turn it all around."

How can some people who are handed lemons make them into lemonade? In his book *The Resiliency Advantage*, Al Siebert, PhD, points out that hundreds of research studies "show people who cope best in difficult situations score high on measures of 'internal control' beliefs. They feel personally responsible for how well their lives go, and know that they have some control over events and their responses to events." We can approach life with the idea that the things that happen in our lives are under our control, or we can approach it by seeing ourselves as pawns to outside forces beyond our control. We can focus on what we may see as uncontrollable events and fail to see how we can effect change, or we can focus on our own ability to create the best solution possible for the problem. Resilience comes from taking responsibility for ourselves, and for our decisions that go awry, and for working to make every situation the best is can be.

Try not only to learn from every bad experience, but also to be *enriched* by it. When you fail at something, recognize that it is not an ending but a beginning. Nietzsche was right: You *will* be stronger moving forward, *if* you adapt. You may acknowledge that there were times over the past 10 weeks when you fell short of the plan. That happens to everyone. Look back at the path you took: Where did you go off track? What small decision did you make that seemed so minor, meaningless, or harmless at the time, but which ultimately led you far off your course? You can never go back and change what has been done, but you can use it, learn from it, and dedicate your efforts to doing things differently and better the next time around. Often it takes many attempts, or two steps forward and one step back, but that is the cyclic nature of life. Put the detour behind you immediately and get back on track right away.

OPTIMISM CAN BE LEARNED

Facing life's changes with a positive outlook is essential to resilience. Optimism can mean the difference between life and death. Research at Duke University Medical Center aimed at developing a resilience scale to assess the coping skills of different groups of people showed that being optimistic about the effects of life's changes is a key to surviving stress. Daniel Goleman, in his book *Emotional Intelligence,* cited a study of 122 men who had their first heart attack and were assessed on their degree of optimism or pessimism. Eight years later, 21 of the 25 most pessimistic had died, but only 6 of the 25 most optimistic had passed on. Goleman found that mental outlook proved a better predictor of survival than any medical risk factor.

How can you suffer through life's most

difficult experiences and remain optimistic? Put these thoughts foremost in your mind in times of trouble.

- Accept that change is a natural and even very beneficial part of life! Setbacks, pitfalls, and lapses will often occur. Things change, and change can certainly be uncomfortable, stressful, and challenging, but without change, there would be much less adventure in our lives.
- Pay attention to the thoughts that are related to your reactions or responses to change and life's disruptions. What are you telling yourself about the change and your ability to deal with it? Challenge those self-defeating thoughts.
- Setbacks and problems are temporary and they can absolutely be solved! Bad times never last forever. If you weather the storm, you will ultimately sail into calmer waters and clearer skies. Tell yourself, "This too shall pass."
- When one door closes, another that offers better opportunities is bound to open. Look for the opening, because sometimes the door may only be half open and you could miss it.
- You must believe that if you stay committed to your goals and tasks you can succeed. Use new thoughts and words that acknowledge the problem, but see it as solvable with your new positive efforts.
- Create a new solution from this opportunity to learn, and immediately put it into action.
- Start responding to situations rather than reacting to them. This one small change can be incredibly life altering. People who are successful and resilient acknowledge that nothing stays the same, good or bad, that when one thing goes bad it does not mean that everything will; and that they have the primary role in their own destiny. They know

that time passes, things change, and they, in fact, control their ultimate fate more than external forces do. They have mastered their mental myostatin. Their inner monologue is, "This is one thing, for a short time, and I can handle it. I won't give up." They are the true Alpha Males.

NOW WHAT?

Now you choose. You can retreat to your old patterns and practices, or you can integrate the Challenge into the rest of your life. By now you're used to three workouts per week and to integrating Work Heart/Play Heart into your everyday life. By now, following the Fuel Rules of the Alpha Fuel Solution has become quite natural for you. Eating healthy Fuel Foods in Man-Hand portions is easy, and it's something you can do for *life*. The Handshake Diet can nourish you during intense physical training and help you get even leaner. And if you revisit the Spartan Diet, you'll have the chance to experience even more dramatic fat loss.

Your enhanced commitment, confidence, courage, and conscience can stay with you for life—but only if you continue to exercise your Alpha Attitude! After all, your attitude muscles—just like your biceps and triceps—will atrophy and shrink from disuse unless you keep them pumped!

We believe that the changes you've seen in the past 10 weeks aren't an end—they're a beginning. You can continue to make beneficial changes to your life by following the plans and principles of the Challenge. So ask yourself: Why stop now? Think how much leaner, stronger, faster, and more powerful you'll be in 10 *more* weeks! Why not up the ante by setting new goals, pushing even harder, and continuing to improve in all aspects of the program? Why let your attitude drills recede into memory? Why not weave them into your regular routine and keep flexing these important muscles? You'll be better for it, and so will the world around you.

You have a choice. You can look at the past 10 weeks as a program you did, and move on. Or you can recommit to the Pledge. If you're stronger and leaner, you feel better about yourself, then doesn't it make sense to stick with the program? If you need inspiration or ideas on how to take your Alpha Factor to the *next* level, visit us online at www.alphamalechallenge.com. We'll be there to support you!

After all, in the grand scheme of the 2.5-million-year life span of our collective existence, each of our individual life spans is fleeting. We can spend our brief time in weakness or in strength. We can face the world with fear or with courage. We can be content to be who we were, or we can become the men we want to be. The *Alpha Male Challenge* is more than just a 10-week plan, if you believe in it like we do. It's a way to live your life in strength and honor—for yourself, and for those around you.

APPENDIX A
EXERCISES

These are the exercise movements you will perform during your 10-week Challenge. Most require some type of resistance training apparatus, such as a machine, bench, dumbbells, or resistance tubing, but others require only your body weight, such as many Power Boost movements. We've selected a collection of exercises that we believe will maximally develop muscular size, strength, and power over the next 10 weeks. The exercises are carefully rotated within the Challenge for optimal effect. For the Warmup section, see page 299.

The Chest: Stronger, Thicker Pecs

What else can be said about this bulk of muscle that sits on the front of your upper body than that it is what every guy wants and what most women desire on a man—a strong-looking chest! The chest muscles are used in many everyday activities, such as tightly holding on to stuff to carry, pushing yourself up from a sitting position, and climbing out of a pool. The stronger your chest is, the more effortless your ability to lift, carry, and actively perform.

The chest muscles are made up of two muscles: the pectoralis major and the pectoralis minor. They are both located on the front of your rib cage. The pec major (for short) attaches to the humerus (upper arm bone) close to the shoulder joint and originates in the center of the chest, on the breastbone. The pecs are fan shaped, which allows your arms to move in a variety of different directions. The pec minor is located underneath the pec major. It originates on the middle ribs and attaches to the coracoid process of your scapula.

The function of the pec major is to bring your upper arm bone (the humerus) across the midline (chest) of your body. A great example of this is having both arms completely opened up as if to wrap your arms around someone in a big bear hug. The function of the pec minor is to bring the shoulder forward, like when you shrug your shoulders in a forward direction.

When you take an exercise such as a bench press, most guys don't think about how different grips can greatly affect their chest training results. Many guys would rather use a narrow grip, which will usually help them lift heavier weights because of greater involvement of the triceps and front shoulders. The positive thing about the narrow grip is that it increases your range of motion, extending your time under tension. The wider grip, however, may be more effective because it places more emphasis on the chest and lessens the involvement of the triceps and shoulders. The wider grip also allows a greater stretch at the bottom portion of the exercise, even though the range of motion might not be as great as one that the narrower grip provides.

One way to put the brunt of the force on the pec muscles, rather than the shoulders, is as follows: When you lie on the bench or sit upright against a bench to perform your chest exercise, bring your shoulders back (retract the scapulae) as far as they will go. You will notice that the chest rises higher than normal and rises higher than the shoulders, thus taking the shoulders out of the equation to a greater degree and transferring the stimulus to the chest—exactly where you want it!

CHEST

Flat Barbell Bench Press

TARGETED MUSCLES: Pectoralis major and minor (midchest)

SECONDARY MUSCLES: Anterior deltoids, triceps

This exercise is often considered the foundation piece for developing the chest muscles. However, many guys complain that the exercise hurts their shoulders. Any pain may be due to the lifter's individual mechanics and the fact that the barbell's fixed-bar hand placement may inhibit the lifter's natural range of motion. The best advice is to see whether it feels good for you; if it does, continue with it. If it does not, there are plenty of other exercises that are just as effective at building powerful pecs.

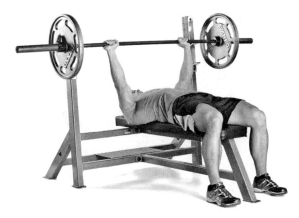 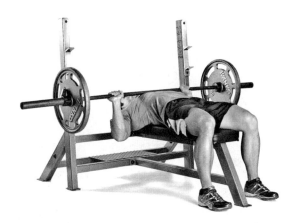

Lie back on the bench and center yourself under the barbell. Plant your feet flat on the floor. Grasp the bar in an overhand (pronated) grip with your hands slightly wider than shoulder-width apart. Arch your chest high, as if you were trying to touch your sternum to the ceiling, and simultaneously retract your shoulder blades. (Bring your shoulder blades back.) This will help isolate the chest muscles and, to a degree, keep your anterior deltoids from being involved during the exercise. Inhale and tense your chest muscles and lats. Exhale as you extend your arms to push the bar up and unrack it. If you're using very heavy weights, have your training partner help you with this part so that you don't injure your shoulders. You should be holding the weight with your arms extended straight toward the ceiling. If you have a shoulder injury or are lifting heavy weight, use your training partner for a spot lift.

Inhale as you slowly lower the barbell toward your chest. The descent should be slow and controlled. As your elbows come down, don't let them go straight out to the sides—angle them toward your hips a bit. This will recruit the strongest part of your chest instead of your shoulders.

When the barbell is within an inch of your chest, squeeze hard with your chest muscles and press it back up. You may touch the bar to your chest, but absolutely no bouncing or momentum. Exhale as you press it back up to the starting position. Don't lock your elbows at the top of the press; that will take stimulation off your chest muscles. Keep your chest muscles contracted throughout the exercise. Once you reach the top of the press, momentarily contract your chest muscles as hard as possible. Then inhale as you start lowering the bar for the next repetition.

Flat Dumbbell Bench Press

TARGETED MUSCLES: *Pectoralis major and minor (midchest)*

SECONDARY MUSCLES: *Anterior deltoids, triceps*

This is the ultimate exercise for creating powerful pecs. Each arm works independently, requiring more stabilizer muscles in the arms and shoulders. The motion is almost exactly like a punch, so it's great for building your punching strength for self-defense. Like the flat barbell bench press, the flat dumbbell bench press uses all the major muscle groups of the upper body and is capable of high intensity energy output. However, the extra stabilization strength required means you won't be using as much weight as you could with a barbell.

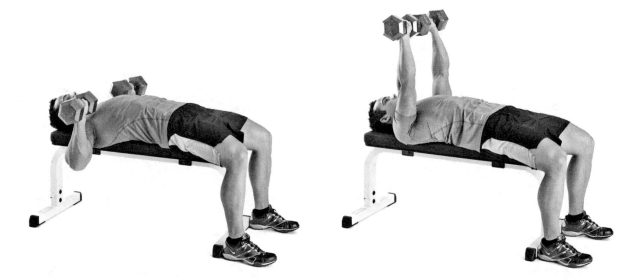

Either take a pair of dumbbells from the rack or squat down and pick up the dumbbells, using your legs. Do not bend over at the hips to do this, as it can injure your lower back. Stand up and place the dumbbells in front of each thigh and sit down on the end of the bench.

Holding the dumbbells on top of your thighs, independently thrust each up into place as you lie back on the bench. (The whole sequence should be one smooth move, i.e., thrust left leg/dumbbell up, move quickly right into thrusting right leg/dumbbell up, and sit back and position the dumbbells in the starting position.) Plant your feet flat on the floor. With your elbows out to the sides, hold the dumbbells at chest level in an overhand (pronated) grip as shown. Arch your chest high, as if you were trying to touch your sternum to the ceiling, and squeeze your shoulder blades back into the bench.

Tense your pecs and press the dumbbells straight up toward the ceiling.

Inhale as you slowly lower the dumbbells toward your chest. The descent should be slow and controlled. As you approach the bottom of the movement, allow your chest muscles to get a good stretch before contracting and pushing back up to the starting position for the next repetition.

> *True Alpha Tip: If you have an existing shoulder injury or are using heavy a weight, let your training partner assist you in getting the dumbbells into the overhead position. At the top of the press, you'll be able to contract your pecs extra hard by touching the inner dumbbell plates together. Don't lock your elbows, which will take the stimulation off your muscles and put pressure on your elbows.*

Incline Dumbbell Bench Press

TARGETED MUSCLES: Pectoralis major and minor (upper chest)

SECONDARY MUSCLES: Anterior deltoids, triceps

This exercise targets the upper chest muscles. You may want to position the bench to the incline position as it uses less of your shoulder muscles while still principally targeting your upper chest. This permits you to use slightly heavier dumbbells to stimulate more muscle fibers in the upper chest. If you don't feel your upper chest being stimulated, you may raise the seat back, but just make sure that you're not allowing your anterior deltoids to play a major role during the exercise.

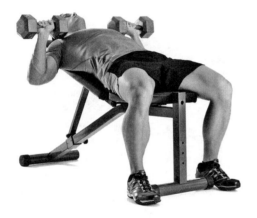

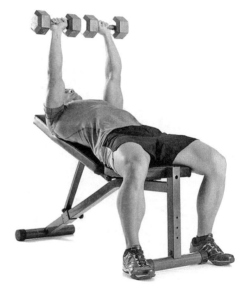

Set the incline position of your bench to about 23 degrees (try for halfway between 0 and 45 degrees). Pick up a dumbbell in each hand and take a seat. Lift each dumbbell on top of your thighs and independently thrust each up into place as you lie back on the bench. With your elbows out to the sides, hold the dumbbells at chest level in an overhand (pronated) grip. Arch your chest high, as if you were trying to touch your sternum to the ceiling and remember to retract those shoulder blades to raise the chest higher than the anterior deltoids.

Tense your pecs as you press the dumbbells straight up toward the ceiling. Exhale as you press. At the top of the press, you'll have an opportunity to contract the pecs extra hard by touching the inner plates of the dumbbells together. Don't lock your elbows, which will take the stimulation off of your muscles and put pressure on your elbows. Keep your upper chest muscles contracted throughout the exercise.

Inhale as you slowly lower the dumbbells toward your chest. The descent should be slow and controlled. As you approach the bottom of the movement, allow your chest muscles to get a good stretch. Without resting, slowly and smoothly begin contracting your chest muscles and push those dumbbells back up for the next repetition.

Incline Barbell Bench Press

TARGETED MUSCLES: Pectoralis major and minor (upper chest)

SECONDARY MUSCLES: Anterior deltoids, triceps

Performing barbell presses on an incline will stimulate the muscles across the top portion of your chest. When you fully develop your upper chest, your overall chest will look larger than it really is. Nothing looks better in an open-collar shirt than thick upper pecs.

The front shoulders (anterior deltoids) come into play more in this exercise than in the flat barbell press, so you won't be able to use as much weight. However, because fewer stabilizer muscles are needed, most guys are able to lift significantly more weight compared to the dumbbell versions.

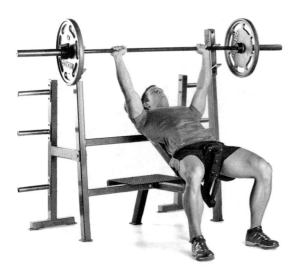
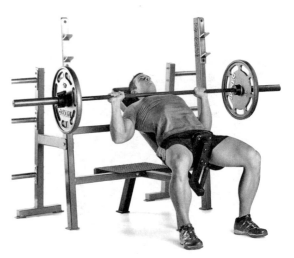

Lie back on the incline bench and center yourself under the barbell. Plant your feet flat on the floor. Grasp the bar in an overhand (pronated) grip with your hands slightly wider than shoulder-width apart. Arch your chest high, as if you were trying to touch your sternum to the ceiling and remember to bring your shoulder blades back. Inhale and tense your chest muscles. Exhale and extend your arms to push the bar up and unrack it. You should be holding the weight with your arms extended straight toward the ceiling. If you have a shoulder injury or are lifting heavy weight, ask your training partner for a spot lift.

Inhale as you slowly lower the barbell toward your collarbone. The descent should be slow and controlled. When the barbell comes within ½ inch of your collarbone (or briefly touches you, as long as you feel no shoulder pain), contract your chest hard and press it back up. Exhale as you press. Don't lock your elbows at the top of the press, which will take stimulation off your muscles and put pressure on your elbows. Once you reach the top of the press, contract those pecs as powerfully as you can. Inhale as you start lowering the bar back toward your chest for the next repetition.

True Alpha Tip: You can play around with your grip width to see which stimulates your chest muscles more.

Pec Deck Fly

TARGETED MUSCLES: *Pectoralis major and minor (midchest)*

SECONDARY MUSCLES: *Anterior deltoids*

The machine fly will allow you to get a great pec contraction at the top portion of the exercise. This is often difficult to accomplish with dumbbells, as the majority of resistance is distributed to the shoulder and elbow joints when you reach the top portion of the exercise. The fly is essential for lifting and carrying large objects you have to wrap your arms around.

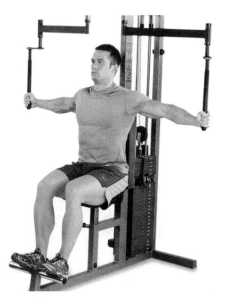 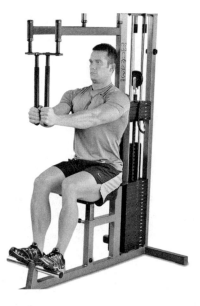

Sit in the machine with your feet on the foot rest and your entire back—especially your lower back—pressed firmly to the seat back. **For the hand bar option:** Position the seat so that your outstretched arms are at the same height as the handles. Sitting too low or too high can put undue stress on your shoulders. **For the forearm pad option:** Set the arm pads for pressing movements, positioning them out to the sides rather than in front of or behind the seat back. Open your arms out to the sides, with your upper arms parallel to the floor, elbows bent at right angles, and hands approximately level with your head. Place your forearms against the pads and grasp the handles.

Inhale and tighten your chest and abdominal muscles. Squeeze your chest muscles and follow the directions for the machine you're using.

For the hand bar option (shown): With a closed neutral grip on the handles and your arms out to the sides of your body, bend your elbows slightly and keep them bent throughout the exercise. Exhale as you begin to contract your chest muscles and bring the bars toward one another, imagining that you're giving a bear hug. The bear hug imagery will help keep the emphasis on your chest muscles. When you reach the top position, momentarily contract your pecs as hard as possible. Inhale and slowly return the bars to the starting position. Just before the weight hits bottom, contract your chest and start the next repetition without pause or momentum.

For the forearm pad option: Using your forearms to apply pressure to the pads will ensure maximum pec involvement while minimizing front shoulder activation. Follow the same execution guidelines for the hand bar option, as described above.

Flat Dumbbell Fly

Dumbbell flies are a great exercise to further develop your chest. They deliver an excellent pump that triggers the pec muscle fibers. Although dumbbell flies don't develop as much strength as machine flies do (because you use lighter weight), they are better for developing joint strength and stability. Make sure to contract the pecs hardest in the top portion of the exercise.

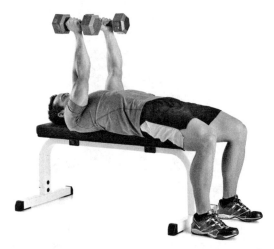

Pick up a dumbbell in each hand and sit on the end of a flat bench. Hold the dumbbells to your chest, using the independent thigh thrust and lie back on the bench. Plant your feet flat and firmly on the floor. Press the dumbbells straight up toward the ceiling, holding the dumbbells in one of the following ways:

Palms facing: Your palms face each other. This is the traditional fly grip.

Palms away: Your palms face away from the front of your body. This grip might feel a bit strange at first, but give it a chance. If you feel any stress on your shoulders, stop and go back to the palms-facing grip.

Press the dumbbells straight up toward the ceiling, holding them parallel to each other. Contract your chest muscles and inhale as you allow the dumbbells to arc out to the sides and down. The motion is as if you were open-

ing a pair of wings. Allow your elbows to bend very slightly to keep the biceps from getting overstretched. Stop lowering the dumbbells before they are level with your chest. At chest level and below, you will be using more deltoid (shoulder) muscle than chest muscle and may risk injury.

Just before the dumbbells reach chest level, contract your chest muscles and reverse the direction of the dumbbells, bear hugging them back up to the top. Touch the dumbbells together just briefly at the top (don't rest them against each other), then slowly and smoothly begin lowering them for the next repetition.

After the last repetition of the set, instead of lowering the dumbbells out to your sides, bring them straight down to your chest. You can thrust your thighs down for momentum to help get you back up to a sitting position.

Incline Dumbbell Fly

This version of the fly focuses on the upper chest muscles. Use much lighter weights for this exercise than you would for presses, because holding a weight at arm's length multiplies its effective resistance. Working with dumbbells that are too heavy can easily result in injury.

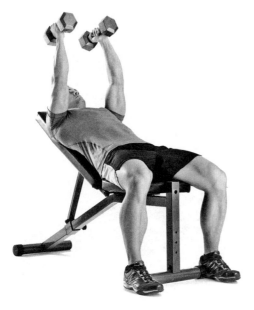

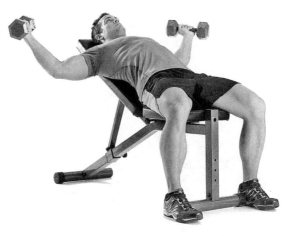

Set your bench at an incline of about 45 degrees. Pick up a dumbbell in each hand, place them on the fronts of your thighs, and take a seat. Press your entire back firmly against the seat back and put your feet flat on the floor. Lift the dumbbells to your chest, using the independent thigh thrust. Press the dumbbells straight up toward the ceiling, holding the dumbbells in one of the following ways:

Palms facing: Your palms face each other. This is the traditional fly grip.

Palms away: Your palms face away from the front of your body. This grip might feel a bit strange at first, but give it a chance. If you feel any stress on the shoulders, stop and go back to the palms-facing grip.

The palms facing away grip might feel a bit strange at first, but give it a chance. If you feel any stress on your shoulders, stop and go back to the palms facing grip.

Contract your chest muscles and inhale as you allow the dumbbells to arc out to the sides and down. The motion is

as if you were opening a pair of wings. Allow your elbows to bend very slightly to keep your biceps from getting overstretched. Stop lowering the dumbbells before they become level with your chest. At chest level and below, you will be using more deltoid (shoulder) muscle than chest muscle and may risk injury.

Just before the dumbbells reach shoulder level, contract your chest muscles and slowly, smoothly, and deliberately reverse direction, arcing (bear hugging) the dumbbells back up to the top as you exhale. Touch the dumbbells together just briefly at the top (don't rest them against each other). Then slowly and smoothly begin lowering again for the next repetition.

After the last repetition of the set, instead of lowering the dumbbells out to the sides, bring them into your chest and down to your thighs. Then sit up and set the dumbbells on the floor. Although not as difficult a position as the flat bench, you can thrust your thighs down for momentum to help get you back up to a sitting position.

Chest Dumbbell Pullover

TARGETED MUSCLES: *Pectoralis major and minor (mid- and upper-chest)*

SECONDARY MUSCLES: *Triceps, latissimus dorsi*

Before the invention of forklifts and winches, man used to lift heavy objects using a rope and pulley. That's the kind of strength this exercise develops: massive pulling power. Dumbbell pullovers will really thicken your chest and strengthen the serratus muscles along your ribs; those muscles are responsible for much of your vertical pulling power.

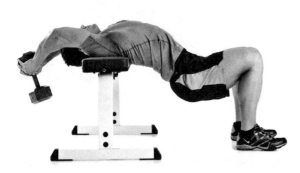 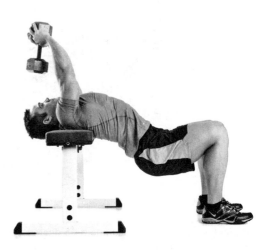

With a dumbbell in hand, lie with your shoulders and upper back across a flat bench and place your feet flat on the floor. Your body and the bench should form a T. Lower your hips so they are below the height of the bench seat. Make sure the plates on your dumbbell are secure, then hold it vertically in both hands by placing your palms in an overlapping position against the inside of the dumbbell's top plate. The handle of the dumbbell should pass between the thumb and first finger of both your hands held in a butterfly grip. Press the dumbbell straight up and fully extend your arms. The dumbbell should be directly over your face. Inhale and tighten your abdominals and glutes.

Keep them tight throughout the exercise. Lower the dumbbell behind your head while keeping your arms as straight as possible. (If you bend your elbows too much, this becomes a triceps exercise rather than a chest exercise.) Do not let your hips rise up as you lower the weight as far back as you can without losing control, and make sure to inhale. Let the weight stretch your muscles.

Contract your chest and pull the dumbbell back overhead in an arcing motion. Exhale as you pull the dumbbell up. Once the dumbbells are overhead again, contract your chest muscles as hard as you can. Then inhale and slowly and smoothly start lowering again for the next repetition.

Chest Dip

TARGETED MUSCLES: Pectoralis major and minor (midchest)

SECONDARY MUSCLES: Anterior deltoids, triceps

The chest dip is an essential climbing exercise—it's like pushing yourself out of the deep end of a swimming pool. If you go for sports like rock climbing, this exercise paired with pullups are great for strengthening your arms for pulling and pushing yourself from one ledge to another. Roofers, carpenters, and construction workers will also find many uses for the strength developed through chest dips.

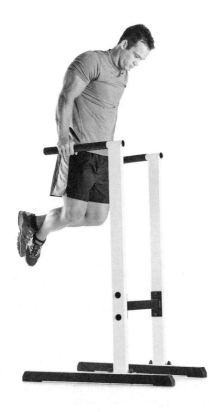
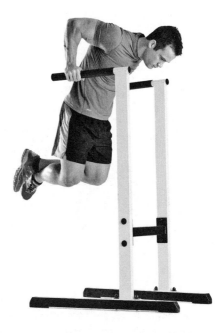

Situate yourself on a parallel dip station so that each hand is on a dip bar and your arms are fully extended with your elbows locked. Your body should be hanging between the dip bars. Bend your knees and cross your ankles behind you.

Inhale and contract your chest and triceps muscles, then lean as far forward as gravity will allow and lower your body between the dip bars. (Note that failure to lean forward makes this more of a triceps exercise than a chest exercise.

To help you lean forward, look down throughout the exercise.) Stop lowering yourself when your chest is level with the dip bars. In the lowered position, no part of your body should touch the floor—remain suspended at all times. Then push through your lower chest and raise yourself back up as you exhale. Just before your elbows lock, start lowering yourself for the next repetition. To add more resistance to your body weight, see Alternate Weighted Dip on page 278.

Pushup

Nothing is more functional than resistance training using your own body weight. Every guy should include pushups in his chest workout, even if it's just as a warmup or cooldown. If you need to make pushups tougher, place your hands farther from your body (either out in front of you or out to the sides) or elevate your feet. Doing pushups between two benches (a hand on each bench with feet elevated to a similar height) so that you can go deeper into the stretch will also increase the difficulty and help build thicker, fully developed chest muscles.

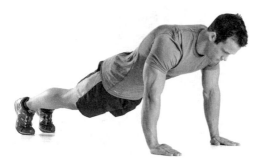
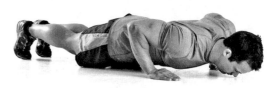

Assume the classic military pushup position in which you support your body on hands and toes. Your arms should be as straight as possible without locking your elbows, and your palms should be flat on the floor. Look up slightly and keep your eyes fixed on a spot just in front of you. If you have a weak lower back and find it difficult to maintain a straight body, let your butt come up just a little bit and allow your hips to have a slight bend. Contract and tighten every muscle in your body from shoulders to ankles. You should be completely rigid throughout the movement to avoid stressing your lower back.

Inhale and bend at the elbows to lower yourself to the floor. Descend slowly and in control as you lower your body. Stop descending when your chest is about 2 inches from the floor, but do not let your chest hit the floor. Contract your chest muscles hard and push yourself back up to the starting position, exhaling. Stop the ascent just before locking your elbows. Start immediately into the next repetition.

True Alpha Tip: If doing pushups on your palms aggravates a wrist problem, you can perform them on the knuckles of your closed fists or on the popular Perfect Pushup handles.

THE PUSHUP CHALLENGE

Inspired by the martial arts and *sometimes* used as a training test for black belt status, this test requires you to perform as many consecutive full repetition (You'll bring your chest to about 2 inches off the floor on each rep) pushups as you can without stopping.

To pass a black belt test, the minimum number of pushups required is 75 consecutive repetitions. By all means, if you can perform more than 75 pushups in one shot, go for it. Not only would that be an awesome feat, but based on the statistics of how many consecutive pushups a man can do (see chart below) within his age bracket, performing more than 60 consecutive pushups for any man is an extraordinary feat!

Level C trainers will perform one set only, for as many as you can get using great form. Level's A and B will perform two sets, separated by a one minute rest interval. *Set a goal:* Shoot for 40 pushups on your first set and 35 pushups on your second set. Although you've got a 1.5 minute rest in between sets, it's still very challenging, especially for men who are not used to doing pushups.

It takes confidence to get down on the floor and meet the Pushup Challenge, but don't back down! Keep going until you can't do one more. Try your hardest to get as many reps as you can.

(Refer to the chart below to see how well most guys do.)

Pushup Test

AGE	17–19	20–29	30–39	40–49	50–59	60–65
Excellent	>56	>47	>41	>34	>31	>30
Good	47–56	39–47	34–41	28–34	25–31	24–30
Above average	35–46	30–39	25–33	21–28	18–24	17–23
Average	19–34	17–29	13–24	11–20	9–17	6–16
Below average	11–18	10–16	8–12	6–10	5–8	3–5
Poor	4–10	4–9	2–7	1–5	1–4	1–2
Very Poor	<4	<4	<2	0	0	0

RESISTANCE TUBING EXERCISE

TARGETED MUSCLES: Pectoralis major

SECONDARY TARGET: Anterior deltoids

Band Bench

Here's a great shoulder exercise for your Home Body Routine or for training while traveling.

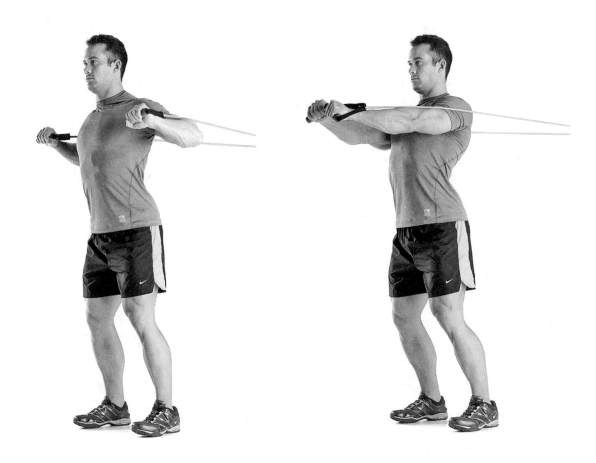

Affix resistive tubing or a resistance band around a pole or firm object so that the handles or loose ends are available. Standing with your back to the pole, grab the handles and assume a starting position similar to a bench press. Keeping your feet firmly planted and your chest and head up with little bend at the waist, press both tube ends away from your chest. Fully extend your arms, then bring them back to the starting position under control before beginning the next repetition.

POWER BOOST MOVEMENTS/ PLYOMETRICS

TARGETED MUSCLES: *Pectoralis major and minor*

SECONDARY MUSCLES: *Anterior deltoids, triceps*

Power Pushup

This Power Boost movement is a great upper body exercise. It's one thing to be able to do a strict pushup, but it's another thing to be able to thrust your body into midair and catch yourself. This movement will absolutely produce a powerful upper body. Remember that it's not just important to get as high as you can; you also want to reduce the time it takes for you to transition from your landing right back into the next power pushup repetition. Focus on staying strict with your form, progressively increasing the height of your air time and rebound as quickly as possible!

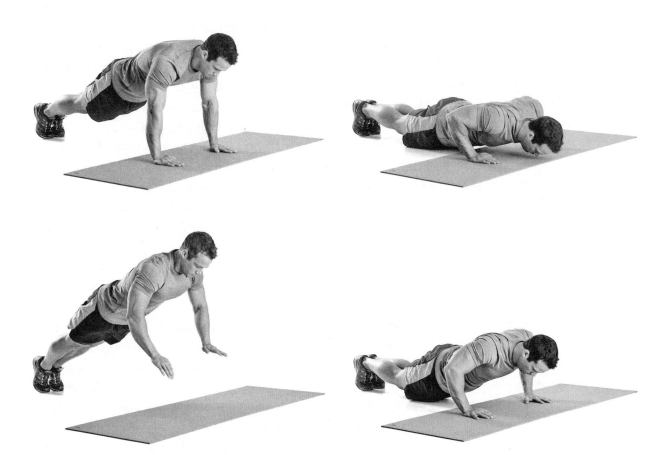

Assume the top position of a pushup, with your hands just wider than your shoulders, your feet together, your back flat, and your face pointed at the floor. Rapidly descend into the bottom position.

When your chest is 2 inches from the floor, reverse your direction and push yourself up as quickly as possible. Try to accelerate all the way through the pushup so that your hands leave the ground when you reach the top.

When your hands return to the ground, catch your body with a slight bend in your elbows and without pause, go right into your next pushup. Reset and perform again. It is essential to keep your abs tight and back flat throughout this exercise. Any sagging of your trunk or shoulders will make it more difficult to get off the ground and will increase your chance of injury.

THE BACK: GETTING THE V-TAPER

The back comprises the largest muscular area of the upper body. Training the back's muscles will greatly improve your overall body training efforts, which is one reason why you should be really focusing on this fat-burning and muscle-building arsenal.

The back is made up of five superficial muscles known as the latissimus dorsi, the rhomboid major, the rhomboid minor, the trapezius, and the levator scapulae. They are also made up of deep muscles known as the erector spinae.

The latissimus dorsi are the monster muscles of the back. They are known by most guys as the wings, or what makes up the V in the V-taper look. These large fan-shaped muscles, like the pecs, allow you to perform a wide range of movements. Even more multifaceted than the chest muscles, the lats (for short) can perform movements in a variety of positions, including standing, leaning back, and many others. They are attached to the upper end of the upper arm (the humerus), with the muscle fibers running in a fan shape down the vertebral column and the pelvic girdle. Obviously, the lats are *huge* muscles—even more reason to really focus on developing them.

The teres major muscle is located on the outside edge of the scapula and is attached to the upper arm (the humerus). Its function is to move the upper arm to the posterior (back behind you).

The rhomboids are rectangular-shaped muscles, and their function is to bring the shoulder blades (scapulae) back.

The teres and rhomboids together are great for developing superior posture. Many guys suffer from internally protracted shoulders. This can be caused by genetics, but in most cases it's due to an obsession with training only the chest and front of the shoulders while neglecting to train these very useful back muscles. The good news is that you can usually reverse rounded shoulders and bring the shoulders back. By training these muscles you'll get the superior posture that conveys confidence and a strong disposition.

The trapezius, along with the levator scapulae muscles, allow you to shrug your shoulders. The trapezius muscles are located on the tops and rear of your shoulders, while the levator scapulae are located at the back and sides of your neck. Many people mistake the trapezius muscles for shoulder muscles, but they are, in fact, part of your many back muscles. They are named the trapezius muscles (traps for short) because of their trapezoid shape. The traps begin at the base of the skull, run down the upper part of the spinal cord, and then extend down to the middle of the lower back.

The function of the deeper erector spinae muscles is to help keep your body erect. The erectors help extend the trunk and rotate it. The erectors are known as the strongest muscles of all the back muscles because they take on most of the work.

It should be no surprise how important these muscles are in helping you perform everyday movements. Without them, your ability to sit, stand, turn, and ultimately function effectively would be impeded. You can also imagine just how hard these muscles are always working to keep you upright. It's a good thing they get their rest while you sleep!

As you can clearly see, the back muscles are like a fleet of soldiers, all working for a great cause: to protect your spine, give you greater physical presence, and keep you tall and upright. They are used in just about any activity you can think of. Exercises like pullups and chinups are staples in military training because they are the most effective and efficient exercises for developing the muscles whose strength could easily mean the difference between life and death. Think about scaling a wall, pulling yourself up from a rock ledge, picking up a heavy sack of cement, or leisurely hopping out of a pool—the benefits of a strong back are endless!

BACK

SECONDARY MUSCLES: *Biceps, trapezius, rear deltoids, rhomboids, teres*

T-Bar Row

The T-bar row develops massive power in the lats and upper back. It has the same advantage of a barbell row, but it allows a greater range of motion.

This rowing exercise uses a bar that has barbell plates loaded on only one end while the other end is locked into a hinge that allows the bar to tilt up and down while keeping the end from rolling. If your gym doesn't have a secure hinge to lock in one side of the barbell, you can tuck one side into a secure metal framed corner and have your training partner stand on the end to hold it in place. The weight-loaded end has a crossbar attached just below the collar. Our favorite machine of this kind has a chest pad, so you can lean forward for added lower back support. The traditional machine provides only a metal platform where you stand, and there's nothing else between you and the barbell end/weights.

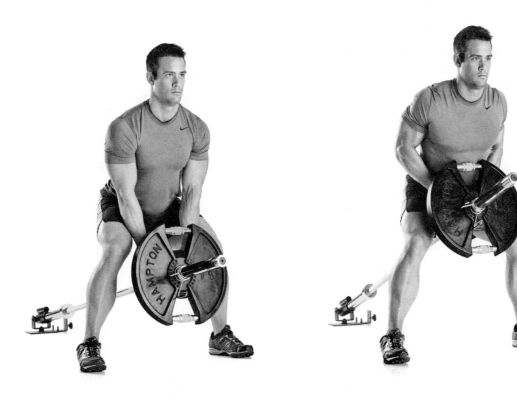

Stand over the bar with a foot on either side. (Machine T-bars usually have a platform for each foot.) Bend over and grasp the crossbar handles. Now lower your hips and butt until your knees are bent at a 90-degree angle or slightly less.

With your chest out, shoulders back, and head up, tense the muscles in your abdomen, butt, and back. Exhale and pull the weight toward your sternum. Drive your elbows back and up as far as you can, attempting to touch the crossbar to your sternum. Squeeze the shoulder blades together at the top of your movement. Pause before inhaling and lowering the weight.

Machine Row (Neutral Grip)

This close, two-hand grip exercise simulates practical, everyday pulling actions. The neutral grip targets the upper portion of the lats and the teres major (under the back side of your shoulder) more than some of the other rows.

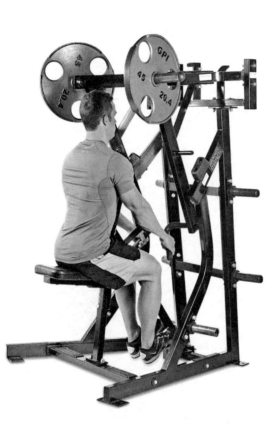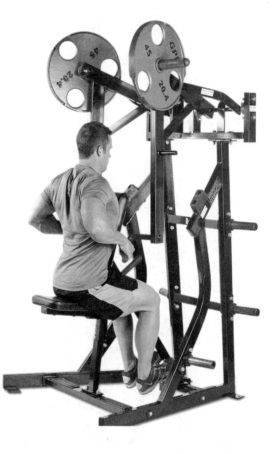

Take a seat on the machine and face the handles. Place your feet on the platforms. If the handles are adjustable, adjust them to a vertical position so that you can grasp them with a neutral grip. Keep your torso as vertical and straight as possible. Your gaze should be straight ahead.

With your chest against the pad, shoulders back, and head up, tighten your abs, exhale, and pull the grips toward your belly. Really drive your elbows back as far as you can go, concentrating on the pull of the lats. During the pull, do not think about your arms. Instead, focus on

pulling with your lats and upper back muscles. Squeeze those shoulder blades and try to touch them together.

Your final position should have your elbows reaching behind and past your back. (Don't lie back as if you're on a lounge chair like some folks at the gym do. That puts a strain on the lower back.)

Once you've pulled the grips as far back as you can, contract your back muscles as hard as possible, and return to the starting position. Inhale as you resist the weight on the way back. Prepare for the next repetition.

One Arm Machine Row

TARGETED MUSCLES: Latissimus dorsi

SECONDARY MUSCLES: Teres, trapezius, rear deltoids, biceps

Nothing conveys strength and power like a broad back—the kind of back men used to get by heaving boulders, rowing boats, and swinging sledgehammers. In the modern age, most men don't have to do that kind of work. They turn to the gym for a safer, more effective workout. Rows of all kinds are key to building that strong, powerful, broad back. The one-arm row with pronated grip is great because it allows a more powerful pull.

Performing rows one arm at a time can also help you correct or prevent muscle imbalances in your upper back. You know you're getting an equal workout on both sides.

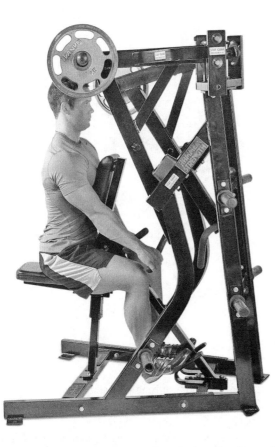

Take a seat on the machine and face the handles. Depending on the style of machine, either place your feet on the platforms or flat on the floor. Grasp the neutral grip handle and with your nonworking hand, grab a stationary handle or other nonmoving part of the machine to maintain your balance. Keep your torso as vertical and straight as possible. Keep your gaze straight ahead.

With your chest against the pad, shoulders back, and head up, tighten your abs and glutes, exhale, and pull the grip toward your shoulder. Really drive your elbow back as far as you can go, concentrating on the pull of the lats.

During the pull, do not think about your arm. Instead, focus on pulling with your lats and upper back muscles.

Once you've pulled that grip as far back as you can get it while keeping your torso straight, hold momentarily, and then return to the starting position. Inhale as you resist the weight on the way back. Prepare for the next repetition.

One Arm Dumbbell Row

TARGETED MUSCLES: *Latissimus dorsi*

SECONDARY MUSCLES: *Trapezius, rear deltoids, biceps, rhomboids, teres*

For those of you still using a push mower to mow your lawn, this exercise will quickly get your arms in shape for pulling that starting cord. It's the exact same movement. Rowing with one arm at a time allows you to focus on developing those back muscles while the support of the non-working arm reduces the risk of lower back injury.

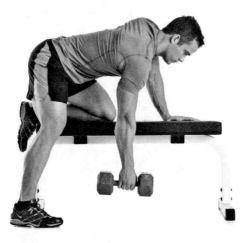
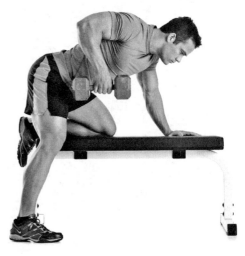

Place your left hand and left knee on the long edge of a flat bench. Position your right foot flat on the floor with enough bend in the knee to keep your hips level. Your hips should be even with or slightly lower than the shoulders. With your right hand, pick up a dumbbell with a neutral grip so that the dumbbell is parallel to your body. While allowing your arm to hang straight, lift the dumbbell high enough off the floor that you can keep your hips level.

With your chest out, shoulders back, and head down, inhale. Exhale and tighten the abdominals. Focus on pulling with your lats as you pull the dumbbell up and close to the side of your body, driving your elbow toward the ceiling. Keep pulling until your elbow is slightly higher than your back.

Hold the maximally contracted position for just a moment before inhaling and slowly lowering the dumbbell toward the floor. *Do not* set the dumbbell on the floor! Only lower the dumbbell far enough to fully extend your arm and stretch the lat without leaning forward or tilting the hips. Once you reach the fully extended position, exhale and pull hard on the lat and start the next repetition.

Lat Pullup

TARGETED MUSCLES: *Latissimus dorsi*

SECONDARY MUSCLES: *Trapezius, rear deltoids, biceps,rhomboids, teres*

This is, without question, one of the greatest back exercises available to you. Pullups are sometimes confused with chinups. They are a classic and very functional exercise for developing the muscles of the back and arms. They are popular in military training because of their direct application to pulling yourself up over fences and walls in a combat situation. If you are not strong enough yet to do a pullup, you can use a Gravitron machine to assist you. Instructions for using a Gravitron are usually on the machine. For more of a challenge, add resistance. See alphamalechallenge.com.

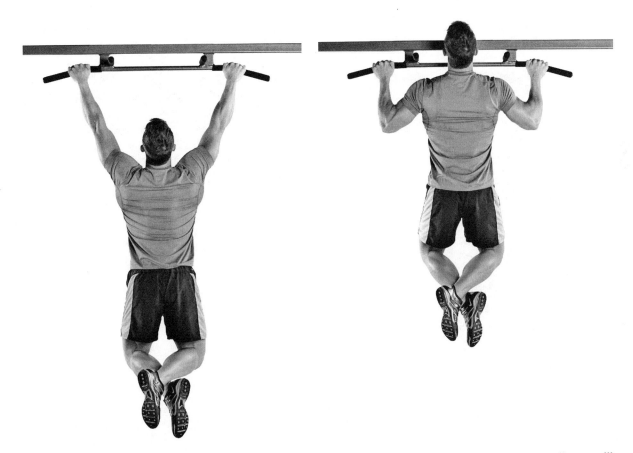

Stand under a pullup bar, reach up, and grab hold of it with an overhand grip with your hands 30 inches apart (slightly wider than shoulder-width) or more. Now hang by your hands. Bend your knees, cross your ankles, and hold your feet up behind you; or, for a more difficult exercise, lift your feet off the ground in front of you and let your abdominal muscles hold them up.

Begin by tensing all the muscles in your arms, back, and abdomen. Take a breath and get ready to pull your chest to the bar as you exhale. Ideally, you should be able to touch the bar to your collarbone, but don't worry if you

can't get all the way up there yet—eventually you will. When you pull up, concentrate on pulling with your lats—those big, thick muscles across the middle of your back. Don't think about your biceps, just your back.

As you reach the top of the pullup, hold the position for just a moment and really contract those back muscles as hard as you can before lowering yourself to the starting position. Inhale as you descend, but make sure that you descend at a controlled speed, and keep your lats tense. That extra muscle tension directed at your lats during your descent will really pump up those back muscles.

Narrow-Grip Pullup
Alternate: Narrow-Grip Pulldown

Executing pullups with a narrow grip attacks the lats and some of the underlying muscles from a different angle than the wide-grip pullup does. Combining narrow-grip pullups with wide-grip pullups will lead to more complete development of the lats. Using a neutral grip instead of just moving your hands close together helps keep your forearms out of the equation so you can fully engage the lats.

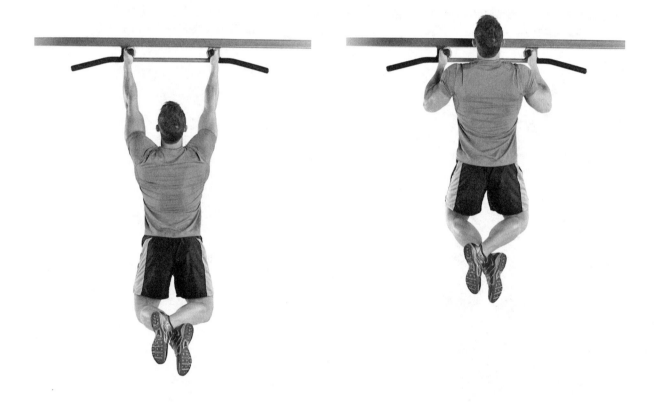

Some pullup stations have stationary parallel (neutral grip) pullup bars. You can either use them (as shown in the photos) or use a V-bar. Simply place the V-bar over the pullup bar so that one handle is on either side.

Stand under a pullup bar, reach up and grab the handles. Now hang by your hands. Bend your knees and hold your feet up behind you.

Tense all the muscles in your arms, back, and abdomen. Take a breath and exhale as you pull your chest as close to the bars as possible while exhaling. As your head nears the pullup bar, keep your head tilted slightly back, to avoid hitting your head on the bar.

When you pull up, concentrate on pulling with your lats. Don't think about your biceps, just your back.

When you reach the top of the pullup, hold the position for just a moment as you contract your back muscles as hard as you can before lowering yourself to the starting position. Descend at a controlled speed and keep your lats tense throughout the exercise.

Lat Pulldown

TARGETED MUSCLES: *Latissimus dorsi*

SECONDARY MUSCLES: *Biceps, rear deltoids, rhomboids, teres*

This is an excellent alternate to pullups if you are not yet strong enough to do a pullup. It is also excellent if you've already done as many body-weight pullups as you can but still want to reach your rep target. Pulldowns require a cable pulley system in which the pulley is higher than your head, as with a lat pulldown machine.

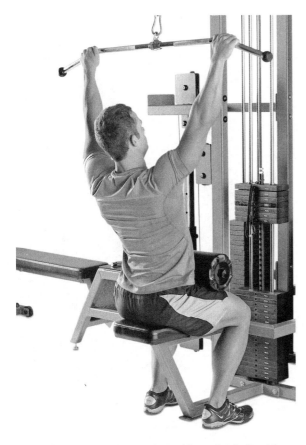
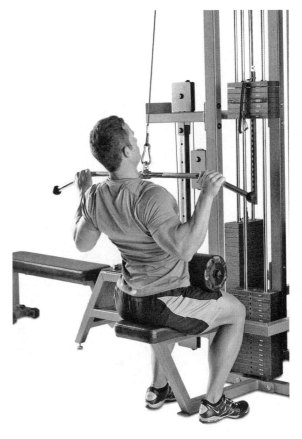

Attach a wide-grip bar to the cable and grip it with an overhand grip. You can use either a straight bar or a bar with angled grips. A bar with angled grips puts less stress on your wrists in the lowered contracted position. Sit directly under the pulley with your arms extended overhead. If the pulley isn't high enough to allow you to fully extend your arms while keeping the cable tight, try leaning back to accommodate the shallow distance.

Lean back slightly from your hips, stick your chest out, bring your shoulders back, and gaze at an angle at the wall in front of you. With elbows wide, exhale, and pull the bar down to your chest. Drive your elbows down as far as you can, concentrating on the pull of the lats.

Ideally, you should be able to touch the bar to your chest. Once in that final position, hold momentarily as you contract your lats as hard as possible, and then return the bar back to the starting position. Inhale and resist the weight on the way back. Start the next repetition just before the weight touches bottom.

TARGETED MUSCLES: *Latissimus dorsi, biceps*

SECONDARY MUSCLES: *Biceps, rear deltoids, rhomboids, teres*

Chindown

Chindowns are an excellent alternate to chinups when you can't pull up your own body weight and still want to reach your target repetitions. This seated exercise will allow you to lock your thighs underneath a lap bar, which allows you to do chindowns with either more or less weight than your body weight.

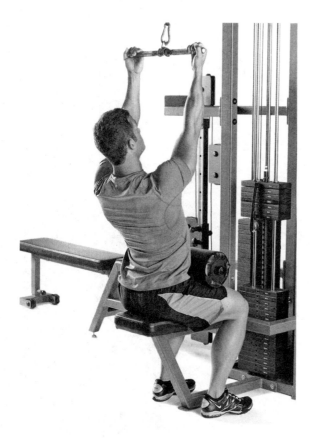
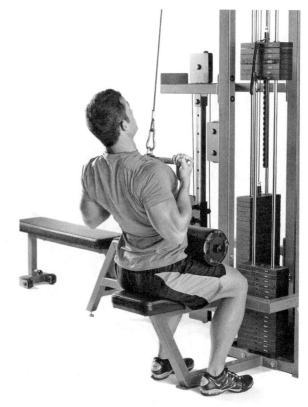

Attach an E-Z bar to the cable and grip it with an underhand grip. Sit directly under the pulley with your arms extended overhead. If the pulley isn't high enough to allow you to fully extend your arms while keeping the cable tight, lean back slightly to accommodate the shallow distance.

Lean back from your hips, stick your chest out, bring your shoulders back, and gaze up at an angle at the wall in front of you. Pull the bar down toward your chest. Drive your elbows back as far as you can, concentrating on the pull of the lats.

Ideally, you should be able to touch the bar to your chest. Once in that final position, hold momentarily, as you contract your lats as hard as possible and return the bar back to the starting position. Inhale as you resist the weight as it pulls your arms up. Start the next repetition just before the weight touches bottom.

Chinup
Alternate: Weighted Chinup

TARGETED MUSCLES: *Lower latissimus dorsi*

SECONDARY MUSCLES: *Biceps, teres major, lower trapezius, serratus, core*

Chinups employ more of the biceps and serratus muscles than do the overhand-grip pullups. This particular exercise helps develop complete vertical pulling power of the back and torso. For more of a challenge, add resistance. See alphamalechallenge.com.

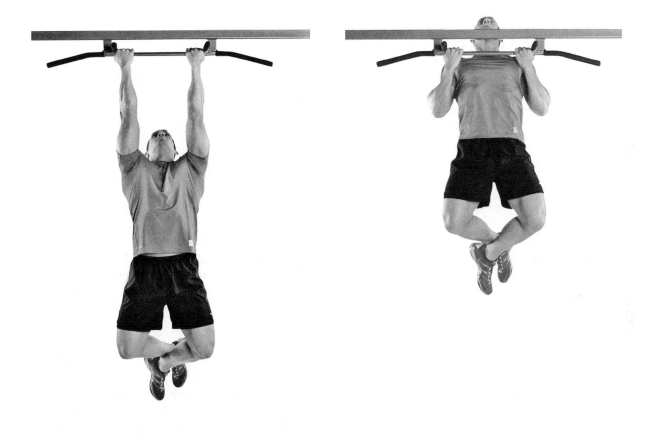

Stand under a pullup bar. Reach up and grab the bar with a shoulder-width underhand grip. Now hang by your hands, bend your knees, cross your feet, and hold them up behind you.

Tense all the muscles in your arms, back, and abdomen. Take a deep breath and begin by exhaling as you pull yourself up, striving to get your head over the bar. Ideally, you should be able to raise your chin up over the bar and even touch the bar to your collarbone or chest. When you pull up, concentrate on pulling with your lats.

As you reach the top of the pullup, hold the position for a brief moment and contract those back muscles and biceps as hard as possible before lowering yourself back to the starting position. Descend at a controlled speed and keep your lats tense.

Seated Cable Row (Neutral Grip)
Alternate: Underhand Grip

TARGETED MUSCLES: Latissimus dorsi

SECONDARY MUSCLES: Trapezius, rear deltoids, erector spinae, rhomboids, teres major, biceps

Just like rowing a boat, this exercise really targets the back muscles. To perform it you need a machine with a low pulley that is located near your feet when you're seated; most gyms have this specific machine. However, a cable crossover machine is an excellent alternate.

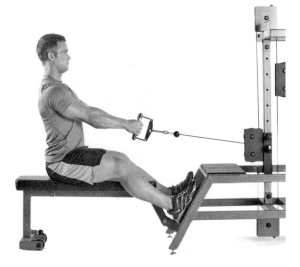
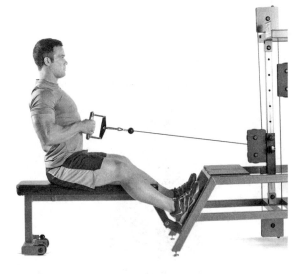

Take a seat on the machine and face the weight stack. Place your feet on the platforms provided. If using a cable crossover machine, sit on the floor with your knees bent, and feet flat on the floor or braced against the toe stop. Attach a close-grip V-bar attachment with vertical grips to the cable. Grip the V-bar with a neutral grip.

Your torso should be leaning slightly forward, but the lean should not be exaggerated and your spine should not be rounded. Keep your gaze straight ahead, rather than down, to prevent rounding your spine. Stick your chest out, pull your shoulders back, and keep your head up.

Tighten your abs and glutes, exhale, and lean back to an upright posture while pulling the bar to your belly. Really drive your elbows back as far as they can go. (Sticking out your chest will help you get your elbows back as far

as possible while adding a more powerful contraction in the back muscles). Concentrate on the pull of the lats.

Avoid lying back, which puts strain on your lower back. The heels of your hands should be touching your stomach. Once in that final position, hold, while really contracting your back muscles *momentarily*. Inhale and slowly return to the starting position, resisting the bar on the way back. Prepare for the next repetition.

> *True Alpha Tip: You can experiment with the areas to which you pull the bar. If you don't feel maximum latissimus dorsi stimulation from pulling the bar to your upper belly, try pulling the bar a little higher to your chest or to your lower belly. Everyone is different—and that goes for body mechanics, too. Experiment to figure out what works best for you.*

Lat Dumbbell Pullover

TARGETED MUSCLES: *Latissimus dorsi*

SECONDARY MUSCLES: *Serratus, chest, triceps, abdominals*

If you want to train your back muscles with an unorthodox exercise that really isolates your lats, this is *the* exercise to fire up those muscle fibers. The straight-arm pullover is off the beaten track because you're not doing as much of a row. The motion of pulling over on an arch will give you a renewed back-training experience. The first thing that you should know about this exercise is how easy it will be for the secondary muscles (chest and triceps) to take over during the exercise. It's crucial that you concentrate on making sure that your back muscles (lats) are the primary muscles working.

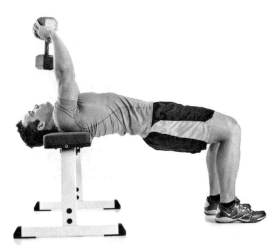
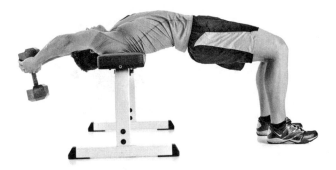

Take hold of a dumbbell and squat down on the long side of a bench. Hold the dumbbell on one thigh and lie back as you draw the dumbbell up to your chest. Your shoulders and upper back should be supported by the bench.

Place your feet flat on the floor. Your body and the bench should form a T. Keep your hips up so that they are even with your torso. Make sure the plates on your dumbbell are secure, then hold it vertically in both hands by placing your palms in an overlapping position against the inside of the dumbbell's top plate. The handle of the dumbbell should pass between your thumb and first finger on both hands in a butterfly grip.

Press the dumbbell straight up and fully extend your arms. The dumbbell should be directly over your face.

Inhale and tighten your abdominals and glutes. Keep them tight throughout the exercise. Lower the dumbbell behind your head while keeping your arms as straight as possible. (Bending your elbows could transfer the stimulation to the triceps and chest muscles.)

Do not let your hips fall as you lower the weight as far back as you can get without losing control. Let the weight stretch your latissimus dorsi muscles.

As you begin to pull the dumbbell back up to the overhead position, exhale and start contracting your back muscles as you bring the dumbbell up. Once the dumbbell is overhead, contract the lat muscles as hard as you can, and then slowly lower the dumbbell back to the starting position and get ready for your next repetition.

POWER BOOST MOVEMENTS/ PLYOMETRICS

Power Row
Alternate: Power Tubing Row

TARGETED MUSCLES: Latissimus dorsi

SECONDARY MUSCLES: Rear deltoids, mid trapezius, rhomboids, teres, biceps

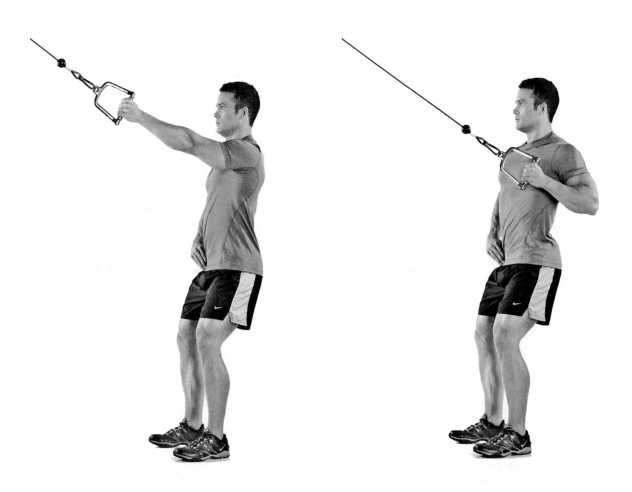

Using a cable pulley system, grab the handle, and stand facing the machine with your arm fully extended. Keep a solid posture with your feet hip-width apart, knees slightly bent, head and chest up and your shoulders pulled back. Begin to pull toward your body between chest and abdom-inal height. Pull through a full range of motion before returning your arm back to the extended position. This is an explosive exercise and should be performed as fast as possible without creating momentum or improper body mechanics.

THE SHOULDERS: BROADER, ROUNDER DELTS

What would your body look like without the brawn and width of well-developed shoulder muscles? Without them, your body would be shaped more like a triangle. The shoulder muscles, also known as the deltoids, are responsible not just for great looks, but also for just about any activity involving your arms.

The deltoid muscles have three heads that cover the shoulder. They are the anterior head, the medial (lateral) head, and the posterior head. All three muscles attach to your upper arm bone (the humerus). The anterior and medial head both connect (originate) on your collarbone, while the posterior head connects to your scapula.

The function of the deltoids is ultimately to bring your arm away from your body. The anterior head brings your arm away from the body toward the front. It's easy to see how the anterior deltoid is greatly involved with movements such as bench press–type exercises because of its forward motion and position right next to the pecs. The medial head is responsible for bringing your arm out to the side of the body. The posterior head brings the arm away from the body toward the rear.

Based on these three very important motions (arm directions), it should be apparent just how much your deltoids are involved in everything you do while you're awake—well, aside from lying on the couch and watching television. But if you're eating popcorn, guess what? Those delts are working!

Whether you're throwing a ball, reaching in any direction for a file, giving your wife a hug, or employing a bear hug to restrain a thug, your shoulders are a huge part of your life.

Unless you take care of your deltoids through proper and regular training, not only will they become weak, but they will also have a greater chance of injury because they're always in use.

If you want to function better in all upper body activities and you have a desire to build a physique with that amazing V-taper, you must fully develop all three heads of the shoulders.

SHOULDERS

Dumbbell Shoulder Press (Seated)
Alternate: Standing Position

TARGETED MUSCLES: Anterior deltoids

SECONDARY MUSCLES: Mid deltoid, triceps, trapezius

The dumbbell shoulder press is one of the most functional exercises for your upper body. It prepares your shoulders and arms for placing heavy boxes on a high shelf, holding up lumber as you nail it in place, and other sorts of manual labor and repair jobs that guys frequently find themselves doing. Using dumbbells strengthens stabilizer muscles in your shoulders and arms so you can safely lift objects overhead.

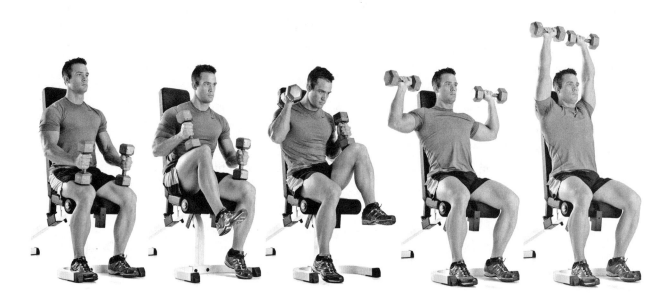

With a dumbbell in each hand, take a seat on a bench, preferably one with an upright seatback. (If you have trouble with trunk stability or are using very heavy dumbbells, you may want to select a bench with an upright seat back and press your back firmly against it.) Place your feet flat on the floor.

Contract your abdominals and lift the dumbbells to your shoulders. It's best to first place the dumbbells on your thighs and thrust each one up to the shoulder/starting position.

Hold the dumbbells in an overhand grip with your elbows thrust out to the sides. Sit up straight. The dumbbells should be positioned level with your head. Do not let the dumbbells go lower than your shoulders. You should gaze straight ahead throughout the exercise.

Inhale and tense your shoulders and triceps. Exhale as you press the dumbbells straight up overhead and extend your arms. Concentrate on using your deltoids to push your upper arms into a vertical position. Thinking about pulling instead of pushing will engage the deltoids more than the triceps.

Do not lock your elbows at the top. Stop just before locking and hold the extended position momentarily before lowering the dumbbells back to your shoulders again. Inhale as you lower the dumbbells. When you reach the starting position (do not let the dumbbells go below your shoulders), pause for a very brief moment (just one second) and let your muscles fill with blood before pressing into the next repetition. This slight pause gives the deltoids a good pump and increases the work they have to do.

Shoulder Press Machine

TARGETED MUSCLES: *Anterior deltoids*

SECONDARY MUSCLES: *Mid deltoid, triceps, trapezius*

The shoulder press machine is great for switching up your shoulder routine. The one thing you must be careful with when it comes to any machine is the predefined range of motion that most machines limit you to. Machines only allow you to move the fixed bar up or down. The problem occurs when a joint wants to arc out or follow something other than what a machine can offer. If you're moving a lot of weight and simultaneously creating forces against your free range of motion, it can wreak havoc on your shoulder joints. Try a few different shoulder machines. Many provide different movement patterns, and you may find that one is actually a great fit.

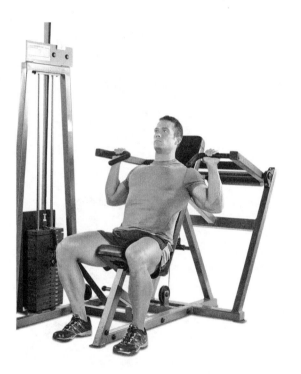 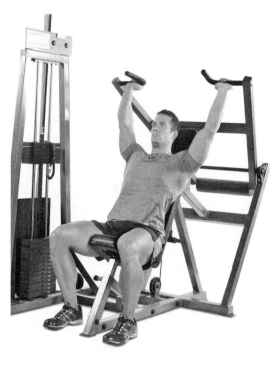

Sit with your back firmly against the machine's pad. Put your feet flat on the floor and keep them straight. Keep your abs tight, your chest relaxed, and your shoulders back and down. Be sure to keep your head straight; do not move it as you're pressing and lowering the weight stack. Doing so can harm your neck region.

Take a firm overhand grip on the outside handles, about shoulder-width apart. Go too narrow and you'll hit more of your triceps. Grab too wide, and you'll put your shoulders in a compromised and potentially harmful position.

Inhale and prepare to push the handles up overhead. As you push, exhale and allow the shoulder muscles to do all the work. Use a fluid yet forceful motion.

Push to the point where your arms are fully extended, but stop just before your elbows are locked. Don't pause. Come right back down in a slow and controlled motion. When the backs of your upper arms reach a point slightly lower than parallel to the floor, immediately begin pushing back up for your second repetition.

Arnold Press

The Arnold press is a great shoulder exercise that hits all three heads of the deltoids. This is another very functional shoulder exercise because the overhead pressing and turning movement is common in your everyday life.

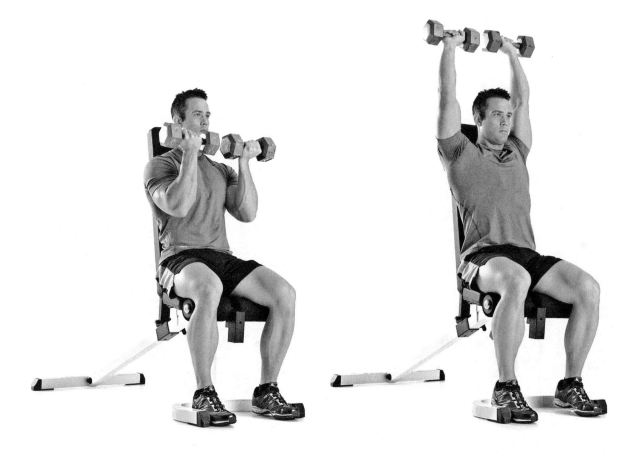

Place your feet flat on the floor and keep your back straight and your head up with your gaze straight ahead.

Begin by pressing the dumbbells up, and simultaneously rotate the forearms/dumbbells throughout the ascent until both hands are facing forward at the fully extended overhead position. Make sure you don't lock your elbows; instead, maintain a slight bend.

Don't rest at the top position. Instead, slowly reverse the movement and bring the dumbbells back to the curled starting position. Again, without rest, smoothly transition right into your next repetition.

Standing Barbell Shoulder Press

TARGETED MUSCLES: Anterior deltoids

SECONDARY MUSCLES: Mid deltoid, upper chest, triceps, trapezius

Almost as functional as the dumbbell shoulder press, the barbell shoulder press (aka military press) permits you to use more weight than dumbbells allow. This builds strength and power in your arms so you can safely handle fairly heavy loads like when you push something overhead. Standing presses develop extra torso stability.

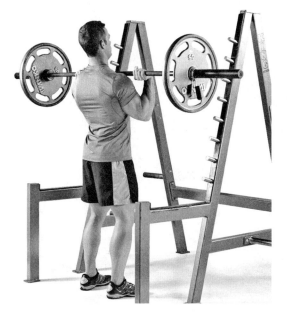
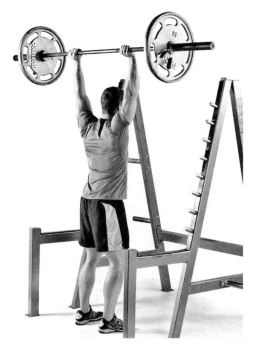

Place a barbell in an upper squat rack position, at about chest height. Be sure to keep your knees bent and abs tight to protect that lower back region. Maintain strict posture, form, and technique during this exercise. Take an overhand grip with hands slightly wider than shoulder-width apart.

Move close to the bar, and with elbows tucked at your sides and palms facing forward, lift the bar from the rack. Step a few inches away from the rack, as you will want to avoid hitting it when you hoist the barbell up. The barbell will be resting on your upper chest. Your elbows will now be sticking out slightly to the sides. Your gaze should be straight ahead or at a slight upward angle (to help avoid hitting the bar against your chin when you lift), and it should remain there throughout the exercise.

Inhale and tense your shoulders and triceps. Exhale as you press the barbell straight up overhead and extend your arms. Concentrate on using the deltoids as you push your upper arms into a vertical position.

Do not lock your elbows at the top of the movement. Stop just before locking and without pausing slowly lower the barbell back to your upper chest. Immediately begin pressing into the next repetition.

Bent-Over Dumbbell Lateral Raise

TARGETED MUSCLES: *Rear deltoids*

SECONDARY MUSCLES: *Mid deltoid, rhomboids, teres, triceps, mid trapezius*

Although you won't be able to use very heavy weights for this exercise, don't underestimate the impact of this rear deltoid exercise. Because the weights are held far from the pivot point (your shoulders), their effective weight is multiplied. Bent-over lateral raises will strengthen your upper back and shoulders in preparation for many kinds of lifting activities. Building strength in these areas will also keep your strong chest muscles from pulling your shoulders forward and your spine into poor posture.

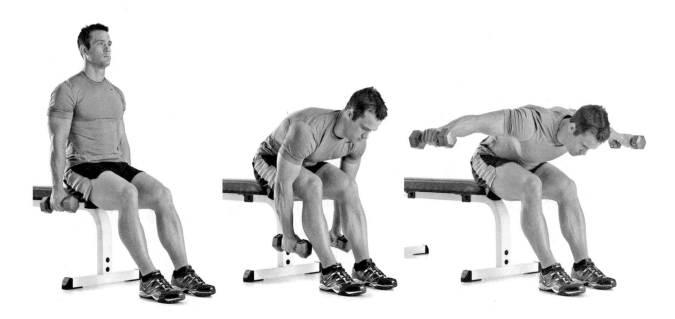

With a dumbbell in each hand, take a seat on a bench. Place your feet flat on the floor and bend over at your waist to rest your stomach and chest on or near your thighs.

Let the dumbbells hang from straight arms down to the floor. Hold the dumbbells in a neutral position so they are parallel to each other and your palms are facing each other. Inhale and tighten your abdominals and glutes.

With straight arms, exhale and raise the dumbbells out to the sides so that they arc upward. Pull with your shoulders and upper back. The motion is like spreading your wings. Raise the dumbbells as high as you can, keeping your arms fully extended and your upper back muscles clenched tight.

Pause for a moment at the top position, as you forcefully contract the rear deltoids. before slowly lowering the dumbbells back down to the starting position. Inhale as you lower your arms. Don't let your arms relax at the bottom of the motion, and transition right into the next repetition in a smooth and controlled movement.

Rear Deltoid Machine

TARGETED MUSCLES: *Deltoids (posterior and middle heads), trapezius*

SECONDARY MUSCLES: *Triceps, mid trapezius, rhomboids, teres*

The rear deltoid machine works the same muscles as the bent-over lateral raise, but it permits heavier, more consistent resistance with stricter form, which can result in better rear deltoid stimulation. This exercise is good for people working through a minor shoulder or upper back injury, as you can more effectively maintain proper form.

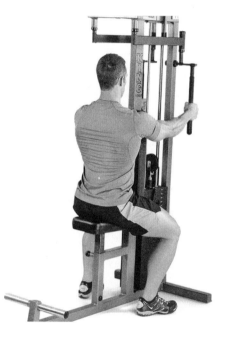 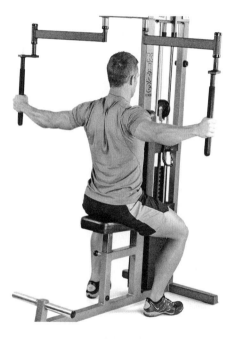

Sit in the machine and place your feet flat on the floor. Grasp the handles in front of you with a neutral grip so that your palms are facing each other. Your arms should be fully extended with a slight bend at the elbows.

Take a deep breath and exhale as you pull the handles apart so that they arc outward and back. Pull intensely with the rear deltoids until your arms are spread as wide as they will go.

Pause for a moment in the fully extended position and contract the rear delts hard before slowly bringing your arms back in front of you to the starting position. Inhale as your arms return. Before the weight touches bottom, contract the deltoids hard and transition right into the next repetition in a smooth and controlled movement.

Dumbbell Lateral Raise (Standing)
Alternate: Dumbbell Lateral Raise (Seated)

Lateral raises will transform your shoulders into cannonballs. This exercise will pile on the muscle mass if performed correctly. You can also perform this exercise seated to better control mementum and leverage.

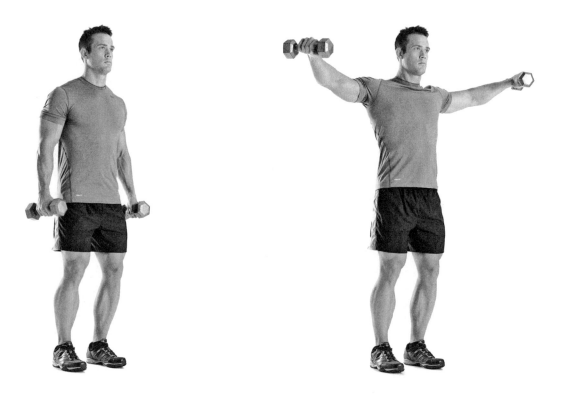

With a dumbbell in each hand, stand with feet shoulder-width apart and toes pointed straight ahead. Let the dumbbells hang straight down at your sides. Hold the dumbbells in a neutral position so they are parallel to each other and your palms are facing your thighs. Inhale, bring your shoulders back tight, and hold. Squeeze the triceps hard and lock them with just a slight bend at your elbows.

Exhale and raise the dumbbells directly out to the sides so that they arc upward. Pull intensely with your mid shoulders. The motion is like spreading your wings. Raise the dumbbells until your hands are slightly higher than your shoulders.

Pause for a moment and contract those medial delts hard at the top position before slowly lowering the dumbbells back down to the starting position. Inhale as you lower your arms. Note that the dumbbells should not come to rest against your legs, nor should you let your arms relax. Before the dumbbells touch your legs, contract the deltoids hard and with a smooth and controlled motion, transition into the next repetition.

Lateral Raise (Cable)

Doing lateral raises with a cable crossover unit permits you to use heavier resistance while keeping your form strict. For most people, form deteriorates quickly when doing lateral raises with dumbbells, which takes the focus off the deltoids and places it on other muscles, particularly the trapezius. To build shoulders with true strength, you should stick to doing lateral raises with dumbbells. Lateral raises, however, are a great way to mix things up for consistent results. Focus on those medial deltoids, as this will help keep the movement focused where you want it, rather than transferring it to other secondary muscles.

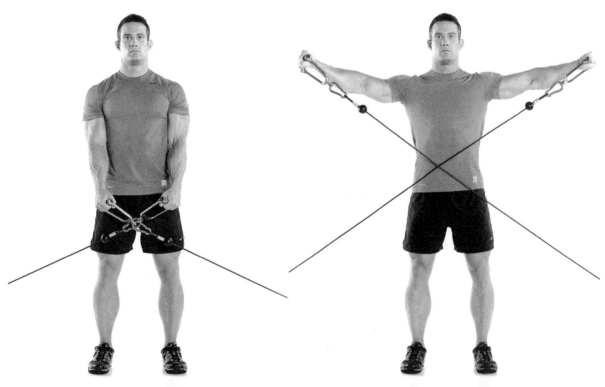

Stand up straight in the middle of the cable crossover unit and place your feet about hip-width apart. Grasp the handles with opposing hands. In other words, take the left handle with your right hand and the right handle with your left. This will form the letter *X* with the cables. Grab the handles using a neutral grip so that your palms are facing each other and keep your arms straight with a slight bend at the elbows. Stick your chest out and pull your shoulders back and down. Take a deep breath and then exhale as you lift your arms up and out to the sides of your body in an upward arc. Lead the motion with your elbows, as they are closer to the working muscles and it will help keep the stimulation where you want it. Pull intensely with the medial deltoids and raise your arms until your elbows are level with your shoulders or just a bit higher.

Pause for a moment at the top position and then slowly lower your arms back down to the starting position. Before the weight stack touches the bottom, inhale quickly and begin your exhale as you contract the deltoids hard and transition right into the next repetition.

Barbell Upright Row
Alternate: Barbell Upright Power Row

Upright rows with a barbell are even more functionally beneficial than performing them on a cable. More stabilizer muscles come into play, especially the core muscles. This is a great exercise for developing strength in the shoulders.

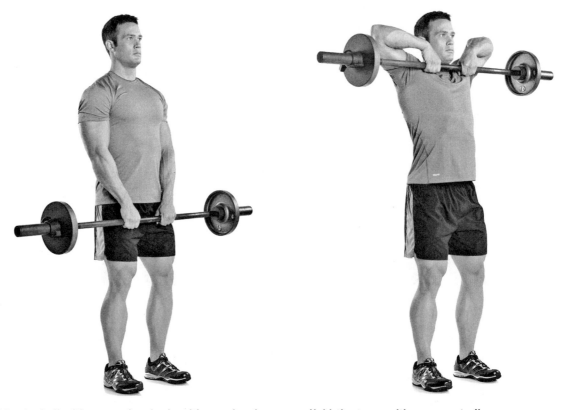

Hold a barbell with an overhand grip with your hands slightly narrower than shoulder-width apart. Stand with your feet shoulder-width apart and toes pointed forward. Start with the barbell in front of your thighs hanging from nearly straight arms. Knees and hips should be slightly bent for stability. Inhale and tighten your abdominals and glutes. Your gaze should be straight ahead during the exercise.

Exhale and raise your elbows straight up so that your upper arms go out to the sides while the barbell hangs from your hands and rises toward your chin. Allow your wrists to flex under the weight of the barbell. Continue pulling the bar up so that it comes level with or just below your chin. Squeeze hard with the deltoids and upper back at the top of the movement.

Hold the top position momentarily, as you squeeze/contract your shoulder muscles, and then lower the barbell to the starting position. As the bar descends, control the weight and inhale. Just before your arms reach full extension, immediately exhale and start pulling the bar back up for the next repetition. Use a smooth and controlled movement to transition into the next rep.

True Alpha Tip: Your objective is to keep the bar about 2 inches away from your body as you pull it up. Holding the bar slightly away from your body will help prevent shoulder impingement and add to the challenging nature of this exercise.

Barbell Upright Power Row

You'll be using much of the same form as you did with the barbell upright row, but with a "power" difference.

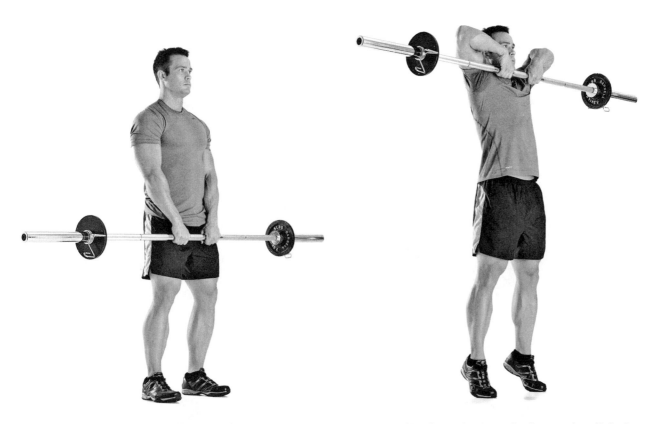

Begin the exercise by holding the barbell with an overhand grip and fully extended arms, down by your thighs. Slightly bend at the knees and over at the hips, like you would at the beginning of a clean and press exercise. This will allow you to generate the force necessary to make this lift most effective.

From this position, in one fluid motion, thrust your legs up and hips forward, as you simultaneously pull the barbell up and in front of your body. The force should be so great that when you reach the top of the movement, when the barbell is in front of your face, you should rise to your tiptoes. This might sound very difficult now, but with the force generated from your legs, hips, and shoulders, coming to your tiptoes will be easier than you might imagine.

Barbell Shrug

The trapezius muscles are the primary muscles for carrying heavy loads, whether that means hauling suitcases through the airport or dragging farm equipment out of a barn. It takes a good amount of resistance to stimulate the trapezius, so don't go light here (relatively speaking, of course). Even if you leave this exercise until last in your routine, chances are that your traps will have a lot of pull left in them.

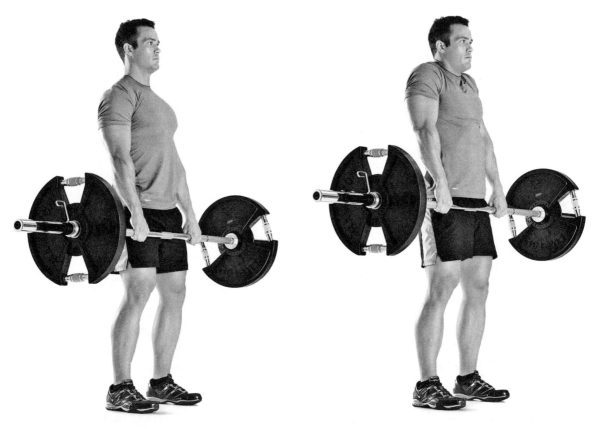

With a fairly heavy loaded barbell or a dumbbell in each hand, stand with your feet shoulder-width apart and your knees bent just slightly. For barbell shrugs, allow your arms to hang straight down in front of your thighs with an overhand grip. For dumbbells, let them hang straight down at your sides and hold them in a neutral position with your palms facing your thighs. Contract and hold your abdominals and glutes tight throughout the exercise.

Exhale as you shrug your shoulders toward your ears, getting them as high as possible without scrunching your head down to meet them—keep your spine tall. Once you reach the top of the shrug, give the trapezius muscles a strong squeeze up and back. Do not roll your shoulders.

After lifting those shoulders as far up as they can go, return the barbell down to your front thighs or the dumbbells back down by your sides. Inhale as you relax. Very briefly let the trapezius get a good stretch before beginning the next repetition, and in a smooth and controlled movement, transition into your next shrug.

True Alpha Tip: In most exercises, you inhale on the relaxation phase and exhale during the exertion phase. However, for shrugs, the more natural and, thus, more effective breathing pattern is to inhale during exertion (shrugging) and exhale during relaxation.

Clean and Power Press

TARGETED MUSCLES: Anterior deltoids

SECONDARY MUSCLES: Quadriceps, erector spinae, trapezius, glutes, abdominals

The clean and press is the ultimate test of muscular strength and power as you forcefully move a barbell from the floor to completely overhead. Although this complicated movement gives the most workout to the shoulders, there are few muscles (if any) that aren't involved to a significant degree, so it is a testament to total-body strength and stability. Because this exercise is technically demanding, you should be relatively fresh when performing it. For this reason, placing it first or second in your routine is a great idea.

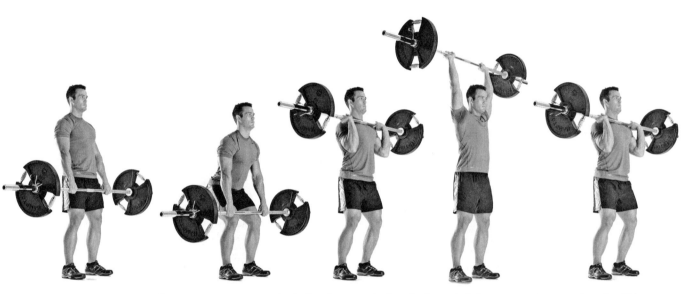

Place a barbell on the floor or, even better, on a barbell rack positioned at a level even with your upper thighs. Stand with your feet about shoulder-width apart and toes just under the bar. (The bar should pass over the balls of your feet.) If you must lift the bar from the ground, keep your back straight or slightly arched (not rounded) and eyes straight ahead, bend at your knees and hips to squat down and grab the bar. Grasp the bar with an overhand grip with your hands slightly more than shoulder-width apart.

Squeeze your shoulder blades and tense the muscles in your legs, abdomen, and back in preparation for a forceful lift.

From this position, take a deep breath, bend over at the hips, then exhale as you thrust through your heels into the floor. Allow momentum to take you up onto the balls of your feet and allow the powerful shrugging and back extension to help you get the bar into the press position. You'll do this by simultaneously upright rowing (not reverse curling) the barbell to shoulder height and quickly shifting your hands under the bar. At the end of the movement, your palms should be facing up with the barbell resting on the heels of your hands. The undersides of your forearms should be facing forward and your bent elbows should be tight to your sides.

Without stopping the motion, quickly press the barbell until your arms are fully extended overhead, just short of locking your elbows. Reverse the motion by lowering the bar with control, until the bar touches your chest. (Palms should be forward and at shoulder-height level.)

Use a slight leg thrust to push the bar up and off your chest. Allow the barbell to drop naturally as you quickly revert back to an overhand grip with your elbows above the bar, letting it drop to your thighs. Absorb the impact by letting your knees and hips bend.

> *True Alpha Tip: Between repetitions, it's okay to stand up and check your stance and form to make sure they are correct. The range of motion and momentum involved in the clean and press can deteriorate your form quickly, so pay attention.*

RESISTANCE TUBING EXERCISE

TARGETED MUSCLES: Anterior deltoids

SECONDARY MUSCLES: Mid deltoid, triceps, trapezius

Resistance Tubing Standing Shoulder Press

This simple exercise is a great shoulder move for your Home Body routine or training while traveling.

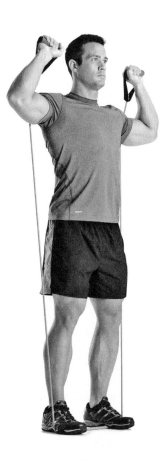
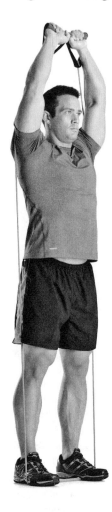

Stand with your feet shoulder-width apart on a piece of tubing with two handles. Step directly in the middle of the tubing and take hold of both handles. One strand of tubing should be on each side of your body. Bring your arms up, so that your upper arms are positioned parallel to the ground and your forearms are positioned vertically. Palms should be facing away from the front of your body. Keep your head up, chest out, and shoulders back. Your back should be flat, with a slight arch at the base.

Press the handles up, just as you would with any shoulder press. The ascent starts with a powerful press up and is followed by a smooth and controlled descent.

POWER BOOST MOVEMENTS/ PLYOMETRICS

TARGETED MUSCLES: *Anterior deltoids*

SECONDARY MUSCLES: *Triceps, trapezius*

Push Press

Here is a great exercise for developing your upper body power. use caution: You may feel like you can push a ton of weight, but remember that this is much more about speed than strength.

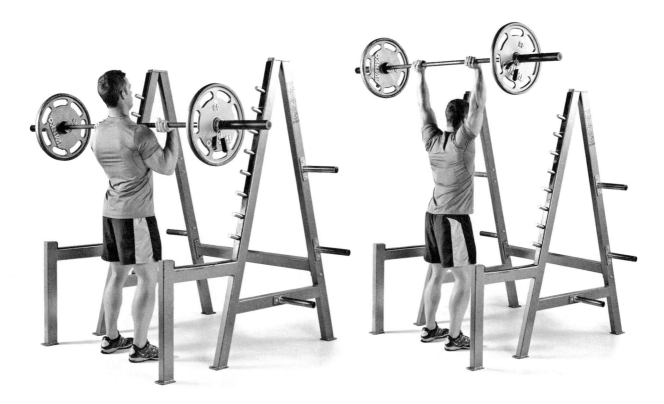

Start by placing the bar in a squat rack or power rack. Position your hands in an overhand grip on the bar. Step under the bar with both feet, and position the bar on your shoulders upper chest. Lift the bar from the rack and take a few small steps back. Your head should be up, your chest out, and your feet shoulder-width apart.

Initiate the movement by flexing your ankles, hips, and knees slightly so your body descends about 4 inches. Then rapidly extend your hips, knees, and ankles so that the body is fully extended. After full extension is reached, quickly press the bar in front of your face. The movement is finished when full lockout of your arms is achieved.

To lower the weight back to the starting position, bend your elbows and control the weight back down to your shoulders. As the weight approaches your shoulders, slightly bend your hips and knees to cushion the weight.

THE LEGS: POWERFUL QUADS, HAMS, AND CALVES

The legs are often the loneliest appendages of the male human body. Why should we waste our time training our legs when we can simply focus more time on building a better upper body? We can simply wear pants and avoid having to reveal our legs at all, right? What other reason could explain why the leg room is always the quietest area of the gym? It should be the busiest. The leg muscles account for the largest muscles in our bodies.

Most men think of the squat as the most effective for creating muscular legs. They refer to the squat as the "king" of leg exercises. Both authors regularly squatted over 500 pounds when in their 20s. Squats are a great and very effective whole body exercise, but more education must be acquired to make gains while avoiding injury. According to the NSCA, "Injuries attributed to the squat may result not from the exercise itself, but from improper technique, preexisting structural abnormalities, other physical activities, fatigue, or excessive training." The majority of guys in the gym doing squats are doing them improperly. Not every body is mechanically equal. What may work for some may not work for others. Have you ever seen a tall person squat? It can be quite difficult for taller guys to maintain proper form. It goes against our body mechanics. If we do an exercise that does not allow us to get into and maintain proper form, we risk great injury. Squats are great, but you must master form and technique and know your limits to make them work for you.

If you're a guy who wants to lose fat, gain muscle, and get more physically fit than most 20-year-olds, training your legs is one of the surest ways to reach your goals. Because your leg muscles make up half of your entire body, with the right sequence of training exercises these bad boys can become your secret weapon to a muscle-producing, fat-burning bonanza! Think of them as the diesel engine of a train. It's the engine that makes the train move, stop, and really go! Without the powerful engine, the train is a wreck.

The legs are made up of many muscle groups, including the quadriceps, hamstrings, glutes, and calves.

Quadriceps

Let's begin with the front thigh muscles typically known as the quads: From the far left to the right are the vastus lateralis (externus), the vastus intermedius, the rectus femoris, and the vastus medialis (internus). They all sit on the anterior (front) aspect of the thigh, with the exception of the rectus femoris, which crosses the hip joint and originates on the pelvis. The overall functional action of the thigh is to extend or straighten the knee.

The rectus femoris not only helps extend the knee but also helps flex the hip (hip flexor) because it crosses over the hip joint. The hip flexors are used for any actions that require lifting your knee. Think about some functional movements where you flex your hips, such as jumping, standing, throwing a knee strike, and so on.

As you can see, the thigh muscles are involved in any activity where you must use knee extension action, including standing up, running, walking, jumping, climbing stairs, and just about any activity you do while standing on your feet. In fact, even standing in place works your thigh muscles; otherwise, you'd just fall down. It should now be obvious how important and beneficial it will be for you to build up the fronts of your thighs, right?

Hamstrings

The other set of muscles of the upper leg are the ones located on the backside, typically known as the hamstring muscles.

From far left to right are the semitendinosus, the semimembranosus, the biceps femoris long head, and the biceps femoris short head. The overall function of the hamstring muscles is to flex (bend) the knee.

The semitendinosus and semimembranosus (aka the medial muscles of the hamstrings) do, however, cross at the hip and knee joints. Besides flexing the knee, they are also involved in extending the hip and turning the knee inward.

The biceps femoris muscles are known as the biceps of the leg. Look at them in a mirror and they look like the leg version of your upper arm! Like the arm biceps, they also have two heads known as the long and short heads. Both heads together help laterally rotate the knee (when the feet are turned outward). The longer head also crosses the hip and knee joints and is involved in flexing the knee and extending the hip (bringing your upper thigh backward). The short head, however, crosses only the knee joint and therefore only helps flex the knee.

Think about all of the activities where the hamstring muscles are responsible for your movement, such as sitting, walking, running, climbing down, and stepping to your left and right. Can you imagine how much more physically active and agile you could become by simply putting more training effort into this other powerhouse muscle group?

A word about training the hamstrings: New evidence is showing that there is an optimum way to train the hamstring muscles. Track and field coaches have known for years that most athletes (and this extends to the average man) naturally have a less dominant set of hamstring muscles, and it's not necessarily on the nondominant hand side. Because of this imbalance, it is good to occasionally include some unilateral training in your hamstring training regimen to help keep balance and avoid injuries. It has been proven through MRI testing that the hamstring muscles must be stretched in order to recruit the maximum number of fibers within the muscles. To do this, the hips must be flexed (forward) and the knee must be extended (back) during each exercise. This can be a little tricky during exercises such as the standing leg curl. To accomplish this, you must bend forward at your waist and begin the exercise with your working leg kept fully straightened. This will improve your hamstring strength and growth like you've never experienced before!

Another way to make the hamstrings work harder is to take the calf muscles out of the equation. The gastrocnemius muscles of the calf are also responsible for flexing the knee, except you don't want them to be if you're trying to most effectively train the hamstring muscles. To take them out of the exercise, during each leg curl, point your toes away from your knees (plantar flex). This will put all of the focus on the hamstring muscles, and believe us, you're going to feel it!

Glutes

This set of muscles is really very interesting. The glutes have been the "butt" of jokes for decades. However, the glutes are no laughing matter. They're not just some fat, clumsy muscles on the back of your body. In fact, they're actually the strongest muscles in your body. That's right! They don't call 'em the gluteus *maximus* for nothing.

The glutes are made up of three muscles: the gluteus maximus, the gluteus minimus, and the gluteus medius. The gluteus maximus is the largest of the three muscles and is responsible for the overall look of the rear end. The function of the glutes is to extend (bring back) and laterally rotate the hip outward from the body, and to extend the trunk of the body.

Think about all of the activities that these muscles are involved with, including walking, standing, climbing, sitting, stepping to the left and right, and stretching back as you reach for the sky. That round rump that was once thought to be a joke is really the star of the show.

The glutes are vitally important to take care of if you want to most effectively make use of your body. If you have lower back pain, there is a very good chance that you may be sitting for too long a period of time. When the glutes are continuously compressed, they begin to atrophy. There is, however, promising new evidence that shows that massaging the glutes can actually help better tone and avoid atrophy in this area of your body. Just don't do it in public, please!

Calves

This set of heart-shaped muscles has become one of the new measures of strength and power. The calf muscles are made up of two muscle groups, the gastrocnemius and the soleus. The gastrocnemius is attached to the heel with its partner, the Achilles tendon. It originates behind the knee on the femur (hip bone), and crosses over two joints.

The gastrocnemius has two heads, the medial head and the lateral head. The soleus muscle can not be when you look at the calf, because it sits beneath the gastrocnemius, but it still adds bulk to the calf because it pushes on the gastrocnemius from the inside out.

The gastrocnemius is activated by keeping the leg straight. The soleus muscle is activated only when the knee is bent. The function of both sets of muscles is to raise the heel. They both do this, but the gastrocnemius does it with the leg straight and the soleus does it with the leg bent.

Think of all of the activities where the calves come into play, such as jumping, walking, running, climbing—virtually every activity you do while standing. It makes sense that training the calves will have you doing what you already do even better, and well-defined calves have really become an icon of true manliness.

LEGS

Smith Machine Hack Squat

Hack squats on a Smith machine allow you to concentrate on the quadriceps without the danger of losing control of the barbell that's typically placed on your upper back. Because the barbell must move on a track, the stance is slightly different than during a regular squat, so pay careful attention. Rather than the barbell being placed on top of your shoulders/trapezius muscles, you will be holding the barbell from below.

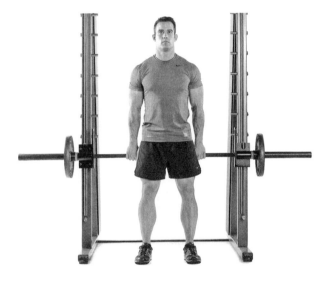 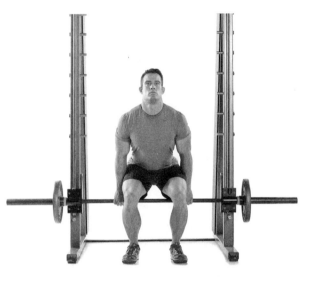

Set the bar at about mid-shin height, and load it with an appropriate amount of weight. Remember, you'll be holding the barbell, so you may not be able to use as much weight as you could with the traditional barbell squat.

Step in front of the bar. Take a hip-width or slightly narrower stance. With knees bent, abs tight, chest out, shoulders pulled back, and head looking up, inhale as you squat down/sit back (mimic sitting in a chair) and take an overhand grip of the barbell. It will be touching very close to your hamstrings. Look straight ahead and maintain a forward gaze throughout the movement.

Begin the ascent (upward movement) by contracting the quadriceps and buttocks and stand up to a fully upright position, using your leg muscles to bring you up.

Note: You must make certain that you are squatting down, allowing your legs to guide you and not your waist; this is a key part of the squat exercise. When you reach the top portion of this exercise, do not pause. Inhale and bend at your knees and hips to lower your buttocks back toward the floor. As you descend, your shoulders will have the tendency to internally round; don't allow this! Keep your chest out and shoulders back and maintain proper form.

Maintain tight abs and buttocks as you descend. Lower your body until your knees are bent at slightly less than 90 degrees.

At the bottom of the movement, exhale as you press through your heels and return to standing.

Dumbbell Squat

Dumbbell squats are a good alternative to barbell squats. If you are concerned about your lower back or balance, this could be a good choice, as the weight will not be placed directly on top of your spine and your center of gravity will be improved.

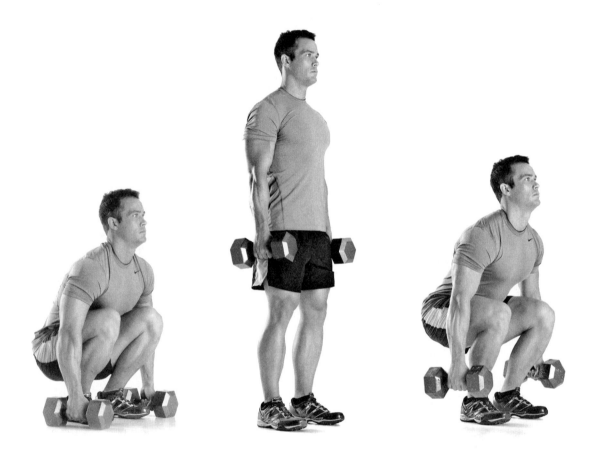

Holding a dumbbell in each hand, stand with your feet approximately hip-width apart. You may certainly play with the width of your stance as everyone's mechanics vary to some degree. Do not lock your knees. Look straight ahead and keep your gaze forward or slightly up throughout the movement. Take a breath and tense your abdominals and buttocks to strengthen your core and lower back. Stick your chest out and keep your shoulders back to help maintain proper postural alignment. Maintain tightness in these muscles throughout the movement.

Begin the movement by bending your knees and folding at your hip (mimicking the action of sitting in a chair). As you descend toward the floor, push your buttocks back and do not let your knees go forward over your toes. If your knees are allowed to go too far forward, they take too much strain and can be injured.

Throughout the movement, keep your arms as relaxed as possible, but arch your lower back and squeeze your shoulder blades together to stabilize your spine and reduce your chance of injury.

When your thighs are parallel to the floor, stop the descent. Thrust through your heels to return to standing. Exhale as you reach the top of the movement.

Leg Extension

TARGETED MUSCLES: *Quadriceps*

SECONDARY MUSCLES: *This is an isolation exercise, so if you're feeling muscles other than your quadriceps muscles working, you may need to either lighten the weight or improve your form.*

The quadriceps on top of the thigh are among the most powerful muscles in your body, capable of generating incredible force. Quads are the key muscles involved in front kicks, whether in martial arts or while kicking a ball. Leg extensions strengthen the quadriceps in a way that amplifies kicking power.

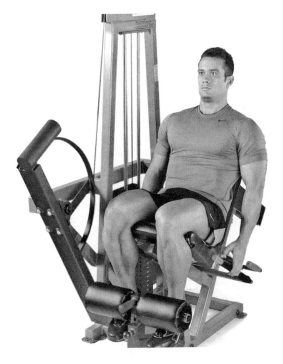
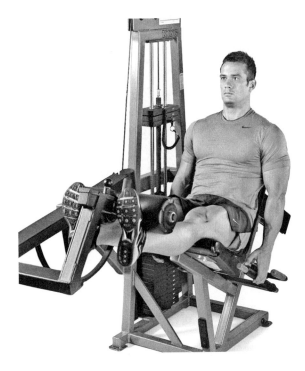

Position yourself by sitting in the machine or on the bench. Adjust the seat and/or position of your body so that your knees are at the edge of the seat. Your knees should also be lined up with the pivot point of the resistance arm. Hook your ankles under the shin pad. Adjust the shin pad so that it is as far down your legs as possible. Sit up straight, bring your back flush against the backrest, and lightly grip the handles.

When properly situated, your toes should be slightly in front of your knees. If they are not, adjust the machine settings or find another machine. When you begin, if your toes are behind your knees, too much strain will be placed on your knees and your chance of injury will be increased.

Take a deep breath and tighten your abdominals and glutes. Begin to exhale, contract the quadriceps on the front of your thigh, and straighten your legs. At the top of the movement, hold a maximum quad contraction momentarily before inhaling and lowering your feet back to the starting position. At the bottom of the movement, don't rest. Immediately begin next repetition.

Lying Leg Curl

TARGETED MUSCLES: Hamstrings, glutes

SECONDARY MUSCLES: Glutes, calves

Leg curls target the hamstring muscles on the backs of the thighs—muscles that play a crucial role in most lifting, jumping, running, and other movements. By focusing on the hamstrings, you can significantly increase power and stability for many leg movements, including climbing stairs and ladders.

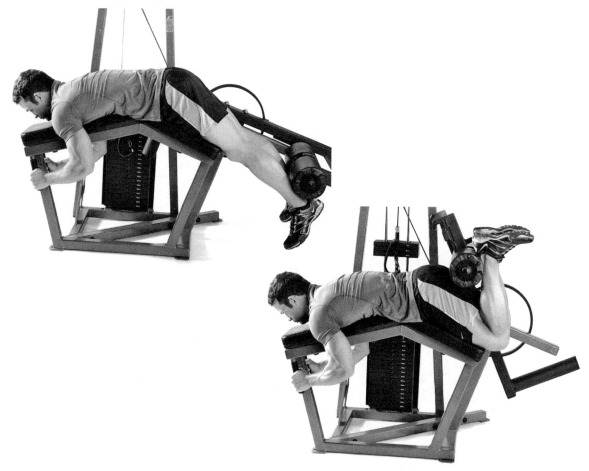

Position yourself by lying face down on the machine's padded surface. Situate your legs so that your knees are in line with the pivot point of the resistance arm of the machine and the heel pad rests across the backs of your lower legs.

Throughout the movement, keep your face down and your upper body relaxed. Most machines have handles you can grip, or you can grip the seat or edge of your bench. If you are using a flat bench with a leg developer, allow your hips to bend slightly and tuck your chin to your chest to reduce lower back strain. Begin by tightening your abdominal muscles and pressing against the heel pad of the machine or leg developer.

Take a deep breath and exhale, flex your feet so that your toes are reaching for your knees, and contract the hamstring muscles to raise the machine's resistance arm. Really drive your heels toward your buttocks, and focus on squeezing the hamstrings or leg biceps. Keep your feet flexed. Your thighs and knees should remain stationary. Once you reach full contraction of the hamstrings, slowly lower your feet back to the starting position. Resist the weight on the way down. Just before the weight stack touches, begin to exhale and slowly and smoothly transition into the ascent of your next repetition.

Seated Leg Curl

The seated leg curl really isolates the leg biceps to build size and enhance their appearance. It's a good alternative to lying leg curls if you have problems with your lower back. This exercise requires the use of a specialized machine.

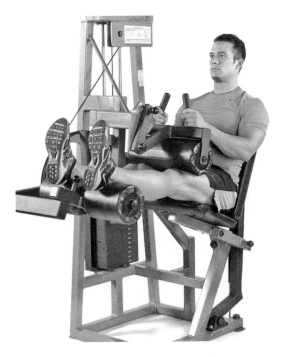

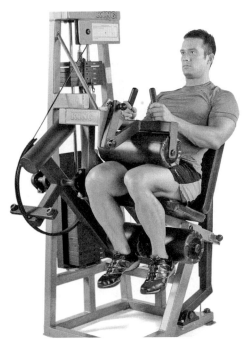

Sit in the machine and adjust it so that you can comfortably rest your back against the seat back while your knees are in line with the pivot point of the resistance arm and your lower thighs are pressed up against the thigh pad. Straighten your legs and rest the backs of your lower legs on the heel pad. Very lightly grip the handles and relax your upper body.

Tighten your abdominals and glutes, exhale, then con- tract the hamstrings and bend at your knees to press the heel pad down. Bring your heels back as far as you can. When you reach the top of the exercise, momentarily contract the hamstrings, inhale, then slowly return to the starting position. When you reach the top of the movement, do not rest. Hold the position, then begin another exhalation as you start the next repetition.

Barbell Lunge
Alternates: Dumbbell Lunge, Cross the River (Walking Dumbbell Lunge)

This is an extremely effective and very functional leg exercise that also builds balance and stability for all kinds of sports, especially football and basketball. Besides building powerful leg muscles, the lunge also strengthens ligaments and joint components in the knee and makes it less susceptible to injury on the field.

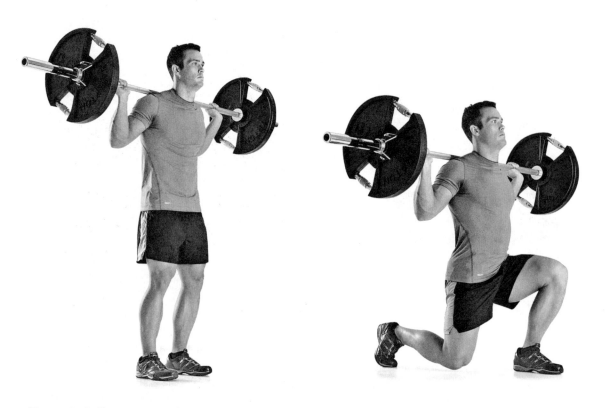

Place a barbell across your shoulders and grip the bar with an overhand grip on each side. Stand straight, with your feet slightly apart and toes pointed forward. Stick your chest out, pull your shoulders back, and look straight ahead. Keep your upper body perfectly aligned throughout the movement.

Inhale and contract your abdominals, then take a long step forward with one foot. (A longer step will target the gluteal muscles more, while a shorter step will target the quadriceps more.) As you step, you want to step/roll from your heel to your toe; this will take the ballistic force off your knee, acting as a shock absorber.

Lower your hips toward the floor. Stop your descent when your rear knee is about 1 inch or less from the floor and your forward thigh is parallel to the floor. (Go at your own pace; if you find going too low hurts your knees or back, don't go so low!) Contract the quadriceps of your forward leg and your buttocks, exhale, then press through the forward heel to return to standing. At the top, inhale and step out with the opposite foot to begin the next repetition.

When pressing back to the standing position, relax the quadriceps of the rear leg and resist the temptation to use the rear leg to assist the movement. Also, keep the motion slow and steady and do not use momentum to spring from the lunge to the standing position.

Alternate: Dumbbell Lunge

TARGETED MUSCLES: Quadriceps, glutes, Hamstrings

SECONDARY MUSCLES: Hamstrings, Glutes, Calves, Forearms

As with barbell lunges, this exercise develops the power, balance, and stability needed for a wide variety of sports. Use wrist straps to help you hang on to the dumbbells if you start using dumbbells heavier than 100 pounds.

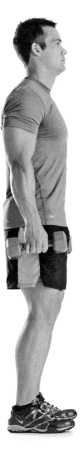

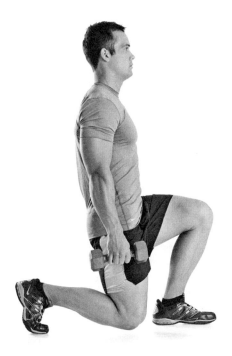

Holding a dumbbell in each hand, stand straight with your feet together, toes pointed forward, and arms hanging at your sides. Stick your chest out, pull your shoulders back, keep the abs tight, and look straight ahead like a soldier at attention. Keep your upper body perfectly aligned throughout the movement.

For execution, follow the same guidelines described in the Barbell Lunge.

Alternate: Cross the River (Walking Dumbbell Lunge)

TARGETED MUSCLES: *Quadriceps, glutes, Hamstrings*

SECONDARY MUSCLES: *Hamstrings, Glutes, Calves, Forearms*

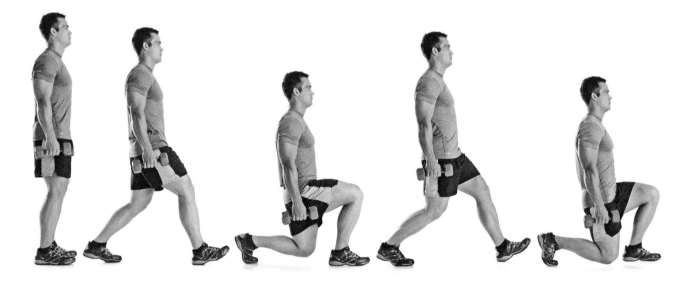

Follow the same setup form as the Alternate Dumbbell Lunge (page 235), but pay close attention to your balance. Instead of pressing back to the starting position, immediately continue lunging forward with the next leg. You will continue lunging and walking, switching back and forth from leg to leg, until you've completed the prescribed number of reps for each leg. Your objective during your walking lunges is to step out far enough on each leg and maintain your balance as you immediately move into your next lunge. These are very challenging and a lot of fun!

Leg Press (Hip Width)
Alternate: Leg Press (Wide Stance)

This is a great exercise for you offensive linemen or weekend warriors who want to develop some real lower body strength. The narrow stance emphasizes strength and power in the quadriceps and outer thighs and provides a strong base for defensive wrestling maneuvers, such as sprawling. Tthe wide-stance leg press will also engage the quads, but will put more emphasis on the inner thigh and hamstring muscles. You may not be able to use as much weight with a narrow stance as with a wide stance, but you can get very close.

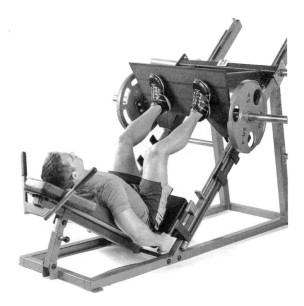
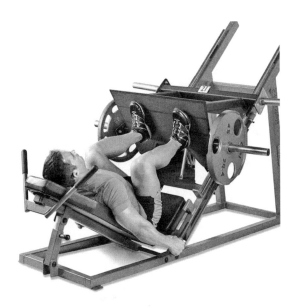

Sit down in the seat of the leg press and place your feet flat on the platform. Your prescribed stance will be indicated in the workout charts. Press your entire back firmly against the seat back, and grip the machine's handles.

When you first sit in the machine, a lock pin of some sort should be holding the weight and platform somewhere in the middle of its range of motion to make getting in and out easy. Tighten up your abdominals and squeeze your glutes, then press the platform an inch or two away and release the lock pin—it's probably connected to the handles in some way. Slowly lower the platform toward you until your knees come close to your chest.

Exhale and press the platform away from you until your legs are fully extended. Focus on pressing evenly through the entire foot. This will help to distribute the resistance to all of the leg muscles. At the top of the exercise, contract the leg muscles, then slowly flex your hips and knees and lower the platform toward your chest. With a very fluid and controlled motion, immediately transition into the next repetition.

On your last repetition, reset the lock pin while your legs are extended. Then let the platform lower onto the lock pin so you can get out of the machine.

Stiff-Legged Deadlift
Alternates: Deep Deadlift, Romanian Deadlift, Dumbbell Deadlift

TARGETED MUSCLES: *Hamstrings, erector spinae*

SECONDARY MUSCLES: *Glutes, core, trapezius, forearms*

The mantra of workplace safety is "bend the knees, lift with the legs." But anybody with any sense knows this isn't always possible. Stiff-legged deadlift will prepare you for those times when lifting with your legs just isn't feasible. You can typically use more weight than you can for the leg curl exercises, because the stiff-legged deadlift targets the hamstring and is a more natural movement. The glutes and lower back muscles are also employed and will become strong and firm as a result of this exercise. This version of the deadlift can be done with any of the tree various deadlift exercises (stiff-legged, Romanian, or deep). The advantage of using dumbbells is that it allows you to customize the movement to your needs. Go to alphamalechallenge.com for more tips.

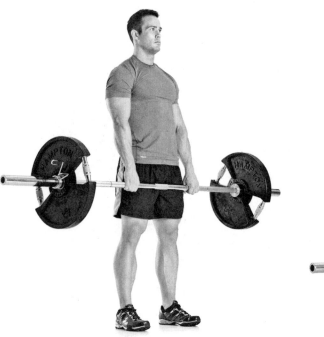
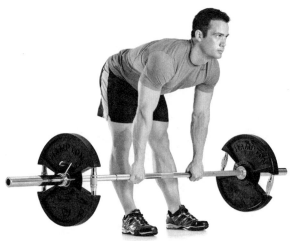

Hold a barbell in front of your thighs with an overhand grip. Keep your arms straight. Stand with your feet shoulder-width apart or slightly closer. Stick your chest out and pull your shoulders back while gazing straight ahead. Maintain a forward gaze with your eyes on the wall in front of you throughout the movement to protect your back. Do not look down.

Tighten your abdominals and squeeze your glutes and hamstrings. Maintain a curve in your lower back (butt out, chest out, shoulders back). Slowly bend forward at the waist while keeping your knees and spine straight. Allow the weight to hang naturally from your arms. As you bend over, keep the bar traveling close to your shins and thighs. Refrain from using any jerking or thrusting movements, which can put you at great risk for injury to your lower back and your hamstrings.

At the bottom of the movement, pause for just a fraction of a second, then contract the glutes and hamstrings, exhale, and slowly return to standing. Inhale at the beginning of each repetition and exhale as you return to standing.

Alternate: Deep Deadlift

TARGETED MUSCLES: Quadriceps, erector spinae

SECONDARY MUSCLES: Full body, including: hamstrings, glutes, core, trapezius, and forearms

Deep deadlifts are the mother of all back exercises—and perhaps the king of all resistance training exercises! They target not only all the muscles of the back, but also the major muscles of the legs, shoulders, and arms. The chest is the only muscle group that doesn't receive much stimulation. As you are getting used to the movement with lighter weights, you may not feel much stimulation in your arms and shoulders, but as you progress to heavier and heavier weights, you'll feel the stimulation in your arms as you struggle to hang on to the bar.

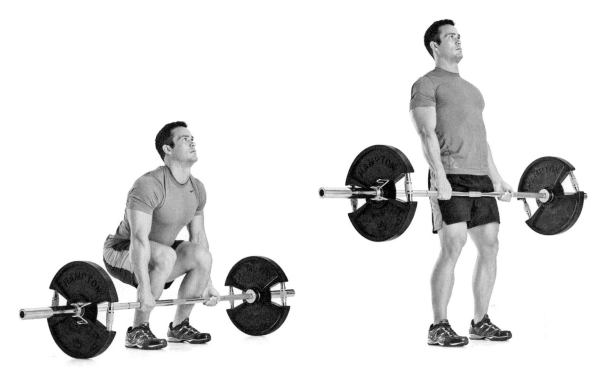

Stand in front of a loaded barbell with your feet less than shoulder-width apart. Your toes and knees should be pointed forward. *Do not* point your toes inward or let your knees buckle!

With your chest sticking out, shoulders pulled back, and abs tight, bend at the knees and hips to reach down and pick up the bar. For increased balance and greater grip strength, take an alternated grip (one hand overhand and one hand underhand) on the bar. Now look up at the ceiling, sink that butt down, straighten your arms, pull your shoulders back, and keep your lower legs as vertical as possible. Tighten every muscle in your body. Maintain this tightness and keep your eyes on the ceiling throughout the exercise to keep a rigid and stable spine that will resist injury.

Take a breath and hold it. Do not look at the bar! If you look down at the bar, you'll curve your spine, ruin your posture, and put yourself at serious risk for injury.

Your upper body must stay upright and rigid as you exhale and drive through your heels and lift the bar. Straighten your hips at the same time that you straighten your knees and forcefully bring those shoulders back. Try your best to keep your upper body higher than your hips and don't make the mistake of straightening your knees or you'll end up lifting mostly with your lower back.

At the top of the lift, thrust your hips forward, stick your chest out, and get your shoulders back to lock out the motion and inhale. Hold for just a second, then slowly reverse the motion by bending at the hips and knees to lower the bar back to the floor.

Do not exhale until the weights have touched the floor again. The intra-abdominal pressure helps keep your spine and core properly aligned and reinforced.

Alternate: Romanian Deadlift

TARGETED MUSCLES: *Hamstrings, Erector Spinae*

SECONDARY MUSCLES: *Full Body including:, Quadriceps Glutes, Core, Trapezius, Forearms*

This is a great version of the deadlift, because it's a cross between a stiff-legged position and a deep knee position. This brings the best of both worlds into play.

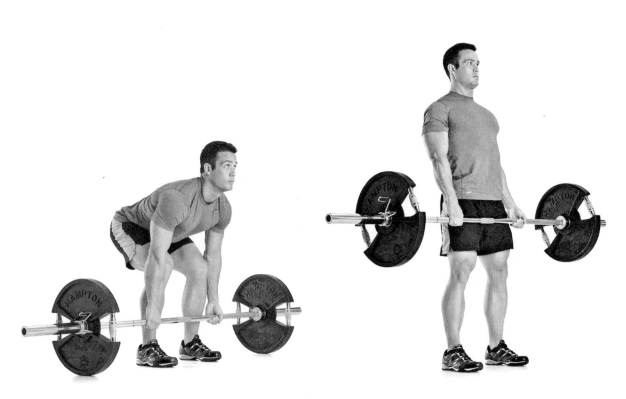

Begin by taking a hip-width stance or even narrower. Bend the knees slightly, and keep your abs tight, your chest out, and your shoulders pinned way back and down. Take your grip on the bar. You may choose either an overhand grip or an alternate grip (one hand is overhand and the other is underhand) for better balance and superior gripping ability.

Simply bend at your knees as you'd imagine a semi-squat to look; but again, make sure you keep those hips low and that chest high. As you deadlift the weight up, push off the bottoms of your feet and simultaneously pull with your lower back/upper back and shoulders, trying your best to keep your upper body higher than your hips. As you reach the top position, pull your shoulders back and bring your posture to an upright position. Pause only for a second as you take a breath, and then begin lowering the bar in full control, keeping the bar traveling close to your shins and thighs.

Weighted Stepup

TARGETED MUSCLES: *Quadriceps, Hip Flexors*

SECONDARY MUSCLES: *Hamstrings, Glutes, Calves*

Stepups on to a bench may appear to be easy and uneventful, but we assure you, that they are amazing leg muscle developers. The high stepup promotes a full range of motion and is actually one of the most functional movements in your leg exercise arsenal. Your quads and hip flexors, the primary muscles engaged, are very important muscles for driving the leg forward during sprinting and jumping.

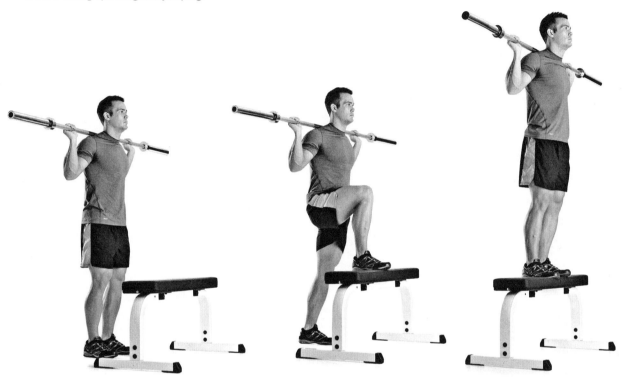

Select a box height between 12 and 18 inches. Start by standing upright with the bar across your back (as you would with the barbell squat) or weights in your hands. Keep your head up and chest out with proper back alignment. Step up so the entire foot is centered on the box. Your thigh should be about parallel to the floor. Your front leg should bend similar to the squat in that the knee should not come over the toe. Force should come from the stepping up leg, so you should not push from the back leg. Stand up, pressing into the bench, and pull the trail leg upward. Without a pause, slowly bring the trail leg back down, staying in control and not coming down too quickly. Maintain proper back alignment during the lift. You can alternate legs or do all your reps on the same leg, then alternate.

Donkey Calf Raise

TARGETED MUSCLES: Calves (primarily the larger part, the gastrocnemius)

SECONDARY MUSCLES: Smaller and deeper part of the calf muscle (soleus)

This calf exercise is a great staple movement and also serves as an awesome alternative for men who have lower back issues and are concerned about performing on the calf raise machine. Perform this calf exercise by using a donkey calf raise machine or a weighted dip belt or by having another person sit on your lower back and hips. Just don't horse around!

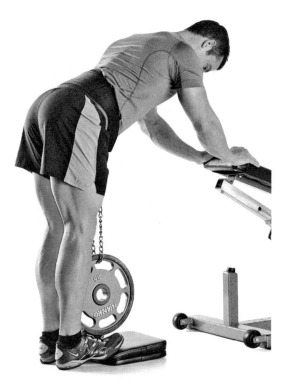
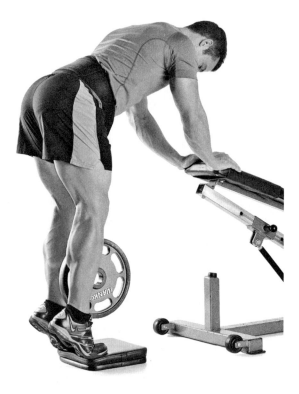

If using a machine, place the balls of your feet and toes on the platform and let your heels hang over the edge of the platform. Bend over and grip the handles so that your torso is parallel to the floor and your lower back and hips press against the resistance pad.

If not using a machine, place a wood block or barbell plates under the balls of your feet and toes (as shown). Let your heels hang off the block or plates. The front of your feet should be elevated 1 to 2 inches. Bend over and keep your torso rigid. Hang on to something solid to maintain your balance. The weighted dip belt should be hang-ing from your waist. If using a partner, have the partner climb onto your lower back and hips *after* you are in the bent-over position.

Contract the abdominal muscles and buttocks to stabilize your lower spine. Exhale as you press through your toes to elevate your heels as high as you can get them. Hold a powerful contraction for a moment before lowering your heels. Inhale and lower your heels ½ to 1 inch below the front of your feet, begin your exhalation, and go into the next repetition.

Leg Press Calf Press

TARGETED MUSCLES: Calves (primarily the larger part, the gastrocnemius)

SECONDARY MUSCLES: Smaller and deeper part of the calf muscle (soleus)

This calf exercise utilizes a leg press machine. Being able to sit down during the exercise takes your mind off maintaining balance, and allows you to focus on really contracting your calf muscles. It also takes some of the pressure off of the lower back, so you can use heavier weights to train these stubborn muscles.

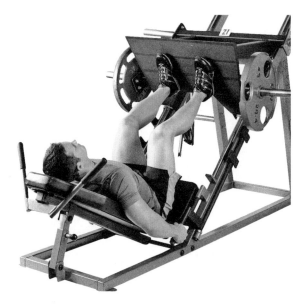

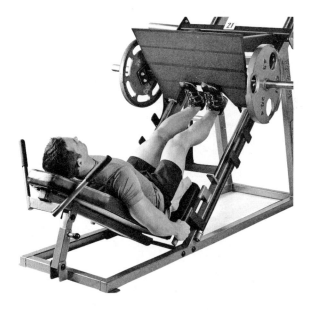

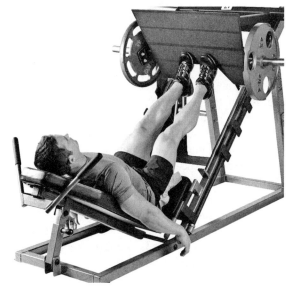

Sit in the machine and place your feet so that only the balls and toes of your feet are on the platform and your heels are hanging off. Exhale as you extend your legs and press the platform away from you. At this point, your heels should be extended beyond the platform so that your feet are in the dorsi-flexed (toes toward knees) position.

Take a deep breath and begin your exhalation while you contract the calf muscles to press your toes forward. Fully extend your feet and push the platform farther away. Get up on those tiptoes! Hold the extended position for a moment with a super squeeze of those calves before inhaling and allowing your feet to return to the starting, dorsi-flexed position. Take another deep breath, get a nice deep stretch (just be sure not to overdo it), and immediately begin the next repetition.

Seated Calf Raise

The soleus is the deep calf muscle, and it is extremely important for walking, running, dancing (for you MC Hammer types), and virtually all sports. In most exercises, it works in conjunction with the gastrocnemius (the calf muscle everybody notices), so it is difficult to isolate. The seated calf raise succeeds in isolating the soleus because the bent knees take most of the gastrocnemius's involvement out of play. Both muscles attach to the heel bone on the bottom end, but the top end of the soleus attaches to the lower leg bones just below the knee, while the gastrocnemius attaches to the thigh bone just above the knee. By flexing the knee, the gastrocnemius has nothing to pull against, but the soleus does.

This exercise is usually performed on a seated calf raise machine, but it can also be done by sitting on a bench with a wood block or a barbell plate under your toes and a barbell across your knees.

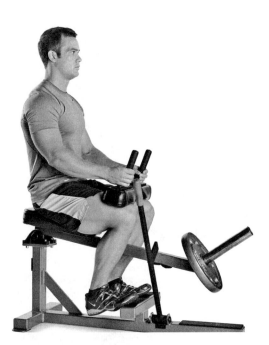 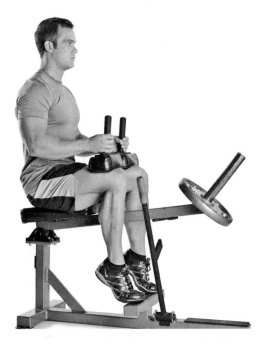

Sit on the machine and place your toes and the balls of your feet on the platform. Your heels should hang off the edge of the platform and your knees should be vertical and directly beneath the machine's knee pad.

You will have the option of adjusting the height of the knee pad so that it does not press your heels too far toward the floor. Your heels should not be able to go more than an inch lower than the platform. You load the machine bar with the appropriate amount of resistance.

Once seated and in position, exhale and press through your toes to raise your heels and knees up and lift the weight. In the up position, unlock the machine so it can go

through its full range of motion. Inhale before beginning the first repetition.

Begin a repetition by slowly lowering your heels toward the floor. Allow your calves to get a good stretch at the bottom, begin your exhalation, then press through your toes to extend the feet and lift the weight back up again. Go as high as possible, for a maximum calf contraction. Slowly and smoothly lower back to the stretch position and, without rest, go into the next repetition.

When you've completed your last repetition, hold the weight in the up position while resetting the lock pin.

RESISTANCE TUBING EXERCISES

TARGETED MUSCLES: Quadriceps

SECONDARY MUSCLES: Glutes, hamstrings, calves

Resistance Tubing Squat

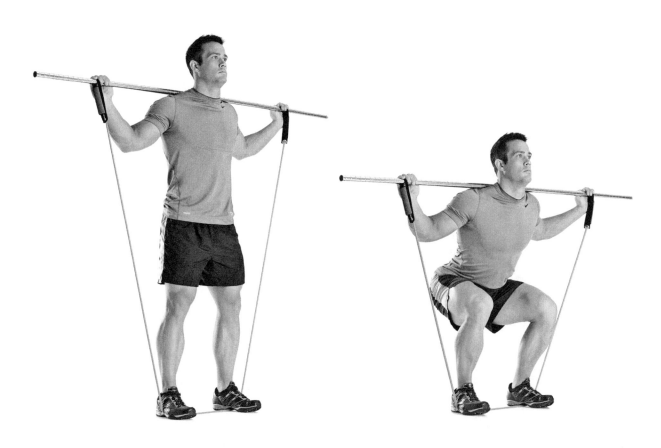

Stand with your feet shoulder-width apart on a piece of tubing with two handles. Slip a broomstick through the handles of the tubing and raise the bar over your head and onto your back, just above your posterior deltoids. One strand of tubing should be on each side of your body. Place your hands just outside your shoulders on top of the handles to prevent them from slipping during the movement. Keep your head up, chest out, and shoulders back. Your back should be flat, with a slight arch at the base.

Point your toes out at an angle of 30 to 35 degrees. Inhale deeply and contract the muscles of your torso to help stabilize your upper body and keep your back flat. Slowly lower your buttocks toward the floor, keeping your hips under the broomstick as much as possible. Descend until the tops of your thighs are parallel to the floor. The ascent starts with an exhalation and a powerful drive to accelerate yourself out of the bottom position. Keep your head looking up to help keep you from leaning forward. Keep the muscles of your torso contracted as you lift. Continue to push with your legs until you come to a full standing position. Take another deep breath, and descend for the next rep.

Resistance Tubing
Single Leg Seated Leg Press

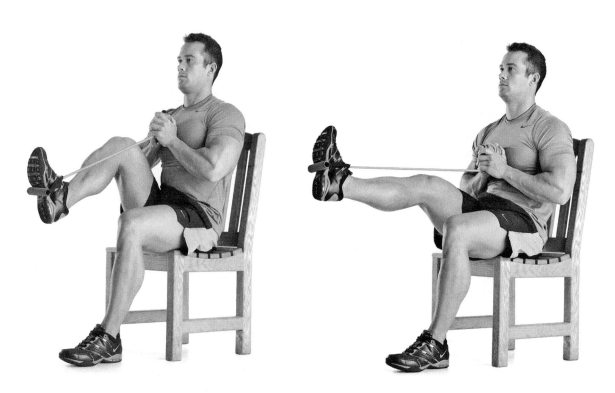

Sit in a straight-back chair and straighten one leg so that it is parallel to the floor. Place the handle of the tubing over your foot so that the ball of your foot is against the handle and your toes point toward the ceiling. Hold the tubing tightly in your hands. Bend your knee so that your thigh moves toward your body. Take a deep breath as you straighten your leg, pressing the tubing handle away from you. Pause for a second and allow your knee to bend toward your body again. Straighten but do not lock your knee during this movement. Do all repetitions with one leg before switching to the other.

Resistance Tubing Standing Leg Curl

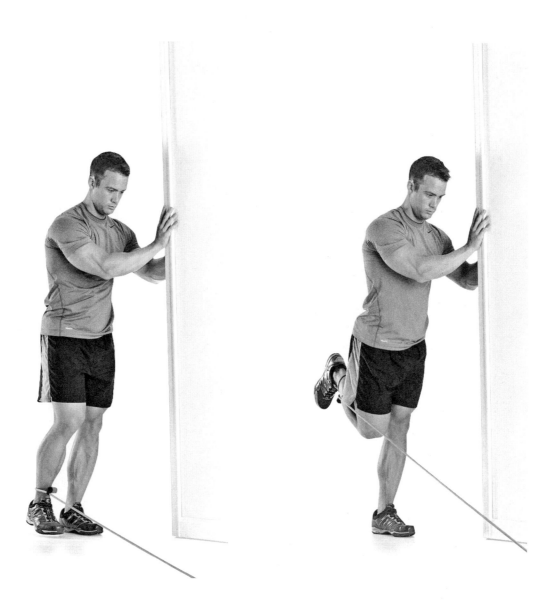

Anchor the tubing under a door or attach it to an ankle-high hook. Slip your foot through the handle or wrap the tubing around your ankle. Step away from the door so that there is some tension on the tubing. Holding on to a broomstick or some other support, such as a wall, to help you maintain your balance, curl your leg and raise your heel toward your buttocks. When you reach the top position, pause and slowly lower your foot back to the starting position. Do all repetitions with one leg before switching to the other.

Resistance Tubing Standing Calf Raise

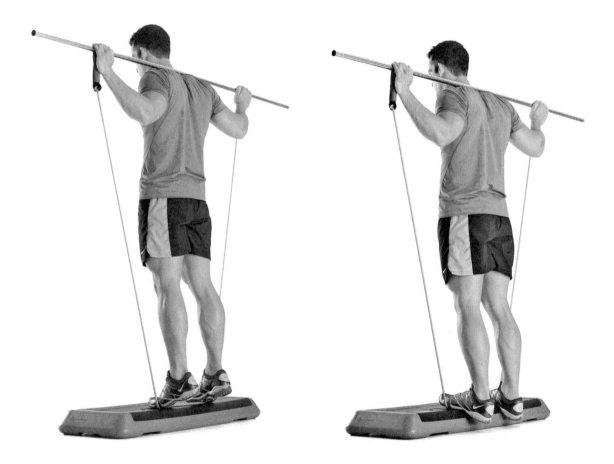

Stand with the balls of your feet on a block 4 to 5 inches high, feet shoulder-width apart, tubing under your feet. Slip a broomstick through the handles of the tubing and raise the broomstick over your head and onto your back, just above your posterior deltoids. One strand of tubing should be on each side of your body. Lower your heels toward the floor as far as possible while keeping the balls of your feet on the block. Lift yourself by rising up on your toes as high as possible, pausing at the top for a second before lowering to the fully stretched position. Keep your legs straight but not locked throughout the movement to make sure the movement is coming from your ankle and that you are not lifting yourself with your other leg muscles.

Standing Calf Raise

TARGETED MUSCLES: Calves (primarily the larger part, the gastrocnemius)

SECONDARY MUSCLES: Smaller and deeper part of the calf muscle (soleus)

Muscular, well-defined calves are the telltale sign of a real man of power. Perform this calf exercise by using a standing calf raise machine. If you have any lower back issues, you may want to swap this exercise for another calf exercise. The heavy load will put pressure on your lower back, so keep those knees slightly bent and keep your abs tensed throughout the exercise. This is a true calf builder!

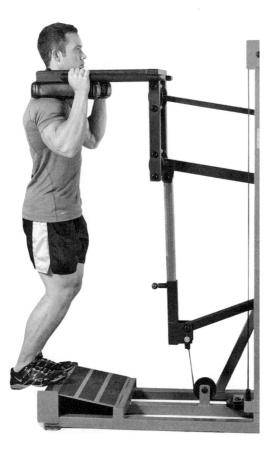 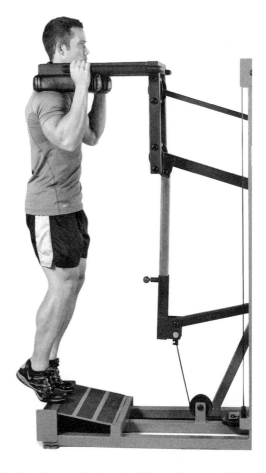

Position the shoulder pads at a height that allows you to comfortably lift the weight stack without having to bend over or squat down too much. You will have to squat down a little bit, and once you are in the starting position, you will continue to keep your knees slightly bent. This position will protect your lower back while allowing you to stretch your calves in the down position of the exercise. Place the balls of your feet and toes on the platform and let your heels hang over the edge of the platform.

Hold the handles or grip the shoulder pads at the sides. Contract all of your muscles to ready your body for the heavy load; especially focus on the abdominal muscles to secure your core. Exhale as you press through your toes to elevate your heels as high as you can get them. Hold a powerful contraction before lowering your heels. Inhale and lower your heels ½ to 1 inch below the front of your feet, begin your exhalation, and begin the next repetition.

POWER BOOST MOVEMENTS/ PLYOMETRICS

TARGETED MUSCLES: *Quadriceps*

SECONDARY MUSCLES: *Hamstrings, glutes, calves*

Squat Jump
Alternate: Resisted Squat Jump

A lack of weights or lifting machines is no excuse for not training your legs. Squat jumps require no equipment at all and develop massive leg power. Squat jumps also build resiliency in the knees, ankles, and hips, making it ideal training for those involved in football, soccer, rugby, and other sports where the leg joints undergo a lot of strain.

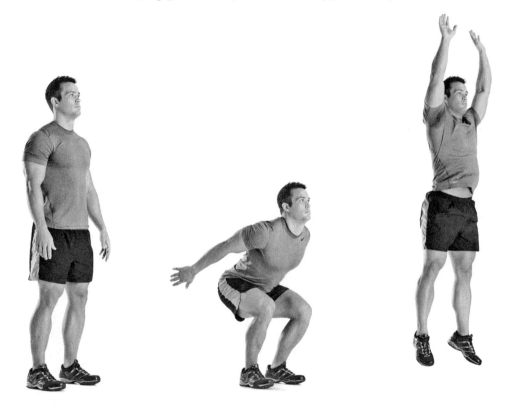

Stand with your feet shoulder-width apart or slightly closer and point your toes forward. Place your arms directly in front of you. Look straight ahead and keep your gaze level throughout the exercise.

Bend your knees and push your butt back to squat down and swing your arms behind you. Lower your hips until your thighs are parallel to the ground. Tense your leg and butt muscles to prepare for the jump. Take a deep breath. Now exhale and explode upward, making sure to push off with your toes. Swing your arms up overhead on the launch.

As you're landing, touch your toes to the floor first, then your heels. Let your knees and hips absorb the impact of the landing by flexing under your weight. Don't lose your balance!

Once you've completed the jump, make sure your feet are positioned properly and assume the squat position for the next jump without any rest in between.

> *True Alpha Tip:* If you hit a plateau in increasing jump height, or if you participate in a sport that requires significant leg power, try the resisted squat jump. Be very careful, though, and start with very light weights or resistance and low jumps so that your joints, tendons, and ligaments can adapt to the extra force.

Alternate: Resisted Squat Jump

This exercise is meant to be done using rubber tubing with handles. It can however also be performed by either holding a medicine ball or a weight plate that has handles. When using a rubber tube (as pictured), secure/anchor one end/handle of tube around the base of a sturdy object. Make sure that there is no chance that the tube can disengage from where it's anchored. Take hold of one handle with both hands (side by side grip) and hold the handle down in front of your waist, with arms straight.

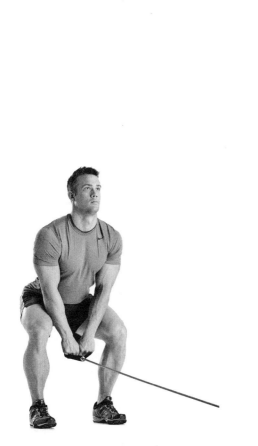
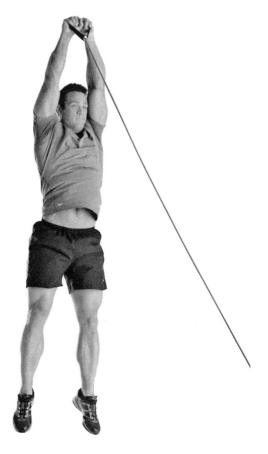

Walk back until you have no slack in the tube. Stand with feet about hip width apart and squat down. Keep the chest out, shoulders pulled back, the head on a slight angle, looking up and keep your abs tight. With arms held down between your legs and in a deep squat position, take a deep breath an than simultaneously swing the arms up while jumping up, exploding upward and extending the knees, hips, ankles and trunk. Focus on completely extending the body, reaching as high as possible. The arm drive is critical for achieving maximum jump height.

The tube will pull you down once you reach the top; quickly repeat the movement.

True Alpha Tip: If you do decide to hold a medicine ball or a weight plate, hold either up to the chest and secure arms tight to body (elbows are tucked into your sides).

Please Note: there must be NO arm raise involved during the exercise, just the jump while holding the ball/weight close to the body.

Tuck Jump

This is an excellent drill for improving hip flexor strength and speed.

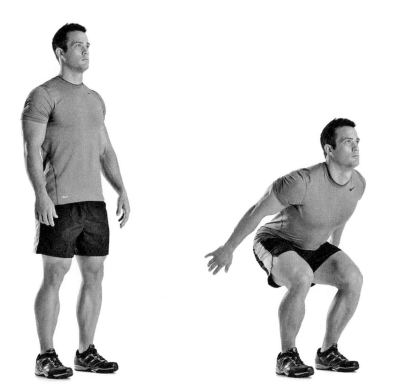
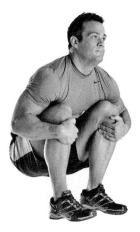

Assume the same starting position as you did for the Squat Jump. Swing your arms back and jump as high as possible, extending your knees, hips, ankles, and trunk. While in the air, quickly pull your knees into your chest, grabbing them with both hands prior to landing.

Jump to Box or Bench

This drill requires a box or set of boxes, varying in height from 24 to 58 inches. If you're using a bench, exercise caution when jumping and landing.

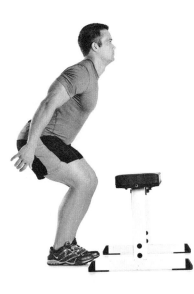

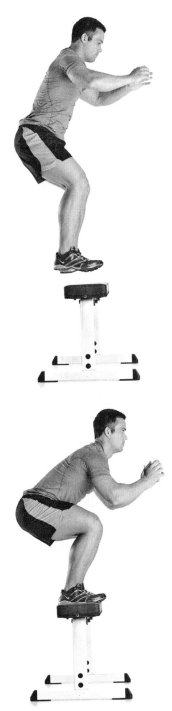

Stand facing the box with your feet hip-width to shoulder-width apart, about an arm's length away from the box. Dip rapidly, swing your arms, drive them upward, and jump onto the box. Jump just high enough to land in a half-squat position. Return to the ground by stepping down or hopping off the box.

Box Landing Two-Step Sprint

This is a particularly good drill for men who play rugby, soccer, basketball, or any other sport where the athlete is required to accelerate into a sprint upon landing.

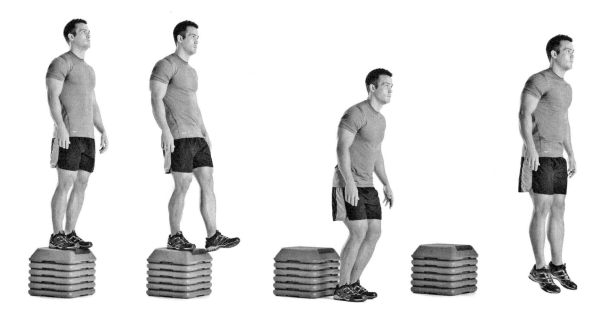

Use the same height box that you would use for Jump to Box. Start by standing on a box or bench, feet shoulder-width apart, hands at your sides. Step off the box. The first step out of the landing will be a short double-leg hop forward, to transfer your weight and momentum from the vertical landing to a horizontal sprint motion. As soon as you land on the ground, sprint forward as fast as possible for 10 yards. Focus on accelerating to your maximum speed as quickly as possible.

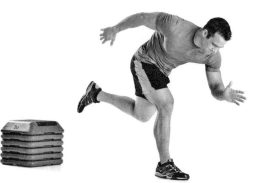

Multidirectional Hop

TARGETED MUSCLES: Quadriceps

SECONDARY MUSCLES: Hamstrings, glutes, calves

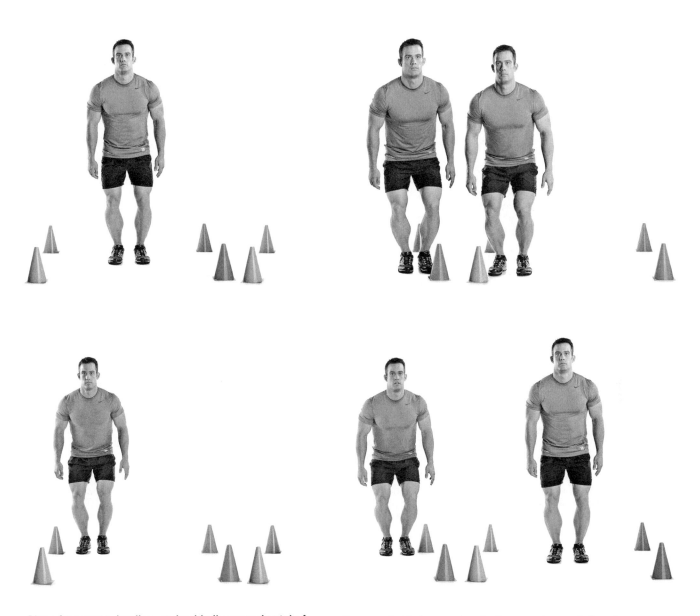

Place four cones, hurdles, or dumbbells approximately 4 feet away from each other to form a box. Stand in the middle of the cones. Take a hip-width stance and keep your hands at your sides. Begin by hopping to each cone, without resting between hops. Begin with the cone to your left, now over to the cone to your right, a backward hop to the cone behind you, a hop to the cone to your left and hop back to the middle. Hop just high enough to reach each cone. The objective is to hop back and forth as fast as possible without stopping. Keep your feet hip-width apart throughout the drill and keep your balance. The sequence of five hops equals one repetition.

Lateral Push-Off Jump

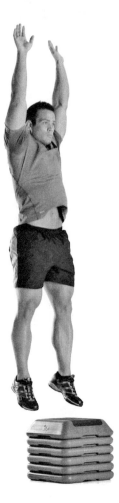

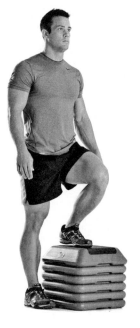

Stand beside a box or bench and place one foot completely on the box; your thigh should be parallel to the floor, creating a 90-degree angle at the knee. Your lower leg should remain on the floor. From this position, swing both arms upward as explosively as possible and push off against the box. Jump as high as you can, completely extending your body and reaching upward as high as possible. Absorb the shock to your knees and hips by landing on your toes with soft knees. You can increase the difficulty by using a higher box.

Forward-Backward Cone Hop
Alternate: Side-To-Side Cone Hop

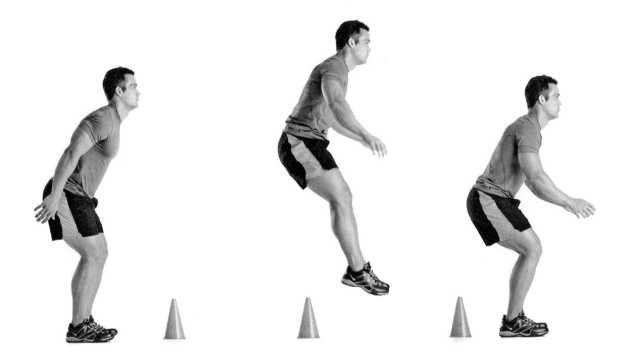

Use a cone, dumbbell, hurdle, or other low object as the object to jump over. Stand facing the cone with your feet shoulder-width apart. Dip down quickly and jump forward over the cone. Land soft, flexing your knees and hips, then immediately jump backward over the cone to your starting position. Use your arms to help you jump, and keep your torso erect and your abdominals tight during every jump. This is a plyometric exercise: Speed is the goal, so keep your hops low and short. Use quick feet and minimize ground contact time.

> **Alternate:** *This same exercise can be done hopping side to side.*

Lunge Jump
Alternate: Lunge Jump, Switch Legs

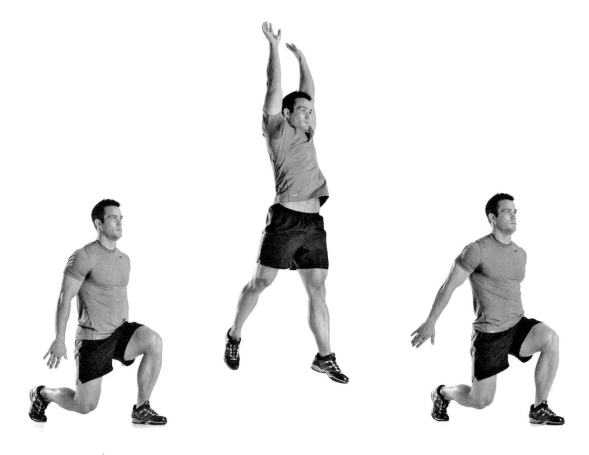

Stand with your feet shoulder-width apart. Step forward into a lunge position, keeping your trunk upright. Jump upward as high as possible, pushing off with both legs and driving your arms upward. As you jump, switch legs in the air, landing with the opposite leg forward. Focus on jumping as high as possible and not just on switching legs quickly. Land in the same split position and take off again.

When stepping forward into the lunge position, remember to step straight forward, maintaining a shoulder-width stance. It is common to bring the feet together when stepping forward, decreasing the width of your base of support and making balance more difficult.

Speed Skater

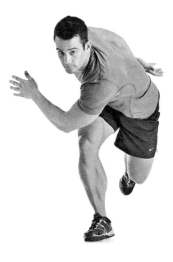 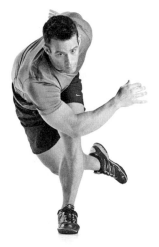

This is an excellent drill for athletes and weekend warriors. Stand on one leg with the other leg bent behind at 90 degrees, hands at your sides, looking straight ahead. Dip until your leg bends to 120 degrees, swinging your arms backward as you dip. Drive your arms forward and sideways, explosively jumping sideways as far as possible. Focus on completely extending your body and drive the opposite leg out to the side to increase your jump distance and prepare for landing. Land on the opposite leg and immediately jump back to the other side.

Long Jump

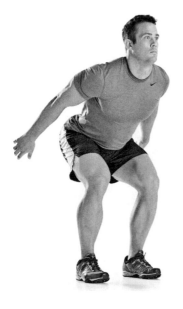

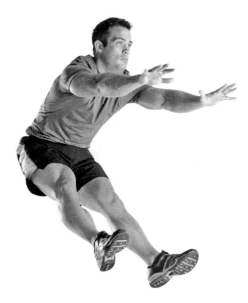

Stand with your feet about shoulder-width apart. Swing your arms back and quickly dip until your knees bend to about 120 degrees. Explode forward, extending your knees, hips, ankles, and trunk while swinging your arms forward as explosively as possible. Focus on completely extending your body, jumping as far forward as possible. Swing your legs forward and land with your heels first, absorbing the impact with your legs, to maximize jumping distance.

Lateral Long Jump

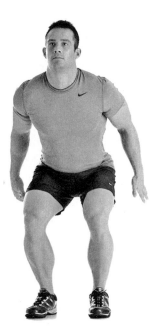

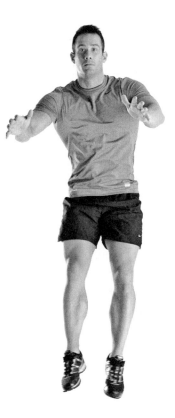

The objective of this drill is to jump as far sideways as possible, taking off and landing on both feet. Start with your feet hip-width apart. Swing your arms back and quickly dip until your knees bend to about 120 degrees. Explode upward and sideways extending your knees, hips, ankles and trunk while swinging your arms forward and slightly sideways, as explosively as possible. Jumps need to be done in both directions since your legs will not contribute evenly to a lateral jump.

ARMS: TWO TICKETS TO THE GUN SHOW

Massive arms are the goal of every aspiring True Alpha Male. Funnyman Will Ferrell's self-deluded character in the film *Anchorman* referred to his spindly arms as "guns" and boasted about doing 1,000 concentration curls. Our goal is a little more in touch with reality.

The arms are made up of the biceps and triceps muscles. The biceps are the rounded muscles on the front of your upper arms. When a person asks you to flex for him, he is usually referring to the biceps flex. The triceps muscles are the horseshoe-shaped (or soon to be!) muscles on the back of the upper arms. Because they make up most of the arm's size, when these muscles are fully developed, they look incredible!

Well-developed arms are without question the gold standard that most men aspire to reach through their fitness training. Think about why: Arms are the most revealed part of the body, period. Why wouldn't a man want to have great looking guns, when they're always just hanging out?

A guy can usually get away with having great looking arms, while letting the rest of his body just sag. It's easy—all he has to do is keep the rest of his body covered up. And don't fool yourself: Many guys do just that! But who wants to be in shape in just one area of the body? Be honest—no one does.

It's just easier to take care of one area of the body than it is to care for the whole body. But here's a secret and a damn good one: When you take the time to care for your whole body through a balanced strength training regimen, your arms will get even bigger. That's right. In fact, you need to gain about 5 pounds of muscle to add 1 inch of size to your arms! That's a lot of muscle, and that's a whole lot of size. Full-body training will add lots of muscle proportionately to your body, and this includes creating the arms that you've only envied on others, up until now. Now it's your turn to turn heads.

Biceps and Forearms

THE BICEPS

On the front of your upper arms are the two head muscles known as the biceps brachii. They make up about one-third of the total upper arm size. The two individual muscles of the biceps brachii are the long head and the short head.

The bicep muscles originate in your shoulder (scapula) in two places, hence the term *bi-cep*. The muscle runs down the front of your upper arm (the humerus) to one of your forearm bones called the radius (which is on the thumb side of your forearm). The function of the biceps is to bring your forearm toward your shoulder. The technical term for this is called *elbow flexion*. The biceps is also responsible for turning (supinating) your forearm from a palm-down position to a palm-up position.

Your objective is to train both heads of the biceps brachii. You can't isolate either one, but with the right mix of exercises, you will develop your biceps to your maximum genetic potential.

The brachialis is the other anterior-located muscle of the upper arm. It also helps flex (bend) the elbow. The brachialis lies just beneath the biceps brachii and is the most powerful flexor of the elbow.

The brachialis attaches from the lower portion on the front of the upper arm right near the insertion point of the deltoid (shoulder muscles). The brachialis does not participate in the pronation/supination of the forearm. It can't, because it does not insert on the radius of the lower arm.

THE FOREARMS

The forearm muscles—the fleshy, muscular masses on the lower arms—like the back and legs, have become even more legendary than the staple body parts of most training regimens. Think again of that Popeye character and how his biceps and triceps paled in comparison to his huge forearms. The muscles of the lower arm are true markers of a remarkably rugged physique. When you see muscular forearms on a man, you know he's worked damn hard to achieve them. You can also guarantee that his strength is diminished throughout the rest of his body. Fully developed forearm muscles are a measure of having reached optimum masculine physical conditioning.

The forearm muscles are divided into two parts: the flexors and the extensors. The flexor group is responsible for pronating (turning the palm from up to down) the forearm. It attaches to the medial epicondyle of the upper arm. The flexors also curl your fingers in toward your palm. Think about activities such as holding and grasping an object; your forearms flexors are responsible for these movements.

The extensors are involved with supination (turning the palm from down to up) of the forearms. Their attachment is on the lateral (outermost) epicondyle of the upper arm.

Grab a weight, hold your hand in a neutral or hammer-grip position, and curl (flex at the elbow) the weight up. Notice how the extensor muscles (brachioradialis) flare out.

The extensor muscles extend and bend the hands and wrists backward. Think of a cop shouting, "Stop in the name of the law!" Think about his hand motion and how his hand extends back. Those are the extensor muscles at work.

The medial and lateral epicondyles are deposits of bone created as attachment points for muscles and ligaments.

The brachioradialis is another forearm muscle, and it is involved in flexing the forearm at the elbow. It also helps with supination (turning the palms from down to up) and pronation (turning the palms from up to down). The borachioradialis is attached to the distal styloid process (another attachment point for muscles) of the radius (on the lower arm) and the lateral supracondylar ridge (a lip that presents itself for attaching the brachioradialis) of the upper arm (the humerus).

When the forearm is pronated (palm down), the brachioradialis naturally tends to supinate (turn the palm from down to up) as it flexes. The opposite is also true: When the forearm is in a supinated position (palm up), it naturally tends to pronate (turn the palm from up to down) as it flexes.

The brachioradialis is at its strongest as an elbow flexor when your forearm is in between a supinating and pronating position (known as a neutral grip or a hammer grip). When elbow flexion is performed in a pronated (palms down) grip, the brachioradialis is much more active than the biceps brachii. The biceps brachii is at a mechanical disadvantage in this particular position.

As you can see, the forearm muscles are a set of intricate and very active muscles in your arms—all the more reason to train them on par with the rest of your body. Think of all the activities the forearm muscles are involved with in your daily life, such as picking up things and flexing the elbow with hands down, hands up, and hands in a neutral (hand held vertically) grip. Think of typing, writing, and eating (fork to mouth). It is imperative that you include these muscles in your training repertoire. If you don't, there is a great chance that you will encounter weaknesses in your arms. Carpal tunnel syndrome, tendonitis, and other repetitive use syndromes are usually nothing more than weaknesses revealing themselves. Avoid them, and reap the awesome rugged look of fully developed forearms!

E-Z Bar Preacher Curl
Alternates: Preacher Curl Machine

Preacher curls emphasize the lower end of the biceps to build mass there and really give the biceps a great isolating movement. The preacher bench almost totally isolates the biceps so they don't get much assistance from the front delts. Although that's good for building biceps strength, it also means you won't be able to use as much weight as with standing curls, so don't go overboard. Do your best not to lean back, as that will bring the deltoids into the exercise, and you want to avoid that. Make sure to contract the biceps as hard as possible in the top position of the exercise. Most people relax here.

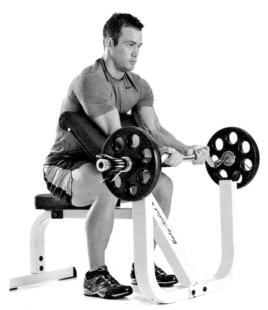
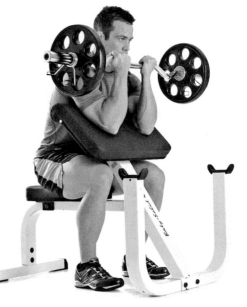

Take a seat in front of the preacher bench. The deck of the preacher bench should be angled with the high edge close to your body. Place the backs of your upper arms on the deck. Make sure you stay seated throughout the exercise or your deltoids will contribute to the curl and cheat your biceps of the full stimulation.

Reach down and grasp the bar with an underhand (supinated) grip and unrack it. Fully extend the arms with a slight bend at the elbows.

Contract the biceps intensely and begin to exhale as you bend your elbows and arc the bar toward your head. Focus hard on those biceps to draw the bar all the way up to a full contraction.

At the top of the curl, contract the biceps good and hard and hold for a moment. Then inhale as you slowly lower the bar to the starting position. Use a full range of motion by coming back into a full extension and immediately begin the next repetition.

Barbell Curl (Shoulder-Width)
Alternate: Wide-Grip Barbell Curl

Barbell curls are the basis of all biceps exercises. This exercise will use more weight than any other biceps exercise because it uses both heads of the muscle and contributes most to powerful, thick biceps. Remember, more weight means more stimulation of the muscle so that it grows bigger and stronger. Make sure you avoid using momentum, and you're best not to raise the shoulders forward.

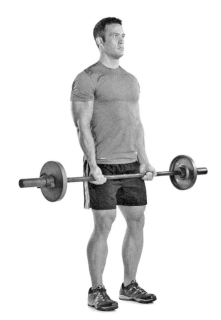 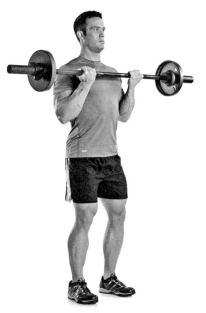

Stand with your feet approximately shoulder-width apart, holding a barbell in both hands with an underhand (supinated) grip. Hands should be shoulder-width apart. Bend your knees and hips just enough to stabilize your posture. Stick your chest out, pull your shoulders back and down, keep your head up, and your eyes forward to keep your back from rounding.

Let your arms hang almost straight down (leave just a slight flex in your elbows) and curl your wrists just a bit. You want to avoid overstretching the muscle, especially for men who tend to overextend their elbows.) Keep your elbows tight to your sides and as stationary as possible throughout the movement.

Take a deep breath and tighten your abdominals and glutes to stabilize your torso. Contract the biceps hard, exhale, and arc the barbell up toward your chest by bending your elbows.

Hold the top position a moment and give those biceps an extra squeeze before inhaling and allowing your arms to straighten and return to the starting position. Resist the weight on the way down. When you reach the starting position, immediately, but without momentum, start the next rep; do not pause.

Alternate: Wide-Grip Barbell Curl

Wide-grip barbell curls put more emphasis on the inside (short) head of the biceps. This puts emphasis on that particular part of the muscle and gives it that cannonball look when flexed.

Use the same form as above, but bring your hands farther apart than the width of your shoulders.

Incline Dumbbell Curl
Alternate: One Arm at a Time

Arnold Schwarzenegger says this exercise develops biceps mass and peak at the same time. Who's to argue with The Oak? Incline dumbbell curls stretch the biceps to their full length while still allowing the use of fairly heavy dumbbells without great risk of injury. Do your best to focus on the biceps, while relaxing the anterior deltoids.

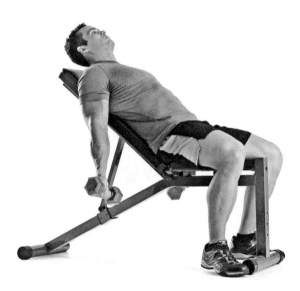
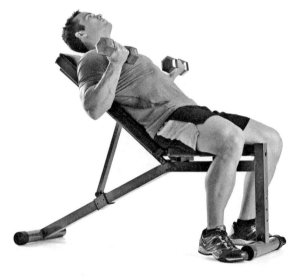

Set an adjustable bench so that the seat back is inclined to 45 or 55 degrees. With a dumbbell in each hand, take a seat and lean back against the backrest. Place your feet flat on the floor. Let the dumbbells hang from straight arms at your sides. To start, hold the dumbbells with palms facing forward.

Take a breath and then exhale as you contract the biceps to bend your elbows and pull the dumbbells toward your shoulders.

Keep your upper arms vertical and your elbows as stationary as possible. This will keep your forearm at an angle during contraction so the biceps are constantly under load. Make sure that you're exhaling as you reach the top, and give the biceps a good, hard squeeze.

After holding the maximum contraction for a moment, inhale and slowly lower the dumbbells back to the starting position. When you get to the starting position, immediately contract the biceps hard and head into the next repetition without pause or momentum.

Alternate: One Arm at a Time

Instead of doing both arms simultaneously, alternate arms so that you do one repetition with one arm, then one repetition with the other arm. There are two advantages to this method: First, each arm gets a brief rest between sets and a good stretch, so you can keep going for more repetitions, and second, it may allow you to use heavier dumbbells because you concentrate on one arm at a time.

Standing Dumbbell Curl
Alternate: Seated Dumbbell Curl

This exercise is the most functional of the biceps curls, developing power and strength for heaving heavy cement blocks, wielding a chainsaw, or hauling a stack of firewood in each arm. Core stabilizer muscles come into play with this exercise, so keep your abs, glutes, and back muscles tight. Use as heavy a dumbbell as you can manage without throwing your back into the exercise. Try doing them seated to remove the possibility of momentum.

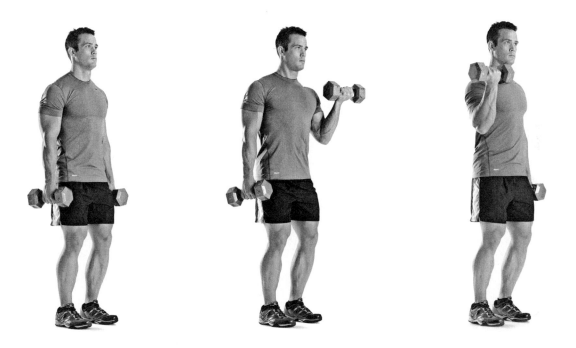

With a dumbbell in each hand, stand with your feet shoulder-width apart and your knees and hips bent just enough to stabilize your torso. Let the dumbbells hang from straight arms at your sides. To start, hold the dumbbells in a neutral position so that your palms face your thighs.

Begin with a deep breath, then exhale and contract the biceps of one arm to bend your elbow and pull the dumbbell in that hand toward your shoulder. As the dumbbell clears your hips, begin rotating it so that your palm faces your shoulder (supinated grip).

Keep your upper arm vertical and your elbow as stationary as possible. This will keep your forearm at an angle during contraction so the biceps are constantly under load. As you reach the top, give the biceps a good, hard squeeze.

After holding the maximum contraction for a moment, inhale and slowly lower the dumbbell back to the starting position. As the dumbbell nears your hips, rotate it back to the neutral position so you can lower it without pulling your arm away from your side. When you get to the starting position, immediately contract the biceps of the opposite arm and do the same movement with that arm. Continue alternating arms until you complete a full set with each arm.

Variation: You can increase the intensity of this exercise a bit by doing both arms simultaneously. However, you may have to sacrifice a little weight because both leverage and concentration will be divided between your arms.

Alternate: Seated Dumbbell Curl:

This is one of the most common exercises on the planet. The seated dumbbell curl will target the biceps and forearms very effectively.

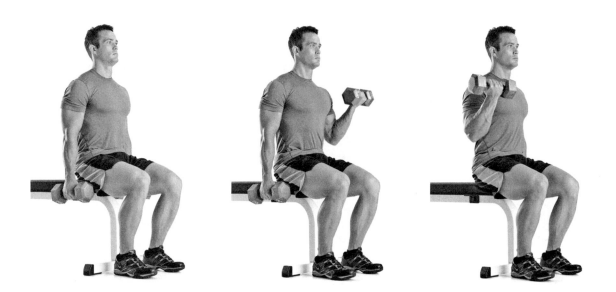

Sit on a bench that has an upright back pad. It's not necessary but it will prevent you from leaning back to gain leverage. Sit up straight on the bench and hold a pair of dumbbells down at your sides with your palms facing your body.

Begin the movement by contracting the biceps muscles and curl the weights up toward your front shoulders. As you begin the curling motion, gradually twist the palms out, so that they face up by the time the dumbbells come close to reaching the shoulder position.

Keep your elbows close to the sides of your body at all times throughout the exercise. Pause at the top for a second, making sure you contract those biceps as hard as possible before lowering. Avoid any swinging motions with your back to get the weight up.

> *True Alpha Tip:* Keeping the palms facing each other throughout the movement will place more work on the forearms.

Dumbbell Hammer Curl

TARGETED MUSCLES: *Brachialis (outer biceps), brachioradialis*

SECONDARY MUSCLES: *Forearm flexors, anterior deltoids*

As the name implies, the motion and wrist position of this exercise are like those used when swinging a hammer, but without the shoulder movement. Hammer curls build a good base of strength and power for the biceps, but they will also thicken your wrists and strengthen your forearms. From a practical standpoint, this is good because your biceps usually work in tandem with your wrists and forearms in the real world.

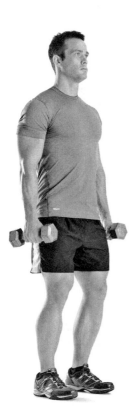
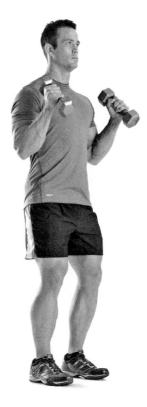

With a dumbbell in each hand, stand with your feet shoulder-width apart and your knees and hips bent just enough to stabilize your torso. Let the dumbbells hang from straight arms at your sides. Hold the dumbbells in a neutral position so that your palms face your thighs.

Take a breath, exhale, and contract the biceps of both arms, as you bend at your elbows and pull the dumbbells up toward your shoulders. Unlike the standing dumbbell curl, *do not* rotate your hands and dumbbells; instead, maintain the neutral-grip position and raise the dumbbells until the top plate comes close to your shoulders.

Keep your upper arm vertical and your elbow as stationary as possible. This will keep your forearm at an angle during contraction so the biceps are constantly under load. As you reach the top, give the biceps a good, hard squeeze.

After holding the maximum contraction for a moment, inhale and slowly lower the dumbbells back to the starting position. When you get to the starting position, immediately contract the biceps and begin the next repetitions.

> ***True Alpha Tip:*** *You can increase the intensity of this exercise a bit by training one arm at a time. This will allow you to lift more weight but could compromise your ability to use proper form.*

Reverse E-Z Bar Curl

TARGETED MUSCLES: *Biceps (especially the long head on the outside)*

SECONDARY TARGET: *Forearm extensors*

Curls with a reverse or pronated grip really blast the long head (outside) of the biceps and top extensor muscles of the forearms. Karate enthusiasts will love this exercise because it really hardens the forearm muscles used for blocking—your opponents will think you blocked their punch with a lead pipe!

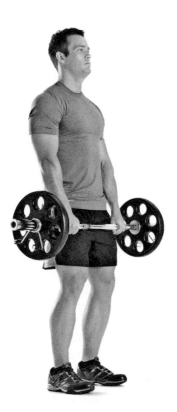
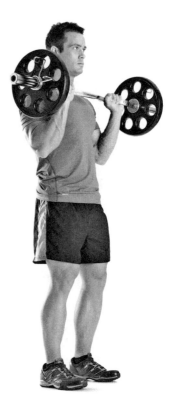

Stand with your feet shoulder-width apart, holding an E-Z bar in both hands with an overhand (pronated) grip. Bend your knees and hips just enough to stabilize your posture. Keep your head up and eyes forward to keep your back from rounding. Let your arms hang straight and keep your wrists straight. Keep your elbows tight to your sides and as stationary as possible throughout the movement.

Take a breath and tighten your abdominals and glutes to stabilize your torso. Now exhale as you contract the biceps hard and arc the bar up toward your chest by bending your elbows.

Hold the top position for moment and give the biceps an extra squeeze before inhaling and allowing your arms to straighten and return to the starting position. Resist the weight on the way down. When you reach the starting position, immediately start the next rep without pausing or allowing your elbows to fully extend. Make sure you avoid using momentum to aid in the lift.

TARGETED MUSCLES: Biceps

SECONDARY MUSCLES: Anterior deltoids, forearms

21 Curls

This variation on the standing barbell curl will totally blast your biceps and help them build superhuman endurance. We have saved these until last in your biceps workout, because you won't be able to do any of the others if you do these first! The exercise is called 21s because it involves three stages with seven reps per stage (3 x 7 = 21).

| STAGE 1 | STAGE 2 | STAGE 3 |

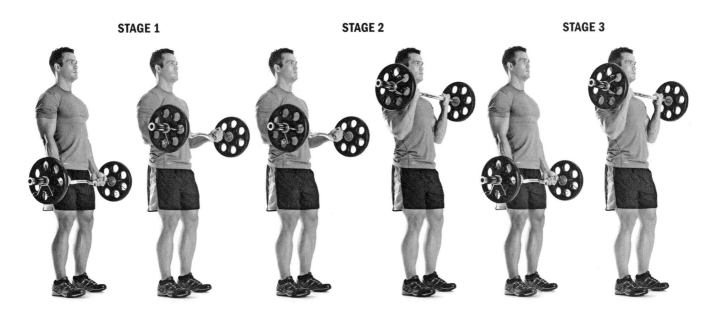

You have an option of using a barbell or you can hold a dumbbell in each hand. Stand with feet shoulder-width apart and your knees and hips bent just enough to stabilize your torso. Let the barbell or dumbbells hang from straight arms, down at your thighs. Hold the barbell or dumbbells in a pronated position.

STAGE 1: Take a deep breath. Exhale as you contract the biceps to bend your elbows and pull the weight up toward your shoulders. Stop contracting when your forearms are parallel to the floor. Repeat Stage 1 seven times before progressing to Stage 2.

STAGE 2: After the last repetition of Stage 1, curl the weight all the way up to your shoulders. Inhale as you lower the weight back down, but stop when your forearms are parallel to the floor. Immediately contract your biceps and raise the weight back to the top. Repeat Stage 2 for a total of seven repetitions before progressing to Stage 3.

STAGE 3: After the last repetition of Stage 2, perform seven full-length curls from full extension to full flexion. At the top of the curl, squeeze the biceps hard before lowering the weight again. Exhale as you raise the weights; inhale as you lower them.

TRICEPS

The three-headed muscle on the back of the upper arm is one of the greatest looking and most helpful muscles you have. When the triceps are fully developed, they resemble the shape of a horseshoe. To bring about that level of development, it is important to train the triceps at various angles.

The three heads of the triceps are the long head, the lateral head, and the medial head. The triceps connects to the upper arm (the humerus) and scapula and runs down the back of the arm to the forearm bone called the ulna (located on the pinkie side of the forearm).

The lateral head, which is the one mostly responsible for the horseshoe shape, is located on the outer side of the upper arm. Look in the mirror, extend your arm down, and contract the triceps; it's the muscle that bulks out of the side of your upper arm. The medial head is located on the inside of the upper arm (closest to your body). It's the smallest of the three heads and is located down under the long head. The long head is the largest of the three triceps heads. It is located on the underside of the upper arm. If you extend your arm out from the side of your body, with palms facing toward the front, the long head is the one that hangs down from your upper arm.

The function of the triceps is to straighten the arm. The long head of the triceps is also involved with bringing the arm down toward the side of the body, known as shoulder adduction.

You should get an idea of all of the activities you do where the triceps participate. Think about things like using your arms to stand up from a sitting position, pushing a broken-down car, pulling yourself up a ledge, pushing a box up into the attic, and throwing your kid up in the air.

TRICEPS

Dumbbell Skull Crusher

TARGETED MUSCLES: Triceps

SECONDARY MUSCLES: Anterior deltoids

The lying position of this exercise lets you concentrate on using heavier weights to build thick, strong arms that your loved ones will have fun hanging on to. Using dumbbells ensures that each arm is doing equal work and that one arm is not compensating for weakness in the other.

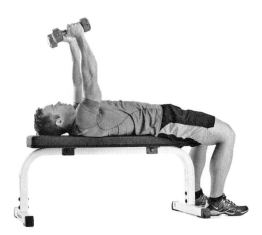

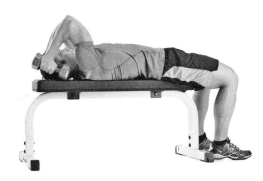

Hold a dumbbell in each hand. Place them on top of your thighs and sit on the edge of a flat bench. Hold the dumbbells tightly to your chest and thighs, and thrust them up as you lie back on the bench. Once you are lying down, place your feet flat on the floor. If your thighs feel stretched or you can't put your feet flat on the floor, then the bench is too high and your back will be arched in a way that could lead to injury. Place some blocks or weight plates under your feet until you can comfortably reach the floor.

Hold the dumbbells in a neutral grip with the pinkie-finger end of your fist pressed against the bottom dumbbell plates. This will make it easier to control the dumbbells. Press your lower back against the bench to support your lower spine, and push the dumbbells straight up toward the ceiling. Angle your arms slightly overhead and toward the back of you, to take stress off your elbow joint and to emphasize the triceps muscle more.

Tighten your abdominal muscles and inhale. Contract the triceps hard, and slowly lower the dumbbells toward your shoulders. Keep your elbows completely stationary throughout the movement.

Just before the dumbbells touch your shoulders, stop the descent, exhale, and squeeze the triceps hard to extend your arms and return to the starting position.

TARGETED MUSCLES: Triceps

SECONDARY MUSCLES: Anterior deltoids

Overhead Single Arm Dumbbell Extension

This is a great isolation exercise for the back of the arms. With this one, you'll not only stimulate the triceps, but you'll also work on your core stabilizing muscles. Remember that in sports or physical labor of any sort, the core is essential to safe movement and functional strength, so it's important to include exercises that strengthen the core in combination with other strength-training movements.

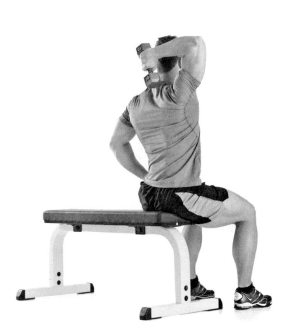
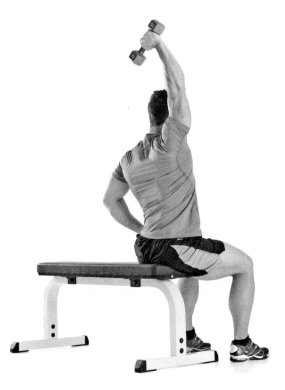

The overhead dumbbell extension can also be done standing, but sitting increases stability and reduces the opportunity to cheat by using momentum.

After selecting a dumbbell that's not overly heavy to use with one hand, sit on the edge of a flat bench. Place your feet flat on the floor. Using both hands, hoist the dumbbell up and bring it behind your head. Hold the dumbbell upright, with your working hand's pinkie finger pressed against the upper inside part of the dumbbell. Direct your working arm's elbow up toward the ceiling, so that your forearm is positioned vertically.

Sit up straight, keep your abs tight, and keep your head straight throughout the entire exercise. Place your other hand on your lap to brace yourself and help maintain good posture during the exercise.

Inhale and contract your working arm's triceps and begin to extend your elbow, lifting the dumbbell overhead. Bring that arm to full elbow extension and contract the triceps muscle as hard as you can. Hold for a moment before bending at your elbow to slowly lower the dumbbell back behind your head.

When your elbow reaches a 90-degree angle, stop the descent, exhale, and immediately begin the next repetition.

When you've completed the set for that arm, quickly switch hands and begin with the other arm.

TARGETED MUSCLES: Triceps

SECONDARY MUSCLES: Anterior deltoids, chest (aka pecs)

Close-Grip Bench Press

The close-grip bench press trains the triceps to generate great strength because it lets you use heavier weights than most other triceps exercises do. The arm motion is also very similar to a punching motion, with the fists starting at the chest and driving straight outward. If you don't have access to an E-Z bar, a straight bar can be used, but it will be harder on your wrists. Let your triceps do the work and not just your chest muscles. The first four photos below demonstrate how to most effectively get the bar into the lifting position.

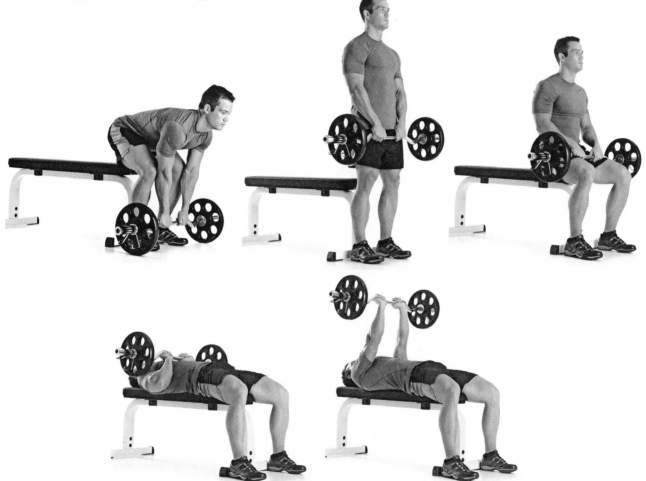

Load an E-Z bar with weight and grasp it with an overhand grip on the innermost angles (about 6 to 8 inches apart). Lie back on a flat bench and place the E-Z bar across your sternum (the bony center of your chest just above the solar plexus). Place your feet flat on the floor.

Inhale and tighten your abdominals and glutes. Exhale as you contract the triceps hard and drive the E-Z bar straight up off your chest until your arms are fully extended. Focus your attention on the triceps so that they do more of the work than your chest. For maximum muscle stimulation, don't lock your elbows at the top—locked elbows put pressure on the elbow joints instead of the muscle. At the top of the movement, contract the triceps.

Hold the full extension for a moment before slowly lowering the bar back to your chest. Resist the weight on the way down to fully stimulate the triceps. Inhale as the bar descends. Just before the bar touches your chest, clench the triceps hard and drive the bar back up for the next repetition in a smooth and controlled movement.

Triceps Pushdown (Rope Attachment or V-Bar)

Here's a great exercise to stimulate the three heads of the triceps. Triceps pushdowns are great for totally burning any remaining energy in those powerful muscles and really pumping them full of blood. The motion of this exercise is similar to swinging a hammer, but without the shoulder movement.

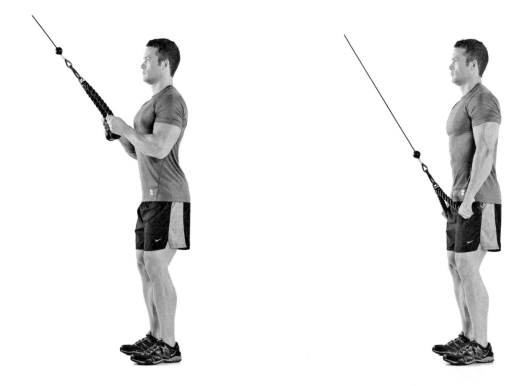

Attach a rope or V-shaped bar attachment to the cable of an overhead pulley. Face the machine and stand close enough to the pulley that the cable pulls down at about a 45 degree angle. Grasp the ends of the rope or bar with an overhand (pronated) grip. The pinkie-finger end of your fist should be against the stops on the ends of the attachment.

Position your body by standing with your feet hip-width apart, knees slightly bent, abs tight, chest out, and shoulders back. Your elbows should be held tightly to your sides and kept locked there throughout the exercise. Bend your elbows to 90 degrees or slightly less. Contract your abdominals and glutes and keep them tight throughout the movement to stabilize your lower back.

Exhale and squeeze your triceps hard to press your hands down and fully extend your arms.

When using the rope attachment, drive your forearms out laterally to really get a great contraction in the triceps. Treat each arm as if you were working it independently from the other one. In other words, don't just go through the motions—really make the triceps muscles work hard. Go ahead and lock your elbows, because the angle of this exercise keeps the pressure on your triceps, rather than the joints. (This only applies, however, to lifting a weight where the triceps are really challenged. If you're using light weight, there is no reason to lock the elbow joints.)

Hold the fully extended position momentarily, making sure that you contract those bad boys as hard as possible. Inhale and allow your arms to return to the starting position. Try to resist the weight on the way up, but don't actually stop it. When you reach the starting position, take a breath. Immediately begin your exhalation, squeeze your triceps hard, and start the next repetition without a pause.

Triceps X-tension

This exercise requires some coordination and serious core stability to perform. Lock your stance in hard, and really squeeze your abs, because you will be fighting resistance pulling you in two directions at once.

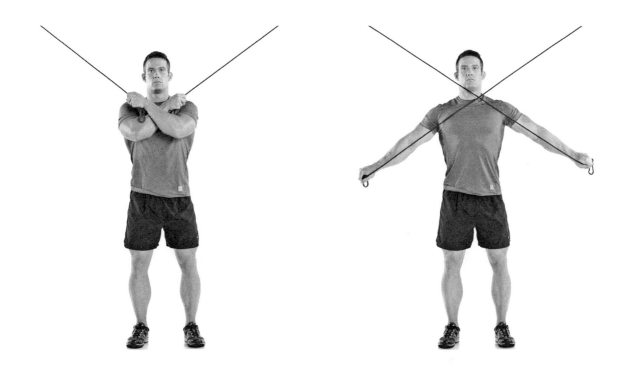

Attach single-hand grips to the high pulleys on both sides of a cable crossover machine. Standing in the middle of the machine (with a weight stack on either side of you), grasp the handle to your left with your right hand and the handle to your right with your left hand. If using the handle grips, grab them with an underhand grip (both palms facing up). If you've done this correctly, the weights will want to pull your arms across each other in front of your body—almost like you're wearing a straitjacket.

Stand with your feet shoulder-width apart with toes pointing forward and knees bent slightly. Look up at the wall in front of you. Maintain tight abs and glutes throughout the exercise to stay stable. Position your arms so that your elbows hang below your chest. Be sure to keep your elbows stationary throughout the movement.

Begin your exhalation, contract the triceps forcefully, and straighten your arms until they are fully extended out to the sides. Go ahead and lock your elbows, because the direction of the resistance keeps the stress on the muscles instead of the joints.

Hold the fully extended position momentarily as you forcefully contract the triceps before slowly returning your hands and forearms to their original positions. Resist the weight on the way back, as you inhale.

Take a quick breath as you reach the starting position and immediately begin your exhalation breath, contract the triceps, and with a fluid motion, begin the next repetition without pause.

Triceps Dip
Alternates: Weighted Dip, Bench Dip

Triceps dips are one of the most effective triceps developers that exist. If you're looking to hit all three heads of this muscle, this is one exercise that you don't want to pass up.

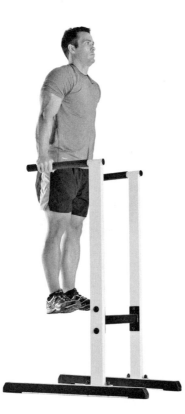
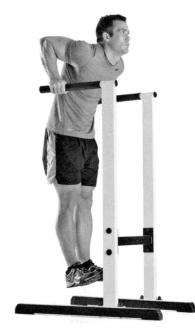

Situate yourself on a parallel dip station so that each hand is on a dip bar, arms fully extended and elbows locked. Your body should be hanging between the dip bars.

Keep your legs and the bottoms of your feet pointed straight down to the ground, tighten your abdominals and glutes, and keep them tight throughout the movement.

Inhale and contract the triceps muscles. Keep those arms pinned close to your body throughout the exercise to keep the stimulation in the triceps. Keep your head up at all times to prevent you from leaning forward. (Note that leaning forward makes this more of a chest exercise than a triceps exercise. To help you maintain an upright posi-

tion, look up throughout the exercise.) Stop lowering yourself when the backs of your arms are parallel to the floor. (Your training partner should let you know how far that is.) In the lowered position, you may quickly touch your flat feet to the ground, but keep the weight on those triceps muscles; don't go too deep and do not rest.

At the bottom of the dip, let your triceps stretch for just a moment, then exhale as you contract hard and allow the triceps to push you back up. Exhale as you push yourself back up. Contract the triceps as hard as possible at the top, but try not to lock your elbows. Slowly lower yourself again for the next repetition.

Alternate: Weighted Dip

Most gyms have a weight belt available to members. Wrap the belt around your waist. Put the chain through the loop, then through the hole in the weight, and then clip back to the loop. Be careful that the chain links don't grab your skin and watch the gems. Make sure you maintain strict form and don't allow the weights to sway from momentum. Start out with a light weight to test yourself and move up from there.

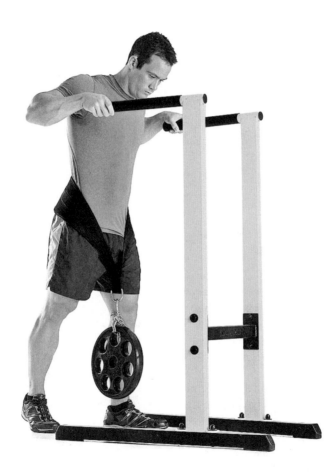

Alternate: Bench Dip

Bench dips provide an awesome exercise to really engage those triceps. Due to the unorthodox angle of this exercise, you may feel the triceps working harder than during some of the other exercises that target the triceps. This is a great thing!

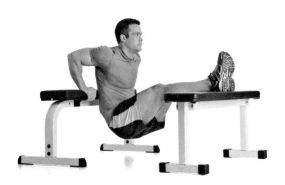

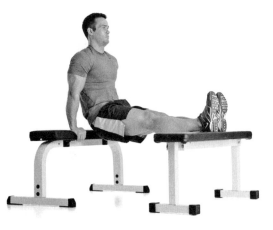

Begin by placing two benches parallel to each other and approximately your legs' distance apart from one another. Place your hands on the inside edge of one bench, about waist-width apart. Your arms are straight at this point in the exercise, and your hands should be positioned right under your shoulders.

Now put your heels on the other bench, preferably toward the middle, so you don't slip off during the exercise. Keep your legs straight—if you feel pain in your lower back, you may bend your knees slightly. If you still feel lower back pain, stop and move on to the next exercise.

At this point, you can either use your body weight only or, for more of a challenge, you can have a training partner place additional weight (barbell plates) on your upper thighs.

Begin the exercise by bending at the elbows and lowering your body down (moving your rear toward the floor).

The lower you go, the more you'll feel a stretch in your triceps. Just be careful not to lower too low, as you will begin to feel an uncomfortable stretch in the anterior deltoids and chest muscles. Lower until the backs of your arms are approximately parallel to the floor. At this point, without rest, exhale as you contract your triceps and lift your body back up to the start position. Begin the next repetition without pausing.

True Alpha Tip: If you don't have a training partner or anyone available to assist with placing additional weight on your upper thighs, you can carefully do this yourself. Begin by sitting on the edge of the bench. Place the weight plate (go light, as this can be a difficult task) on top of your upper thighs before lowerng yourself into position. Make sure that it is well balanced, as you will wobble a bit while getting your body into the proper position.

ABDOMINALS: RIPPED AND ROCK SOLID

We've finally reached the ever-popular abdominal muscles. We call the abs "buried treasure" because most people already have, without realizing it, fairly well-developed abdominals. The abs are involved in just about any movement you make, because one of their functions is to help stabilize your spine. Although you may have decently developed abs, you'd never know it unless you use your hand to dig deeply beneath your belly to feel them. The only way to reveal the abs (the six-pack, as so many men like to refer to them) is through a sound nutrition plan and a vigorous cardio and strength-training regimen. Our goal is help you "unbury" your prize!

A well-developed abdomen is the mark of having reached the highest level of physical conditioning. Most men claim to have a six-pack, but very few actually do. They may have a two-pack or even worse, a keg, but not many actually have a great looking six-pack.

The abdominal muscles are made up of four sets of muscles: the rectus abdominus, the transverse abdominus, the external obliques, and the internal obliques. The ab muscles are positioned on the front and the sides of the torso, from just below the chest down to the pelvis. The muscles originate at the rib cage and attach to the pelvis. The rectus abdominus muscles are the ones you know as the "six pack." The six-pack look is created by thin bands of connective tissue.

The function of these muscles is to flex (bend) the spine, allowing you to bring your rib cage to your pelvis. In exercises such as the abdominal crunch, the crunching movement is the action of these muscles. You can also trigger the rectus abdominus by bringing your legs to your chest (your pelvis toward your chest/rib cage), a movement you use when executing the captain's chair leg lift exercise.

The transverse abdominus (TA) muscles are the deepest of the ab muscles, and they wrap around the core laterally (toward the sides). The TA muscles act like a cummerbund or weight belt around your waist. They're what keeps your insides, inside! This important muscle is what keeps your waist tight and primarily aids in maintaining trunk stability.

The external and internal oblique muscles are positioned diagonally on the torso. Their diagonal position allows you to move at an angle, following the path of the muscles. The obliques' unique diagonal position is also responsible for rotating your torso and, like the rest of the ab muscles but to a higher degree, they are essential for stabilizing the abdomen.

You have to realize by now just how involved and active your abdominal muscles are in your everyday life. The abs are involved in virtually every activity, even while you sleep (unless you sleep like a rock without any tossing and turning).

Think of all the activities that your abs are involved with, such as sitting up, bending down, lifting your legs, maintaining a solid core, and turning you to your left and right. They are involved in any and all movements that require you to just be upright. Imagine how much better you'd feel and how much more incredibly physical you would be if you trained these muscles well.

Don't forget about the very important relationship between those erector spinae back muscles and the abdominals. They completely complement one another, so one can't work efficiently unless the other is working efficiently. Think about it: The abs' concentric muscle action allows you to bend over, while the erectors control your descent downward. The erectors' concentric muscle action allows you to bend backward, while the abdominals control the descent of that action. When you bend forward, the erectors will pull you back up. When you bend backward, the abs will crunch you back up. It's a synergistic relationship. To create this alliance, it is so important to train these sets of muscles directly and consistently. You can either train them together or separately, but make sure you train them.

ABDOMINALS/CORE

TARGETED MUSCLES: *Rectus abdominus*

SECONDARY MUSCLES: *Internal/external obliques, hip flexors*

Floor Crunch
Alternative: Oblique Crunch on Floor

Floor crunches are a great abdominal exercise, as long as you execute them properly.

If you want to truly isolate the abdominal muscles to strengthen them and finally reveal a ripped midsection, we hope you realize by now that the Alpha Fuel Solution is about 80 percent responsible for helping excavate the body fat to reveal the buried treasure we call six-pack abs. This is the most basic of your abdominal exercises, but it's also incredibly effective when combined with the rest of the abdominal exercises here. For the oblique crunch, begin as you did with the standard floor crunch, isometrically contracting the abs even before you begin the oblique crunch; then bring the arm/elbow that's behind your head across your torso toward that arm's opposing knee. Twist as far as you can. Inhale and lower your body back to the starting position. Without rest, immediately switch arm positions and begin your next repetition.

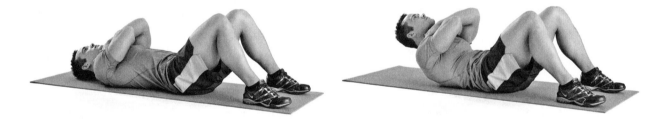

Begin by lying on the floor, facing up. Bend your knees and place your feet flat on the floor. Cross your arms over your chest and place your thumbs on each side of your chin to stabilize your neck. Keep your head in line with your neck and do your best not to flex it forward, as this could strain it.

Begin the movement by first isometrically contracting the abs even before you begin the crunch; focus your concentration on that contraction.

Next, lead with your chest and roll up toward your pelvis. Remember, your objective is not to sit up, but rather crunch the area between your chest and pelvis. Also note that when done correctly, it is actually a very short range of motion to fully contract the abdominals in this position. This knowledge should help you more effectively isolate the abdominal area, while helping you avoid stimulation of the hip flexor muscles.

Once you reach full crunching capacity, momentarily contract the abdominal muscles as hard as you can. Inhale and lower your body back to the starting position. Without rest, immediately begin your next repetition.

Bicycle Maneuver

TARGETED MUSCLES: External obliques

SECONDARY MUSCLES: Rectus abdominus, hip flexors, core

The bicycle maneuver is considered one of the greatest and most effective abdominal exercises in existence according to leading fitness organizations through EMG testing. It's a great exercise for teaching you coordination, it works all areas of the core (abdominals and erector spinae muscles), and it provides a great challenge! Training the abdominals with such a well-rounded exercise ensures that your core will be a strong base for functional strength and athletic performance. This skill is essential for all sports, because abdominal tension keeps the spine stable and reduces your chance of injury.

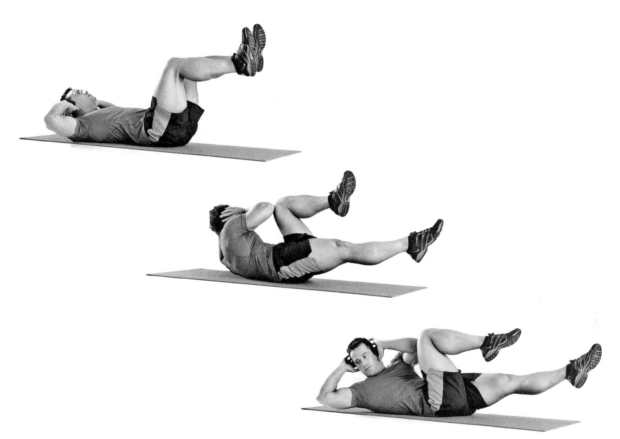

Lie on your back with your legs together. Raise your knees so that your thighs are perpendicular to the floor and your lower legs are parallel to the floor, creating a 90-degree angle. Slightly tuck your chin to your chest and place your interlaced hands behind your neck. *Do not* pull on your neck during the exercise. Placing your hands behind your neck simply gets your arms out of the way and increases resistance on the abdominals.

Contract your abdominal muscles, exhale, and bring your left knee to your chest while simultaneously drawing your right elbow/shoulder toward your left knee. Try your best to touch elbow to knee; but more importantly, really focus on drawing that shoulder across your body, because that's where the abdominal work comes in.

Inhale as you slowly return to the starting position. Do not lower your head to the floor or release tension on your abs. Repeat the procedure on the other side, bringing the right knee to the chest and the left elbow/shoulder to the right knee.

Captain's Chair Leg Lift

TARGETED MUSCLES: *Rectus abdominus*

SECONDARY MUSCLES: *Internal/ external obliques, hip flexors*

Another one of the most effective abdominal exercises, this move not only strengthens the abs but also teaches core stability. Core stability helps with all movement, from athletics to carrying a heavy load.

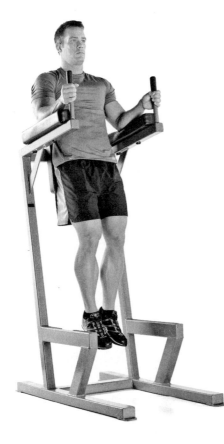 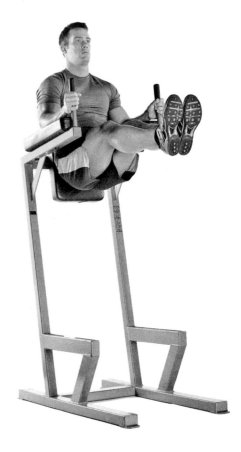

Sit on the chair and press your back to the seat back. If handles are provided, grasp those. Inhale, contract the abdominal muscles, pinch the glutes, and lift your legs up while keeping them together. Keep your knees bent throughout the exercise to keep the abdominals working and to keep the hip flexors from taking over.

Keep your knees together and draw them in toward your chest as far as you can as you're exhaling. Hold the maximum contraction briefly, than slowly lower your legs back to the starting position. Take a breath, and then start the next repetition.

Swiss Ball Crunch
Alternate: Swiss Ball Crunch with Barbell Plate

TARGETED MUSCLES: *Rectus abdominus*

SECONDARY MUSCLES: *Internal/ external obliques*

This is an all-around excellent exercise for core strength and stability; it will help participants in every sport, from swimming to martial arts. It also builds incredible core strength for anyone who frequently lifts or carries heavy loads. Using the Swiss ball stretches the abdominal muscles more than doing crunches on the floor would, so the abs have to work through a greater range of motion. They adapt to this by increasing muscle fiber size and strength. The ball also decreases stability and brings the core stabilizer muscles into play.

Want a challenge? Hold a barbell plate overhead to increase resistance and require your abs to work and contract harder, which builds optimal abdominal strength.

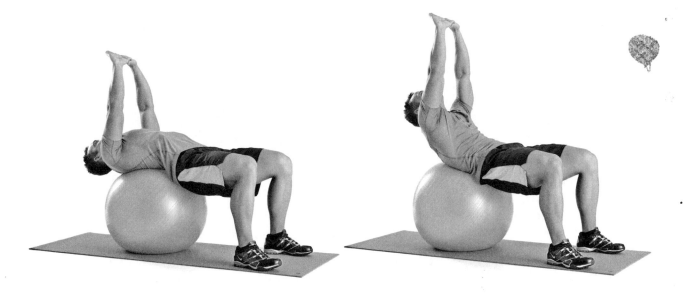

Sit on a Swiss ball and roll your butt down the ball just a bit, until the ball is under your lower back. Lie back over the ball so that your back is arched and you're feeling a comfortable stretch in your abdominal muscles.

Position your legs so that your thighs are parallel to the floor and your knees are bent at 90 degrees or something close to that. In the beginning, start with your feet shoulder-width apart or slightly wider. As the exercise becomes easier, bring your feet closer and closer together. This decreases stability and makes your core muscles work harder.

Bring your fully extended arms overhead, tuck your chin to your chest, tighten your abdominal muscles, and squeeze your glutes. Exhale and contract the abs as you curl (crunch) your spine forward toward your pelvis. It might be easier to think of it as drawing your shoulders toward your hips. Stop when your abs are fully contracted and your upper back is off the ball. Do not sit all the way up or lift your lower back off the ball. Doing so engages the hip flexor muscles, which is not what we're looking to do here.

Hold the top of the crunch momentarily as you contract your abs. Then lower your upper back and shoulder blades back to the starting position, until you feel a comfortable stretch in your abdominal muscles. Take a quick breath, then exhale and begin the next repetition.

Bench Leg Lift

Even more so than the captain's chair leg lift, the bench leg lift develops core stability as well as abdominal strength because there is no chair back or handles to help you maintain balance. If you are very active or play any sports, you need to include this abdominal exercise in your routine!

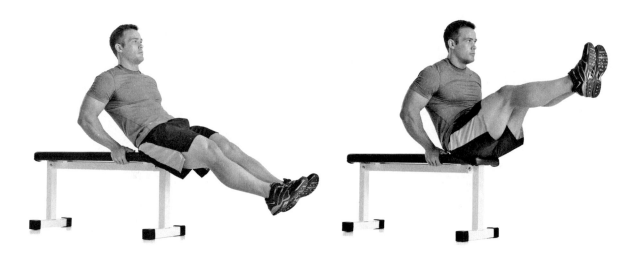

Sit on the bench and grasp the edge of the seat on either side of you. When first starting out, grip the bench directly beneath your shoulders for maximum stability. As the exercise gets easier, move your hands closer and closer to your butt. This decreases stability and causes your stabilizer muscles to work harder.

Take a breath. Exhale, contract the abdominal muscles, pinch the glutes, and lift your heels off the floor while keeping your legs together. Maintain tight abs and glutes throughout the movement.

Keep your knees together and draw them in toward your chest as far as you can. Hold a maximum contraction momentarily, then slowly lower your legs back to the starting position. Without resting, start the next repetition.

Swiss Ball Throw

TARGETED MUSCLES: *Rectus abdominus*

SECONDARY MUSCLES: *Hip flexors, latissimus dorsi, anterior deltoids, internal and external obliques*

You may have seen this exercise used by boxers. It not only develops abdominal strength, but it also conditions the abs to deliver force and power—a very useful skill in any activity. Fortunately for guys who like to train alone in the basement, this exercise can be done by throwing a lighter ball against the wall. It's not as intense, but is still effective!

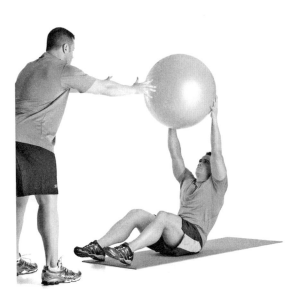
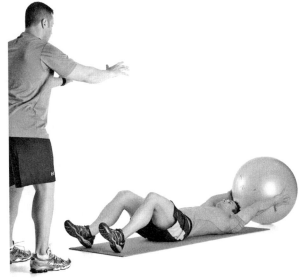

Lie on your back and bend your knees to put your feet flat on the floor. Hold the ball at your chest between both hands. Your partner should stand about 5 feet from your feet and be facing you.

Begin by sitting up with your arms held overhead in anticipation of receiving your first ball throw. Right when you catch the ball, sit back and take a breath.

Next, go all the way back, keeping the arms outstretched, and touch the ball on the floor behind you. Begin your exhalation. Contract the abs forcefully and sit up quickly. At the top of the situp, throw the Swiss ball with outstretched hands back to your partner, who will catch the ball. (Try to only use your shoulder joint to throw the ball, and avoid bending at the elbows when receiving and throwing.) Stay in the situp position until your partner quickly throws the ball back to you. Your partner should aim the ball a little higher, toward the palms of your hands. As you progress with the exercise, you and your partner can discuss increasing the speed of the throw (from exerciser to thrower and vice versa).

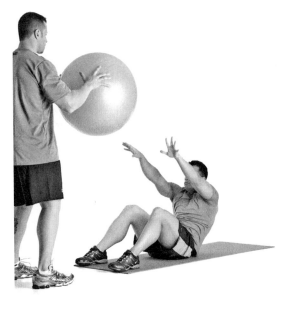

Superman Back Extension

This is a very effective exercise for strengthening the lower back muscles, a commonly vulnerable area.

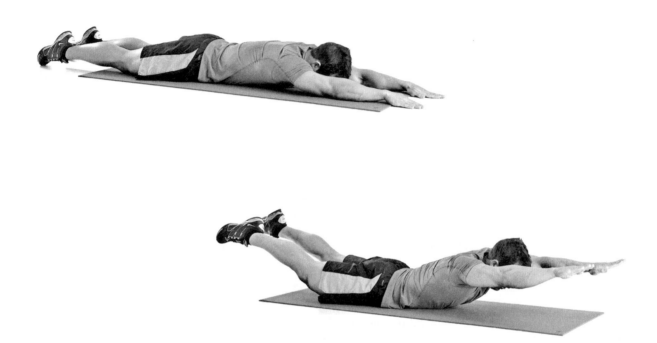

Lie face down on the floor. Extend both your arms and legs. You should look like Superman in flight. Raise both hands and legs off the ground. It is a short range of motion you will be working with, so keep your concentration on squeezing the lower back muscles. Hold at the top for three seconds. Slowly lower back down; don't let your limbs come crashing down. Perform this exercise slowly to ensure its effectiveness.

The Plank

TARGETED MUSCLES: *Rectus abdominus, erector spinae*

SECONDARY MUSCLES: *Anterior deltoids, tibialis anterior, calves*

A very effective core strengthener, the Plank may seem effortless, but it's challenging.

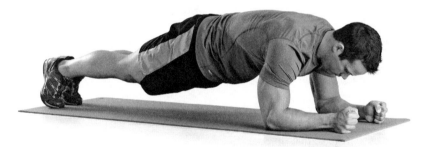

Lie face down on the floor. Raise the front of your body by resting on your forearms, using the sides of your wrists to help stabilize yourself. Raise your lower body, resting on the tips of your toes. Do your best to keep your entire body straight, from head to heels. You can accomplish this by contracting your abdominals and tilting your pelvis forward just a bit. You want to avoid raising your butt in the air or arching your lower back. The plank exercise is primarily a way to build muscular endurance in the abs and back. It is a static, or isometric, exercise for developing core muscular endurance.

Our challenge for you is to hold the plank for at least 1 minute (and up to 2½ minutes) during Week 3, and to add time during Week 4 and Week 9.

POWER BOOST MOVEMENTS/ PLYOMETRICS

TARGETED MUSCLES: *Rectus abdominus, core*

SECONDARY MUSCLES: *Internal/ external obliques*

Please note: For Home Body Training, you can also perform this exercise using rubber tubing. Always make sure that the anchored end of the tubing is securely fastened to a pole or other stable object.

Partner Lying Leg Throw

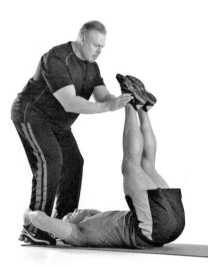
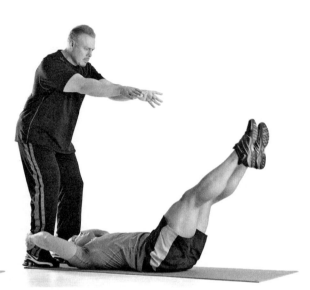
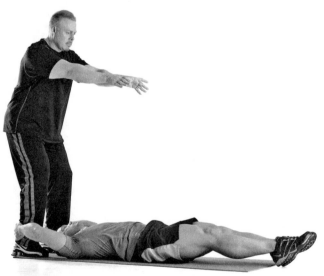

Lie on the ground on your back, legs straight, holding on to your partner's ankles. Raise your legs so that they are perpendicular to the ground. Your partner will push your feet toward the floor. Just before your feet hit the floor, stop the downward movement and explosively raise your legs again. The partner throwing the legs down should adjust the force he uses so that you can stop your feet before they hit the floor. Very strong athletes can do this drill using a bench, allowing the thrower to stand to the side, where he will have better leverage for the throw. In either case, it is essential that the lower back remain in contact with the floor throughout. Keep the abs contracted to accomplish this.

Partner Lying Twisting Leg Throw

TARGETED MUSCLES: *Internal/ external obliques*

SECONDARY MUSCLES: *Rectus abdominus, core*

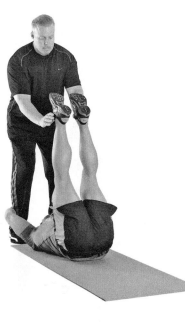

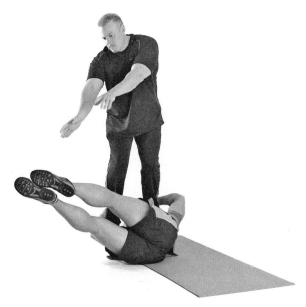

To make the drill even more difficult, rather then throwing the legs straight down, add a twisting throw. Throw your partner's legs down and to the side. This added level of difficulty requires greater activation of all the stomach muscles while incorporating a skill element as well.

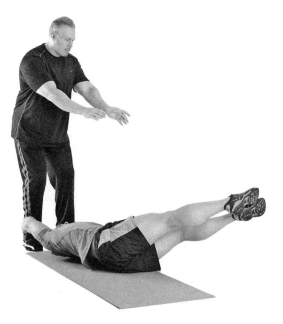

Samurai Swing

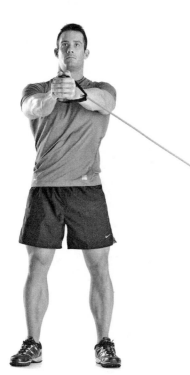

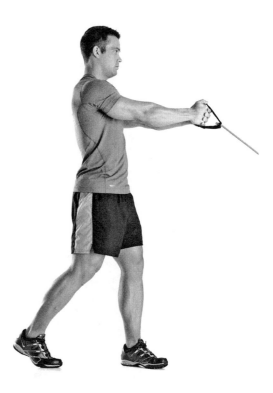

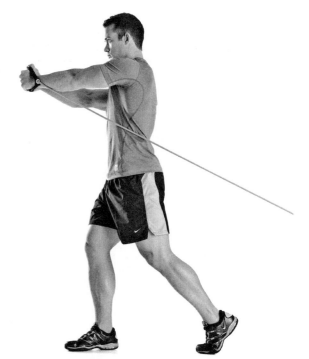

Stand in front of a cable station, such as a cable crossover machine. Adjust the cable swing arm so that it is below chest level. Stand sideways and grab one handle with both hands at chest height. (Reach one arm over and across your body and the other straight out to the side, as if you were holding a sword or a bat, and clasp one hand over the other.) Put a slight bend in your knees, and reach around to your side closest to the cable source.

Twist across your body, pivoting on your feet and rotating at your trunk and hips. Quickly rotate in the opposite direction, driving through with your hips and coming onto your toes. The movement is similar to what you would use in a cross-body samurai swing. Keep your arms fully extended, and move in an arc around your body so that you are only rotating at the waist.

Complete all reps on one side of your body, and then switch to the other side.

Grand Slam

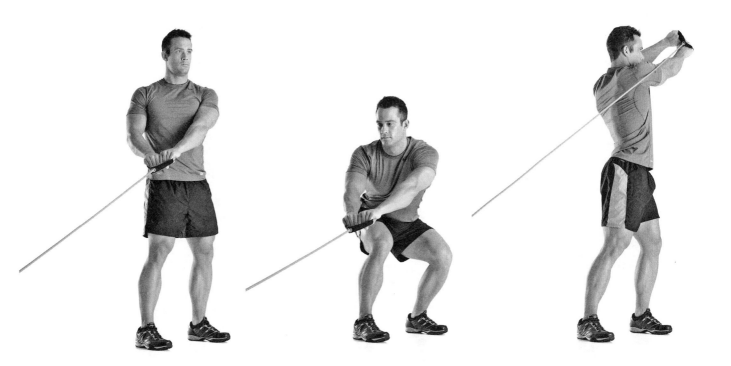

Stand in front of a cable station, such as a cable cross-over machine. Adjust the cable swing arm so that it is positioned down by your feet. Grab the handle with both hands clasped one over the other. Face forward, so that the cable is to the side of your body.

Squat down and turn in toward the cable source, and then rapidly twist your torso up and away from the cable source. Raise your arms up and back as far as possible over the opposite shoulder, as if you were hitting a grand slam in baseball. Use your lower body and torso to aggressively accelerate your arms diagonally and upward across your body. Rapidly return to the starting position and repeat.

Full Body Resistance Extension

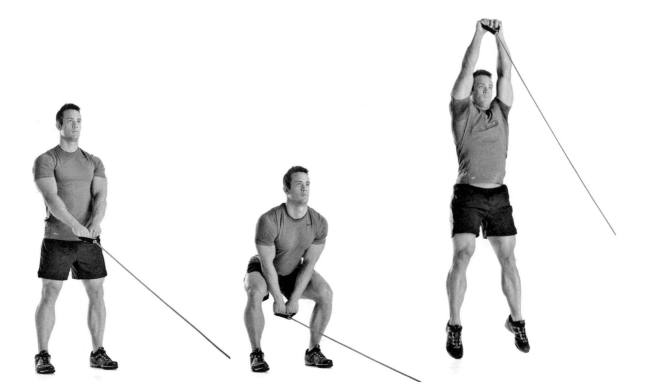

Stand in front of a cable station, such as a cable cross-over machine. Grab a handle with both hands clasped one over the other, and face the cable source.

Begin by squatting down, slightly bending at your waist with your arms hanging down toward your feet. Jump up as high as possible, pulling upward on the cable handle. Be sure to extend up quickly at your waist, driving your hips forward and lifting your arms up as high as possible. If done correctly, your toes should leave the ground during the jump. The cable will pull you down once you reach the top; quickly repeat the movement.

TARGETED MUSCLES: *Chest, triceps, quadriceps, rectus abdominus*

SECONDARY MUSCLES: *Core*

Push Jump to Bench

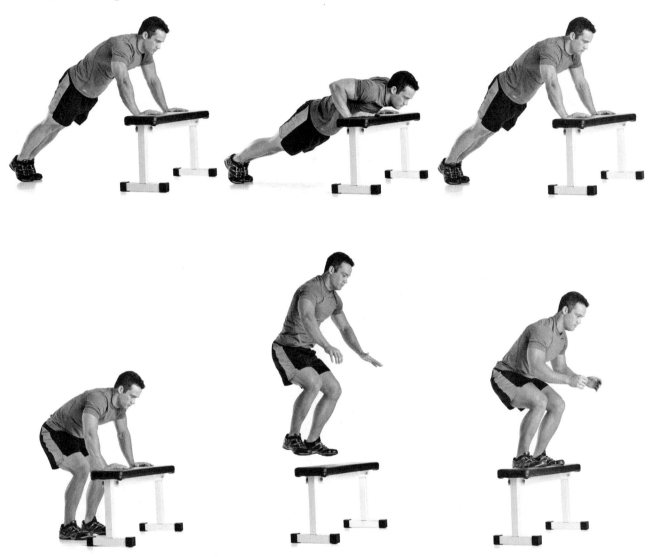

Begin this power-based movement by positioning your hands on a standard bench in a pushup position. Your legs should be fully extended and your feet placed on the ground behind you so that your body forms a 45-degree angle. This is the starting position. From this position, you will do two full pushups, bringing your chest all the way down to touch the bench.

Next, powerfully pull your knees in toward your chest, like you're performing a hopping motion. Land in a squat position with your feet positioned underneath your shoulders.

From this squat position, immediately jump with both feet onto the bench; this is also known as a "jump to box" movement. Remember to land on the bench as softly as possible, with your knees bent, as this will help prevent stress on your knees and back. Be sure to open your hips fully to a standing position.

Without rest, jump back down off the bench to your previous squat position and extend your legs back to the starting position.

Begin your next repetition without resting.

Situp and Pike

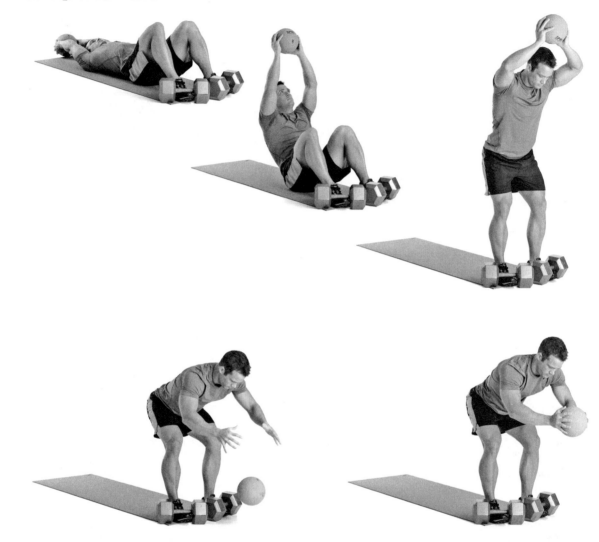

Grab two heavy dumbbells, as these are what will brace you as you perform your situp. Most guys will need at least 60-pound dumbbells. If you weigh more than 220 pounds, go for 70-pound dumbbells or heavier. Have a medicine ball handy.

Place the two dumbbells on the floor, end-to-end horizontally. Take a situp position and place/anchor your feet underneath the handles of the dumbbells. Grab your medicine ball and bring it overhead with both arms fully extended.

Begin the movement by explosively sitting up and moving directly into a standing position. This should be one fluid movement and is accomplished by whipping your arms forward to build enough momentum to get to your feet. Please note: This may take some time to perfect. Just do your best to get to your feet as quickly as possible. The arm-whipping motion should mimic the action of a soccer player throwing a ball back into play.

Once you've gotten to a standing position, the whipping of your hands should have brought your hands and the ball down by your chest.

From here, quickly lift the ball back overhead and slam it to the floor in front of you as hard as you can. The ball will naturally bounce back up to you, so be ready to catch it. Catch it and quickly return to the situp position with the arms and ball extended overhead.

Begin your next repetition without resting.

INTERVAL TRAINING

This is our favorite style of heart-healthy, fat-burning exercise. The alternating combination of fast (intense) and slow (relaxed pace) training has been shown to dramatically improve cardiovascular fitness and fat burning within just a few weeks' time. One study showed that just six sessions of interval training over only 2 weeks *doubled* endurance—even among subjects who were already reasonably fit from jogging and aerobics. Another study published in the *Journal of Applied Physiology* confirmed increases in fitness and fat burning among borderline sedentary subjects and college athletes who began intervals.

Almost any aerobic activity can be performed in an interval training style, by alternating intense activity with a more measured pace. Always warm up first to prevent injury. If you like outdoor training and the weather permits, bleacher runs are a great option.

- Bleacher Runs
  - Many local high schools have stadium bleachers, and they go relatively unused on the weekends, especially on Sundays. Bleachers usually have sets of stairs spaced every 20 yards or so.
- Start at the bottom and ascend the bleacher stairs as quickly as you can to the top, then walk across the top to the nearest adjacent set of stairs and walk briskly down. Repeat 10 times, then briskly walk the track for 15 minutes, followed by 10 more bleacher ascents. Bleacher runs are a great workout!
- The intensity should be based on your current fitness level. At level C, you should try walking, rather than running. Use common sense and don't overdo it—this is just the first week of your Challenge! At level A or B, take each ascent as vigorously and quickly as possible, pumping your arms and driving your knees upward toward your chest with each bound, then walk or jog across the top to another set of stairs and walk briskly down. Repeat 15 to 20 times, then briskly walk the track for 10 minutes, followed by 15 to 20 more bleacher ascents. You'll notice you need to focus intensely as you ascend in order not

SOME TIPS ABOUT SPRINT TRAINING:

◎ Start with a 3-minute warmup walk at the predetermined incline and speed based on your level (see page 65). This will usually have you breaking a very light sweat. This is a sign that you're doing some heart work!

◎ When either increasing or decreasing incline grade and/or speed, always be prepared to grab the handrails if you need to. Your objective is to train without holding on, but sometimes you may find that you need to while catching your breath. If you feel the need, take hold and recover, and then get back at it.

◎ The intensity of this sprint will take a lot out of you, so be ready and stay focused.

◎ Always maintain your form and always be aware of your position on the treadmill. It's easy to get distracted and take an embarrassing and potentially painful fall off the treadmill if you're not fully concentrating during these very intense sessions.

◎ Always be sure to keep up with the speed of the treadmill—if you lag behind, you'll be sorry. Keep up!

to miss a step. Stay focused, and play it safe.

Of course, the vast array of indoor interval training options is limited only by your imagination. Here's a fun one:

- Weighted Stair Climbing
  - If you have access to a building with at least three flights of stairs, climbing with an added 25 to 50 pounds is a rugged and intense way of getting that heart pounding and that excess fat melting. Do three flights at a clip, rest for 1 minute, descend with the weights, rest for 30 seconds, and then climb again. Make 10 climbs. Over time, you'll be able to shorten the rest at the top and eventually work up to 20 climbs.

Want to get your Play Heart done in the gym? Here's a savage training protocol designed to strengthen your lower body muscles, give your heart a great workout, and burn that excess body fat faster than a wildfire.

- Savage Mountain (K2) Sprint Training.
  - In the Himalayan range stand two fearsome mountains, one of which is the second-tallest mountain on Earth. It's known as the "Savage Mountain" due to the difficulty of ascent. For every four people who reach the summit, one dies trying. K1 is the most accessible peak, with the more forbidding K2 somewhat hidden and more remote. You're going to scale them both in an intense bout of interval training. By running on a fairly steep incline, you not only greatly increase the intensity of the workout but also reduce the stress on your knees, hips, and lower back. Leaning forward also helps

you maintain your form and concentration. Keep your core tight, and swing your arms to gain momentum. Your objective is to increase your speed on each successive sprint. The total training time will be about 25 minutes. At about the halfway point, after scaling K1, you'll get 3 minutes to recover; and then you'll do a second round of sprints to climb K2, followed by a cooldown. It may not seem like a long time right now, but this high-intensity training protocol will surely make it challenging for you—trust us! Even better, do it with a partner and make each sprint a race. Not only will the sprints give your heart and lungs a great workout, but the competition can also boost your testosterone levels.

Pay close attention to how you are feeling based on the Borg scale. This simple interval workout is a yo-yo-style training protocol designed to bring your heart rate up for 1 minute (sprint), bring it back down (recovery) for the second minute, and then repeat. You walk, then sprint, walk, then sprint. We recommend that you try to stick to one or maybe two grades of incline throughout this particular workout (begin at a lower grade for a 3 minute warmup and bring it up to a higher grade for the remainder of the session). We want you to focus predominantly on changing your speed rather than worrying about changing grades of incline. Because you will be focused on speed, to make the session challenging enough, you may choose to increase your speed in increments of 0.5. Try to set the speed for each successive sprint a bit faster than the last. For more tips on exciting and varied "outside the box" treadmill training, see www.alphamalechallenge.com.

DYNAMIC WARMUPS

For more information on these warmups, go to alphamalechallenge.com

10 Bodyweight Good Mornings

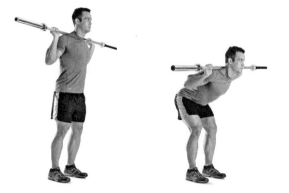

Balance an Olympic barbell on your shoulders, palms facing forward. Stand with feet shoulder-width-apart and a slight bend in knees, torso fully extended with head up and chin forward. Bend at waist until body is parallel with floor by pushing buttocks back. Hold for a brief moment and return to your starting position.

Walking Lunges (Cross the River) (8 lunges on each leg)

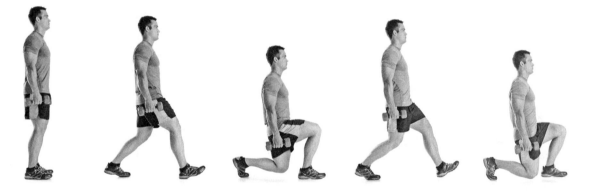

Step out far enough, so that you touch heel to toe and keep the knee from going over the toes. Lunge forward with one leg and without rest, lunge forward with the opposite leg.

Rotational Hamstring Stretch (8 stretches on each side)

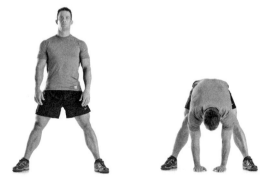
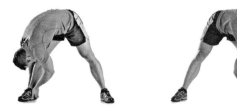

Spread the legs about 3 feet apart from one another and keep the knees just short of lock out. Begin by facing forward. Now bend down at the hips and draw your hands down one leg until you touch your toes. Come back up to the middle, and slide the hands down the other leg.

Trunk Rotations (10 to each side)

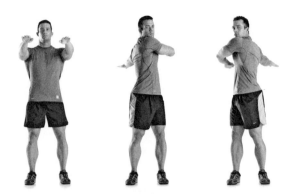

Spread your feet about 5 inches apart, keep a slight bend in the knees; bring arms out to sides, fully extended. Twist your upper body, keeping your head straight.

10 Deep Squats

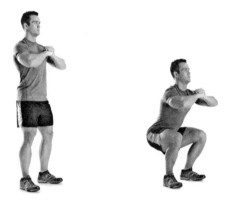

Take a slightly wider than hip width stance, slightly bend the knees, stick your chest out, keep your shoulders back and head up. Squat down and mimic the motion of sitting back as you would in a chair. Stop when thighs are parallel.

Static Quad Stretch
(hold for 15 seconds on each leg)

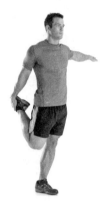

Stand on one leg, grab ankle of other leg and pull up to butt while pointing knee to the ground. Shift pelvis forward and do not lean forward.

Static Lunge Hip Flexor Stretch (hold for 15 seconds on each leg)

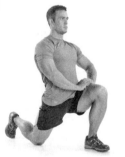

Get into a lunge position, but drop knee to the floor (gently). Lean forward on the front leg; keeping the knee of the back leg on floor, lean forward stretching the hip. Keep torso erect and lean slightly backward.

Static Chest Stretch
(hold for 15 seconds on each side)

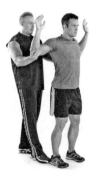

Place hand against a wall or around a pole and turn away.

Static Lat Stretch
(hold for 15 seconds)

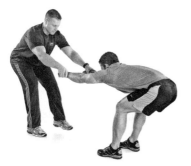

Grab a pole and pull, rounding out your upper back.

10 Pushups (full range of motion)

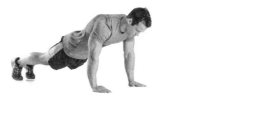
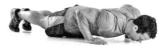

Regular pushups

Stationary Inchworm (8 reps)

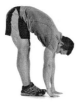
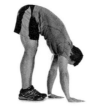
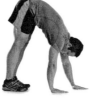
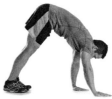

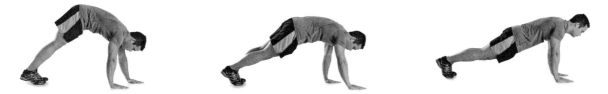

Bend over so that you are on your hands and toes with your butt in the air. Start with hands as close to feet as possible. Walk your hands out until you get to the pushup position. Hold for a moment, than walk your hands back to the starting position.

10 Jumping Jacks

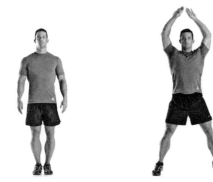

Nothing fancy, just like you did in high school.

Butt-Kickers
(20 total—10 on each leg)

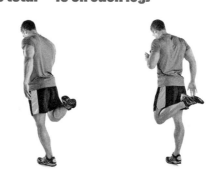

Run in place, driving your heels up until they touch your butt.

Lateral Shuffle (10 total—5 to each side)

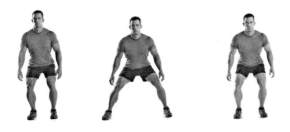
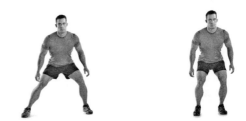

Spread legs about hip-width apart—knees slightly bent, on balls of feet with slight bend at waist. Shuffle sideways but do not allow feet to cross over. Then shuffle back the other way.

APPENDIX B
ALPHA FUEL RECIPES

Most guys are too busy to spend too much time in the kitchen, but they want healthy food that tastes good. The Alpha Fuel Solution is perfectly simple and naturally delicious. Use the Man-Hand portion method and cook by roasting, grilling, broiling, and poaching. Always marinate meats before barbecuing. The George Foreman grill is a handy and worthwhile investment. We also recommend a food processor or an emulsion blender, such as the one by Wolfgang Puck; it has a food processor attachment and an S-blade for chopping.

Colette Nelson, RD, is an experienced dietitian, certified diabetes educator, certified sports specialist dietitian, and cooking whiz who also happens to be a bodybuilding champion. When it comes to health and fitness, Colette is one of the best. She and world-class bodybuilder Dave Palumbo are one of the health and fitness world's most celebrated Alpha Couples. We asked Colette for her tips on basic day-to-day food preparation—no muss, no fuss; stuff that guys can make alone, or as a couple or a family.

SIMPLEST CHICKEN PREPARATION
In a large skillet, boil 6 boneless, skinless chicken breasts in ¼ cup reduced-sodium soy sauce, ¼ cup balsamic vinegar, and enough water to cover the chicken. Cook uncovered until the chicken is no longer pink. Use any of the simple sauces (see page 311), and add steamed vegetables and some nuts to make a complete meal.

SIMPLEST FISH PREPARATION
Place a piece of foil on a baking sheet. Place any type of fish filet on top, and fold the foil sides up to create a pouch for the marinade. Coat the fish with equal parts reduced-sodium soy sauce and vinegar (balsamic, red wine, or raspberry). If you have a lemon handy (or even a bottle of real lemon juice), squeeze on some lemon juice. Then broil in an oven or a toaster oven at 500°F for 15 to 20 minutes, or until done.

SIMPLEST MEAT PREPARATION
Marinate a steak for a couple of hours (or overnight) in reduced-sodium soy sauce, pepper, and lemon juice, turning it over once halfway through. This will soften a very lean cut of meat and add flavor. Then take the steak out of the marinade and just grill or broil it, turning once. Try some homemade Steak Dip (see page 313).

We also asked Colette to work with us to design some specific Alpha Fuel recipes for breakfast, lunch, and dinner. We wanted meals that would give plenty of zing to the taste buds. We wanted each recipe to be easy and quick enough for the least-culinary guy to make on his own, but with enough of a gourmet quality that family and friends would enjoy not only eating it, but also helping to prepare it. The calorie and macronutrient contents are provided; you'll see most of these recipes are strong on protein and light on carbs and fat, which makes perfect sense because your higher-carb fruit and nut snacking will balance out things perfectly. Why not try one or more of our delicious Alpha Fuel recipes once each week? Plan ahead by choosing a specific recipe or two and picking up the necessary ingredients during your shopping run. Take the opportunity to get loved ones involved, but as Colette warns, be sure to make additional servings! And look for more Alpha Fuel recipes at www. alphamalechallenge.com.

BREAKFAST

Alpha Artichoke Scramble

1 tablespoon macadamia nut oil
1 cup artichoke hearts, drained
4 ounces fresh mushrooms
4 ounces spinach
1 tablespoon Dijon mustard
1 tablespoon reduced-sodium soy sauce
1 tablespoon balsamic vinegar
Salt and pepper
2 whole omega-3 eggs
6 egg whites
2 teaspoons paprika

DIRECTIONS

1) In a skillet, heat the oil and sauté the artichoke, mushrooms, and spinach. Add the mustard, soy sauce, and vinegar, and stir well. Season with salt and pepper.

2) In a bowl, whisk together the eggs and egg whites.

3) Spread the vegetables evenly over the bottom of the skillet and pour the beaten eggs over them.

4) Turn the heat to low, cover the skillet, and cook until mostly set, 7 to 10 minutes. Sprinkle paprika over the top and serve.

Yield: 2 servings

NUTRITION INFORMATION PER SERVING
Calories: 270
Protein: 23 g
Carbs: 16.5 g
Fiber: 5 g
Fat: 13 g
Sugar: 4 g

Power Pancakes

4 egg whites
1 cup nonfat cottage cheese
1 scoop vanilla whey protein
1 scoop wheat germ (optional)
1 tablespoon cinnamon
1 teaspoon vanilla extract
4 packets (4 teaspoons) sugar substitute
1 ounce chopped walnuts (optional)
1 teaspoon macadamia nut oil

DIRECTIONS

1) Combine the egg whites, cottage cheese, whey protein, wheat germ (if using), cinnamon, vanilla, sugar substitute, and walnuts (if using). Mix until the batter has no clumps.

2) Heat the oil in a skillet over medium heat.

3) Pour the batter into 4 small silver-dollar pancakes.

4) Cook until bubbles form and the edges of the pancakes look dry, 1 to 2 minutes. Use a spatula to flip the pancakes and cook on the other side, 1 to 2 minutes.

Yield: 4 small pancakes (1 serving)

NUTRITION INFORMATION PER SERVING
(*Note:* Optional ingredients not included in analysis)
Calories: 88
Protein: 16.5 g
Carbs: 2.6 g
Fiber: 0.3 g
Fat: 0.7 g
Sugar: 1 g

Man Made Quiche

1 zucchini, sliced

Salt and pepper

1 teaspoon macadamia nut oil

½ cup shredded broccoli (use a food processor if you have one)

½ cup chopped cauliflower (use a food processor if you have one)

1 clove garlic, chopped

1 teaspoon nutmeg

1 teaspoon cumin

2 cups packaged egg whites

1 teaspoon paprika

DIRECTIONS

1) Preheat the oven to 375°F. Season the zucchini slices with salt and pepper.

2) Heat the oil in an ovenproof skillet over medium heat.

3) Add the zucchini, broccoli, cauliflower, and garlic, and sauté slightly.

4) Add the nutmeg and cumin; sauté over low heat for 5 minutes, then let cool.

5) Whip the egg whites in a blender or with an egg-beater, which will aerate the eggs and create a greater volume for the quiche.

6) Pour the eggs over the vegetables in the skillet. Sprinkle the paprika over the top.

7) Bake for 15 minutes, or until the top is slightly brown. Remove from the oven, cut into wedges, and serve.

Yield: 2 servings

NUTRITION INFORMATION PER SERVING
Calories: 200
Protein: 30 g
Carbs: 13 g
Fiber: 5 g
Fat: 4 g
Sugar: 4 g

A Mean Egg Salad

6 omega-3 eggs

½ cup chopped broccoli

2 tablespoons mild salsa

1 tablespoon Dijon mustard

1 tablespoon paprika

½ teaspoon cayenne pepper

1 pickle, chopped

1 packet (1 teaspoon) sugar substitute (optional)

Salt and pepper

DIRECTIONS

1) Boil the eggs in salted water for 15 minutes. Let cool.

2) While the eggs are boiling, steam the broccoli.

3) Peel the eggs. Discard the yolk from 4 of the eggs while keeping the other 2 whole eggs. Chop the eggs.

4) In a large mixing bowl, combine the eggs, broccoli, salsa, mustard, paprika, pepper, pickle, and sugar substitute, if using.

6) Season with salt and pepper.

Yield: 1 serving

NUTRITION INFORMATION PER SERVING
(*Note:* Optional ingredients not included in analysis)
Calories: 284
Protein: 30 g
Carbs: 12 g
Fiber: 4 g
Fat: 12 g
Sugar: 1 g

SINLESS SALSA

Purchase fresh salsa with no added sugar or high-fructose corn syrup. Salsa is basically just tomatoes, onions, peppers, cilantro, parsley, garlic, and spices. You can even make it yourself in a food processor. Change the flavor of this dish by simply choosing a mild, hot, or spicy salsa.—*CN*

LUNCH

Tough Guy Turkey Burger

1 pound lean ground turkey or chicken

3 tablespoons fresh parsley or cilantro

2 tablespoons Worcestershire sauce

2 tablespoons Dijon mustard

¼ cup chopped red, green, or yellow bell pepper

2 tablespoons reduced sodium soy sauce

1 tablespoon balsamic vinegar

1 teaspoon fresh ground ginger

1 clove garlic

Salt and pepper

1 egg white, beaten

Nonstick cooking spray

3 leaves iceberg lettuce

DIRECTIONS

1) In a large bowl, combine the turkey, parsley, Worcestershire sauce, mustard, bell pepper, soy sauce, vinegar, ginger, and garlic, and season with salt and pepper. With clean hands, squeeze the mixture together until it is well combined.

2) Coat the mixture with the egg white using your hands. (It will appear wet, but once it is cooking it will stick together.)

3) Divide the mixture into three equal portions and form into burgers about ¾ inch thick.

4) Spray a skillet with nonstick cooking spray and place over medium-high heat. Cook the burgers for 5 to 10 minutes per side, or until done. Turkey is a meat that needs to be cooked completely.

5) Serve on a piece of crispy iceberg lettuce. Garnish the burgers with Dijon mustard dressing.

Yield: 3 servings

NUTRITION INFORMATION PER SERVING
Calories: 290
Protein: 29 g
Carbs: 12.5 g
Fiber: 2 g
Fat: 13 g
Sugar: 5 g

True Tuna Salad

12 ounces albacore tuna in water

3 tablespoons Dijon mustard

2 tablespoons reduced-sodium soy sauce

1 tablespoon balsamic vinegar

1 teaspoon lemon juice

½ teaspoon garlic powder

½ teaspoon mustard powder

½ teaspoon paprika

¼ teaspoon garlic powder or 1 clove garlic, chopped

½ red bell pepper, chopped

½ yellow bell pepper, chopped

¼ cup chopped onion (optional)

8 slices high-fiber bran crisp bread

4 leaves lettuce

4 slices tomato

DIRECTIONS

1) Drain the tuna and rinse in a colander.

2) In a large mixing bowl, combine the tuna, mustard, soy sauce, vinegar, lemon juice, garlic powder, mustard powder, and paprika.

3) Add the garlic powder or chopped garlic, peppers, and onion, if using. Mix well.

4) Place leaf of lettuce and 1 slice of tomato on 4 slices of bread and top with 3 ounces of tuna salad. Top with the remaining 4 slices of bread.

Yield: 4 servings

NUTRITION INFORMATION PER SERVING
(*Note:* Optional ingredients not included in analysis)
Calories: 195
Protein: 30 g
Carbs: 8 g
Fiber: 2 g
Fat: 5 g
Sugar: 3 g

Chicken, Nuts, and Spinach

1 (4 ounce) skinless chicken breast

1 tablespoon macadamia nut oil

2 cups spinach

3 tablespoons reduced-sodium soy sauce

2 tablespoons Dijon mustard

1 teaspoon fresh ground ginger

1 ounce sliced almonds

1 ounce cashews

DIRECTIONS

1) Poach the chicken breast in enough water to cover. (Add some reduced-sodium soy sauce to the water for extra flavor, if desired.)

2) Heat the oil in a skillet over medium heat, add the spinach, and sauté until wilted. Add the soy sauce, Dijon mustard, and ginger, and stir to combine.

3) Add the almonds, cashews, and chicken to the spinach, and simmer for another 2 to 3 minutes.

Yield: 2 servings

NUTRITION INFORMATION PER SERVING
Calories: 644
Protein: 65 g
Carbs: 20 g
Fiber: 7 g
Fat: 35 g
Sugar: 4 g

GINGER: THE NEW GARLIC

Ginger is a common ingredient in Asian cuisine. It has a very clean taste and softens the taste of mustard and soy sauce. Ginger is used in Asian medicine and has also been used to help treat rheumatoid arthritis, osteoarthritis, and joint and muscle pain.—*CN*

DINNER

Great Buffalo Chili

1 pound buffalo meat

½ onion, chopped

¼ cup reduced-sodium soy sauce

¼ cup balsamic vinegar

3 tablespoons Dijon mustard

3 tablespoons chili powder

1 tablespoon paprika

1 tablespoon cinnamon

1 teaspoon cayenne pepper

1 can (15.5 ounces) black beans, drained

Salt and pepper

2 cups chopped green beans

DIRECTIONS

1) In a large skillet, combine the meat, onion, soy sauce, vinegar, and Dijon mustard. Sauté until the meat is browned and cooked through.

2) Add the chili powder, paprika, cinnamon, and cayenne pepper, and stir to combine.

3) Drain any excess oil or water from the meat and add the black beans.

4) Meanwhile, bring a pot of water with a pinch of salt and pepper to a boil; add the green beans and boil until tender.

5) Add the green beans to the chili, and stir to combine.

Yield: 2 servings

NUTRITION INFORMATION PER SERVING
Calories: 560
Protein: 60 g
Carbs: 58 g
Fiber: 20 g
Fat: 24 g
Sugar: 16 g

CHILI CHOICES

You can use any type of meat protein, including lean sirloin, turkey, chicken, or even ostrich. Each meat has a different flavor and will give a distinct taste to the dish as well as changing the fat content. Most buffalo is grass-fed, which changes the fatty acid profile and provides a better balance of EFAs.—*CN*

Turbulent Thai Chicken

2 (4 ounce) boneless, skinless chicken breasts
¼ cup reduced-sodium soy sauce
1 tablespoon balsamic vinegar
2 tablespoons natural cashew butter
1 tablespoon sesame oil
1 or 2 cloves garlic, crushed
1 tablespoon lemon juice
1 teaspoon ground cumin
½ teaspoon cayenne pepper
2 teaspoons paprika
2 cups chopped broccoli
1 cup bean sprouts

DIRECTIONS

1) Boil the chicken breasts in 1 tablespoon of the soy sauce and the vinegar until cooked through. When the meat has cooled, slice it into thin strips.

2) In a large skillet, combine the remaining 3 table-spoons of soy sauce with the cashew butter, oil, garlic, lemon juice, cumin, cayenne, and paprika to create a sauce.

3) Add the chopped broccoli and the chicken.

4) Add the bean sprouts and stir; they cook very fast and will give the taste of noodles.

Yield: 2 servings

NUTRITION INFORMATION PER SERVING
Calories: 390
Protein: 42 g
Carbs: 12.5 g
Fiber: 3.5 g
Fat: 20 g
Sugar: 3.5 g

Wild Dijon Salmon

8 ounces fresh wild salmon (or, less favorably,
   farm-raised salmon)
Reduced-sodium soy sauce
Balsamic vinegar
Dijon mustard
½ teaspoon crushed garlic
Lemon
Paprika

DIRECTIONS

1) Preheat the broiler to 500°F.

2) Place the fish on a piece of foil and add enough soy sauce and vinegar to create a steam bath.

3) Using a knife, spread some Dijon mustard over the salmon, and sprinkle with the garlic.

4) Squeeze the lemon over the fish, then sprinkle with paprika.

5) Broil for 20 minutes, of until the top is crispy.

Yield: 1 serving

NUTRITION INFORMATION PER SERVING
Calories: 435
Protein: 50 g
Carbs: 19 g
Fiber: 1.5 g
Fat: 17 g
Sugar: 12 g

Sizzlin' Pepper Steak

½ teaspoon fresh ground ginger
2 tablespoons reduced-sodium soy sauce
½ teaspoon red-pepper flakes (optional)
½ teaspoon salt
½ teaspoon pepper
1 pound top round, top sirloin, or filet mignon
   (leanest cuts of meat), thinly sliced
2 teaspoons sesame oil
1 clove garlic, pressed
1 green bell pepper, sliced
1 medium onion, sliced

DIRECTIONS

1) Whisk together the ginger, soy sauce, red-pepper flakes (if using), salt, and pepper; dredge the steak in the mixture.

2) Heat the oil in a large skillet over high heat for 3 minutes; add the steak and garlic, and sauté for 4 minutes, or until browned. (You can use a George Foreman grill or even an outdoor barbecue grill for this step, but be sure to avoid charring.)

3) Add the bell pepper and onion; sauté for 8 minutes, or until tender. Stir in the broth mixture; reduce the heat and simmer for 3 to 5 minutes, or until thickened.

Yield: 2 servings

NUTRITION INFORMATION PER SERVING
Calories: 367
Protein: 50 g
Carbs: 8 g
Fiber: 2.1 g
Fat: 13 g
Sugar: 4 g

Manly Meat Loaf

1 whole omega-3 egg

1 tomato, chopped

¼ cup reduced-sugar organic ketchup (see note on page 313)

1 tablespoon Worcestershire sauce

2 tablespoons brown mustard

½ teaspoon salt

½ teaspoon pepper

4 cloves garlic, minced

½ cup fresh parsley or ¼ cup dried parsley

2 ribs celery, minced

½ onion, minced

½ green bell pepper, minced

1 pound lean ground sirloin

Nonstick cooking spray

TOPPINGS

2 tablespoons Dijon mustard

¼ cup reduced-sugar ketchup

1 tablespoon red wine vinegar

DIRECTIONS

1) Preheat the oven to 350°F.

2) Combine the egg, tomato, ketchup, Worcestershire sauce, mustard, salt, and pepper. Add the garlic, parsley, celery, onion, and bell pepper, and mix well. Finally, add the meat and mix together with your hands. (If you'd rather use a mixer, just be sure not to overmix.)

3) Spray a loaf pan with cooking spray and spread the meat in it.

4) Top with either the Dijon mustard, ketchup, or red wine vinegar, or use all three.

5) Bake for 1 hour and 10 minutes, then let stand for 10 minutes before slicing.

Yield: 4 servings

NUTRITION INFORMATION PER SERVING
(*Note:* Toppings not included in nutritional analysis)
Calories: 312
Protein: 24 g
Carbs: 9 g
Fiber: 2 g
Fat: 12–19 g, depending on type of meat
Sugar: 5 g

Texan Shrimp

6 ounces shrimp, boiled, shells removed

2 tablespoons chopped fresh cilantro

2 tablespoons mild salsa

1 tablespoon Silver Spring Organic Cocktail Sauce (Or just combine fresh organic tomato paste, organic horseradish, and organic lemon juice to taste. You can also make your own cocktail sauce; see Shrimp Dip on page 309.)

DIRECTIONS

Combine the shrimp, cilantro, salsa, and cocktail sauce in a bowl and mix.

Yield: 1 serving

NUTRITION INFORMATION PER SERVING
Calories: 196
Protein: 36 g
Carbs: 4 g
Fiber: 2 g
Fat: 2 g
Sugar: 2 g

Chick'n Wrapper

6 ounces boneless skinless chicken breast, chopped

1 tablespoon natural cashew butter

2 tablespoons reduced-sodium soy sauce

½ red bell pepper, sliced

1 tablespoon balsamic vinegar

1 low-carb tortilla (5 net carbs)

DIRECTIONS

1) In a food processor or an emulsion blender, combine the chicken, cashew butter, soy sauce, bell pepper, and vinegar; pulse all ingredients together. (This makes the perfect consistency for a wrap.)

2) Place on the center of the tortilla, and fold.

Yield: 1 serving

NUTRITION INFORMATION PER SERVING

Calories: 363
Protein: 51 g
Carbs: 10 g
Fiber: 5 g
Fat: 13 g
Sugar: 3 g

CONDIMENTS

Dijon Salad Sauce

6 ounces Dijon mustard

2 tablespoons balsamic vinegar

2 tablespoons reduced-sodium soy sauce

4 packets (4 teaspoons) sugar substitute

1 tablespoon Mrs. Dash

Any favorite spices to taste: garlic powder, onion powder, paprika, etc.

DIRECTIONS

1) Combine the mustard, vinegar, soy sauce, sugar substitute, Mrs. Dash, and spices (if using) in a squeezable container. Shake vigorously until all ingredients are combined.

2) This dressing can be tailored to your taste depending on what spices and type of vinegar you use.

Yield: 50 servings (1 teaspoon per serving)

NUTRITION INFORMATION PER SERVING

Calories: 7
Protein: 5 g
Carbs: 1 g
Fiber: 0.5 g
Fat: 0.5 g
Sugar: 0.5 g

Pepper-Based Vina-great

½ cup defatted low-sodium chicken broth
   or vegetable broth
¼ cup balsamic vinegar
2 tablespoons reduced-sugar organic ketchup
2 tablespoons mustard
½ teaspoon dried thyme
¼ teaspoon ground red pepper

DIRECTIONS

1) In a small jar with a tight-fitting cover, combine the broth, vinegar, ketchup, mustard, thyme, and pepper. Cover and shake until well combined.

2) Store in the refrigerator for up to 1 week. Shake well before serving.

Yield: 1 cup or 8 servings (2 tablespoons per serving)

NUTRITION INFORMATION PER SERVING
Calories: 17
Protein: 0.5 g
Carbs: 3 g
Fiber: 0.5 g
Fat: 0.5 g
Sugar: 2 g

Tomato Vina-great

½ cup peeled and chopped tomatoes
2 tablespoons white wine vinegar
½ teaspoon dried basil
½ teaspoon dried thyme
¼ teaspoon Dijon mustard

DIRECTIONS

1) In a blender or small food processor, combine the tomatoes, vinegar, basil, thyme, and mustard at a medium to high speed for about 25 seconds, or until well combined.

2) Transfer the vinaigrette to a jar with a tight-fitting lid and refrigerate for up to 2 days. Shake well before serving.

Yield: ⅓ cup or 4 servings (4 teaspoons per serving)

NUTRITION INFORMATION PER SERVING
Calories: 8
Protein: 4 g
Carbs: 1 g
Fiber: 0 g
Fat: 0.5 g
Sugar: 1 g

Steak Dip

½ cup reduced-sugar organic ketchup

2½ to 3 tablespoons Worcestershire sauce

4 drops hot pepper sauce

2 packets (2 teaspoons) sugar substitute

1 tablespoon mustard

1 tablespoon cider vinegar

Pinch each of salt and pepper

DIRECTIONS

Combine the ketchup, Worcestershire sauce, hot pepper sauce, sugar substitute, mustard, vinegar, salt, and pepper, and mix well.

Yield: 12 servings (1 tablespoon per serving)

NUTRITION INFORMATION PER SERVING

Calories: 8
Protein: 1 g
Carbs: 2 g
Fiber: 0 g
Fat: 1 g
Sugar: 0.4

LOW CARB KETCHUP

Most ketchup has high-fructose corn syrup. Look for the varieties with a lower carb count, such as Heinz 1-carb ketchup.

Shrimp Dip

¼ cup prepared horseradish, drained

½ cup reduced-sugar ketchup

1 teaspoon Worcestershire sauce

1 teaspoon hot sauce (we recommend Tabasco)

1 teaspoon chopped fresh cilantro leaves

Salt and pepper

DIRECTIONS

Combine the horseradish, ketchup, Worcestershire sauce, hot sauce, cilantro, salt, and pepper, and mix well.

Yield: 12 servings (1 tablespoon per serving)

NUTRITION INFORMATION PER SERVING

Calories: 13
Protein: 2 g
Carbs: 1 g
Fiber: 1 g
Fat: 1 g
Sugar: 1 g

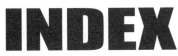

INDEX

Boldface page references indicate photographs. <u>Underscored</u> references indicate boxed text and charts.